Blood Disorders in the Elderly

MEDICINE IN OLD AGE

Volumes already published

Hearing and balance in the elderly
R. Hinchcliffe, *Editor*

Bone and joint disease in the elderly
V. Wright, *Editor*

Peripheral vascular disease in the elderly
S. T. McCarthy, *Editor*

**Clinical pharmacology and drug
treatment in the elderly**
K. O'Malley, *Editor*

Clinical biochemistry in the elderly
H. M. Hodkinson, *Editor*

Immunology and infection in the elderly
R. A. Fox, *Editor*

**Gastrointestinal tract disorders in the
elderly**
J. Hellemans and G. Vantrappen, *Editors*

Arterial disease in the elderly
R. W. Stout, *Editor*

Urology in the elderly
J. C. Brocklehurst, *Editor*

Volumes in preparation

Cardiology in the elderly
R. J. Luchi, *Editor*

Prevention of disease in the elderly
J. A. Muir Gray, *Editor*

Medical ethics and the elderly
R. J. Elford, *Editor*

Skin problems in the elderly
L. Fry, *Editor*

Blood Disorders in the Elderly

Edited by

M. J. Denham MD FRCP

Consultant Geriatrician,
Northwick Park Hospital, Harrow

I. Chanarin MD FRCPath

Consultant Haematologist,
Head of Section of Haematology in the Clinical Research Centre,
Northwick Park Hospital, Harrow

CHURCHILL LIVINGSTONE
EDINBURGH LONDON MELBOURNE AND NEW YORK 1985

CHURCHILL LIVINGSTONE
Medical Division of Longman Group Limited

Distributed in the United States of America by Churchill
Livingstone Inc., 1560 Broadway, New York, N.Y.
10036, and by associated companies, branches and
representatives throughout the world.

First published 1985

ISBN 0 443 02951 2

British Library Cataloguing in Publication Data
Blood disorders in the elderly.—(Medicine in
   old age, ISSN 0264-5602)
   1. Aged—Diseases   2. Blood—Diseases
   I. Denham, Michael   II. Chanarin, I.   III. Series
   618.97′61′5   RC952.9

Printed in Great Britain by Butler & Tanner Ltd,
Frome and London

Introduction

To a great extent the medicine of today and tomorrow is the medicine of old age. In every hospital in the Western World old patients predominate. In the past it was too readily assumed that either the medicine of old age was confined to degenerative disease and was uninfluenced by diagnosis and treatment; or that it was identical to the medicine of young and middle age and required no special study. Neither view is correct. It is now becoming clear that the diseases which strike old people, the symptoms and the signs which are induced, and the response to treatment are distinctive. Years of growth, maturation and decline alter the response of the host to disease and to its management in ways which require special study. As this fact has been grasped medical science and research-minded clinicians have embarked on the study of the diseases of late life and have documented their characteristic features. Progress has been slow, partly because of an initial lack of sense of urgency, and difficulty in attracting research workers and funds; partly because of the complexities of defining normal values in old age and of attributing deviations from the normal to any one cause. Methodological and statistical problems have compounded the difficulties. But over the years there has been a very real and impressive growth of knowledge of the medicine of late life.

Some years ago the idea was conceived of collecting this new knowledge, system by system, in a series of volumes to be entitled 'Medicine in Old Age'. These books were addressed to physicians in all Western countries and in all medical disciplines who dealt with elderly patients. The contributors included physiologists, pathologists, epidemiologists and community physicians, as well as general internal physicians, geriatricians, psychiatrists and specialists in the various systems of the body. The response accorded to the first few volumes in the series was most encouraging, and the publishers are continuing and expanding the series.

This enterprise is supervised by an Editorial Board composed of practising clinicians and academics on both sides of the Atlantic. The Board selects the topics and appoints the guest editors for each volume and have been fortunate in their choice as editors of leaders in each field. These have been able in turn to attract contributions of high merit from many countries, thus putting into the hands of the reader a series of highly authoritative volumes. These bring together a wealth of knowledge and the best of modern practice in the care of elderly patients, retaining the critical spirit in the evaluation of the data which is characteristic of medicine in all age groups. The volumes are intended to stand mid-way between the immediacy of the scientific journal and the urbanity of the standard text book, combining freshness with authority. It is hoped that the profession will find them of value.

Birmingham, 1985   Bernard Isaacs

Preface

Illness in the elderly can present considerable diagnostic, treatment and management problems to the clinician because of non-specific presentation, poor history and blunted symptoms and signs. General ill health and poor diet may compound these problems. Disorders of the blood are no exception and can provide considerable diagnostic dilemmas and, on ocassion, ethical problems in management.

This book concentrates on these aspects of blood disorders which are relevant to the care and management of the elderly and harnesses the views of experts in both fields of haematology and geriatric medicine. The introductory chapters review the changes in blood with age. Later chapters consider the various types of anaemia, leukaemia, myeloma, lymphoma, polycythaemia, bleeding and thrombotic disorders as well as the haematological side effects of drugs. The current state of knowledge, diagnostic techniques, research and treatment are reviewed. Where appropriate ethical aspects of treatment are considered.

We hope the book will be of value to all who treat old people, and will find a place on wards as well as in consulting rooms.

Harrow, 1985

M. J. Denham
I. Chanarin

Contributors

J. David Bessman MD
Assistant Professor of Medicine, Division of Hematology/Oncology, John Sealy Hospital, University of Texas Medical Branch, Galveston, Texas

I. W. Delamore PhD FRCP FRCPath
Physician in Charge, Department of Clinical Haematology, Royal Infirmary, Manchester

Michael L. Freedman MD
Professor of Medicine and Director of the Department of Geriatrics, New York University Medical Center, New York

C. G. Geary MA MB FRCP FRCPath
Consultant Haematologist, Royal Infirmary, Manchester, and Christie Hospital, Manchester

R. G. J. Hayhoe MD FRCP FRCPath
Professor of Haematological Medicine, University of Cambridge Medical School

J. Hirsch MD FRCP(C)
Professor and Chairman, Department of Medicine, McMaster Univerity, Hamilton, Ontario

H. M. Hodkinson MA DM FRCP
Barlow Professor of Geriatric Medicine, University College Hospital, London, and Middlesex Hospital Medical School, London

R. D. Hull MD FRCP(C)
Chief of Medicine, Chedoke Division, Chedoke-McMaster Hospitals, McMaster University, Hamilton, Ontario

J. R. LeClerc MD FRCP(C)
Research Fellow, Department of Medicine, McMaster University, Hamilton, Ontario

David A. Lipschitz MD
Little Rock Veterans Administration Hospital, Little Rock, Arkansas

Sean R. Lynch MD
Professor of Medicine, University of Kansas Medical Center, Kansas City, Kansas

Samuel J. Machin MB MRCPath
Consultant Haematologist, Middlesex Hospital, London

J. S. Malpas DPhil FRCP FRCR
Professor of Medical Oncology and Director, Imperial Cancer Research Fund,
St Bartholomew's Hospital, London

A. M. Middleton MB MRCP
Consulant Physician in Geriatric Medicine, St Mary's Hospital, London

J. K. H. Rees MB MRCP
Lecturer in Haematological Medicine, University of Cambridge Medical School

C. D. L. Reid FRCPath
Consultant Haematologist, Northwick Park Hospital, Harrow, Middlesex

Contents

1. Introduction   1
   I. Chanarin
2. Normal haematological values   4
   J. David Bessman
3. Iron-deficiency anaemia   21
   Sean R. Lynch and David A. Lipschitz
4. Macrocytosis and megaloblastic anaemia   43
   I. Chanarin
5. Normocytic anaemia and anaemias of general disease   64
   I. Delamore
6. Cytopenias due to bone marrow failure: hypersplenism   80
   C. G. Geary
7. Screening for anaemia and its prevention   100
   H. M. Hodkinson
8. Haemolytic disease   109
   Michael L. Freedman
9. Bleeding and coagulation disorders   132
   Samuel J. Machin
10. Clinical management of venous thromboembolism   157
    J. R. LeClerc, R. Hull and J. Hirsh
11. The leukaemias   188
    F. G. J. Hayhoe and J. Rees
12. Multiple myeloma   208
    C. D. L. Reid
13. Polycythaemia and myelofibrosis   234
    A. M. Middleton
14. Lymphomas   245
    J. S. Malpas
15. Drug-induced blood dyscrasias   265
    M. J. Denham

Index   287

Introduction

Do healthy elderly subjects normally show changes in the blood that are due solely to age? This issue is difficult to resolve because the more fully the elderly are investigated, the more disorders are revealed. Thus it is difficult to sample a large number of elderly persons and to exclude accompanying disease as the cause of blood changes that appear. There are some changes, however, that are recognised as being an accompaniment of old age even if the explanation is uncertain.

Cellularity of marrow decreases with age, and an increasing proportion of marrow is occupied by adipose cells. Thus trephine biopsies from the iliac crest suggest that about half the marrow is occupied by fat in adults below the age of 65 and thereafter about two-thirds of marrow is fatty (Hartsock et al, 1965). However, the increase in adipose cells could be the result of loss of bone with osteoporosis rather than to a primary loss of haemopoietic cells.

There is an increased incidence of auto-antibodies in the older age groups. Thus a survey by Whittingham et al (1969) showed that antibodies that are absent or present in low numbers below the age of 20 increase in frequency with age (Table 1.1). Antinuclear factor was present in 18 per cent of females and 15 per cent of males above the age of 61, and antibody against the gastric parietal cell was present in 21 per cent of females above the age of 61 and 16

Table 1.1   Percentage of 'normal' subjects with antibodies (after Whittingham et al, 1969)

Antibody	Female age (years)			Male age (years)		
	0–20	40–60	61+	0–20	40–60	61+
Antinucler factor	0	12	18	0	9	15
Antirheumatoid factor*	0–1	2–7	3–5	0	0–3	1–3
Thyroid cytoplasm	0	18	20	0	6	7
Thyroglobulin	0	2	6	4	2	1
Gastric parietal cell	4	15	21	2	4	16

*Percentage positivity varies with technique.

per cent of males above the age of 61. These may be no more than the accompaniment of disease in the corresponding organ. Thus whereas the gastric biopsy was normal in 78 per cent of subjects below the age of 20, it was normal in only 19 per cent of subjects over the age of 60. That is, 81 per cent of persons over 60 years of age have some degree of atrophic gastritis (Chanarin, 1975). Generally, patients found to have parietal-cell antibodies on further investigation have an abnormal gastric biopsy, and exceptions are rare.

There are some reports that the total lymphocyte count declines in the elderly (Caird et al, 1972), but others have failed to substantiate this. There are no reported changes in the neutrophil count. There is similar disagreement in relation to lymphocyte subsets in the elderly. There are some reports that lymphocyte T-helper cells decrease while B-cells retain their usual numbers (Williams, 1983), but other reports find normal numbers. Lymphocytes from older subjects have been reported by some to show impaired responsiveness to mitogens and to show impaired cell-mediated cytotoxicity. Further, suggestions of impaired cell-mediated immunity in the elderly come from reports of failure to respond to local application of dinitrochlorobenzene as a skin test.

Older subjects have lower immunoglobulin levels than young adults, and levels of IgG and IgA are about 60 per cent of that in younger age groups. Antibody responses, such as that to pneumococcal polysaccharide, are reduced (Ammann et al, 1980) and immunisation with influenza vaccine may be ineffective.

There is a declining haemoglobin level in older people. The mean below the age of 60 is about 15.6g/dl in males and 13.6g/dl in females and at 96–106 years 12.4g/dl. The fall appears to be less in elderly women. It is difficult to be certain that this is not due to accompanying disease. In one study of over two hundred subjects, iron, folate or cobalamin deficiency was found in 23 out of 37 subjects with haemoglobin levels below 12g/dl (McLennan et al, 1973). Changes in red cell count have been reported that correspond to the fall in the haemoglobin concentration. Thus in men 20 years old Giorno et al (1980) found a mean erythrocyte count of 5.3 million dl and in men aged 60 it was 5.05 million dl. In women, however, the red cell count was 4.6 million dl at both ages.

Three studies have reported modest increases in red cell size (MCV) with age. Croft et al (1974) found an increase of 0.4fl for every decade, Okumo (1972) that the MCV was 3.5 fl greater in the over-50s than in the 16–19 age group, and Giorno et al (1980) an MCV of 89 at 20 years and 93 at 60 in males, but the corresponding values in women were 89 and 90 respectively. Kelly & Munan (1977) in a survey of a population sample of over two thousand individuals found an increase of 1fl in the MCV with age in males and no change in women. The highest MCV was in those over the age of 75. There are many causes of a raised MCV in the older population (Chapter 4). Smokers have an MCV that is about 1.5fl above that in non-smokers, and even modest alcohol consumption has a similar and additive effect (Chalmers et al, 1979). Thus the effect of age, if present, is small.

There are at least six studies reporting a fall in the serum cobalamin level with age (Chanarin, 1979) and another five studies failing to show any such fall. There are reports that as many as 30 per cent of elderly persons have low serum cobalamin levels, but the very high incidence of simple atrophic gastritis in the elderly population implies that, if correct, the low cobalamin level is the result of the atrophic gastritis and not a normal age change.

Other variables in age are discussed in the appropriate chapters.

REFERENCES

Ammann A J, Schiffman A, Austrian R 1980 The antibody responses to pneumococcal capsular polysaccharides in aged individuals. Proceedings of the Society for Experimental Biology and Medicine 164: 312–6

Caird F I, Andrews G R, Gallie T B 1972 The leucocyte count in old age. Age and Ageing 1: 239–244

Chalmers D M, Levi A J, Chanarin I, North W R S, Meade T W 1979 Mean cell volume in a working population: the effects of age, smoking, alcohol and oral contraception. British Journal of Haematology 43: 631–636

Chanarin I 1975 The stomach in allergic diseases. In: Gell P G H, Coombs R R A, Lachman P J (eds) Clinical aspects of immunology, 3rd edn. Blackwell, Oxford, p 1429–1440

Chanarin I 1979 The megaloblastic anaemias, 2nd edn. Blackwell, Oxford, pp 126–146

Croft R F, Streeter A M, O'Neill B J 1974 Red cell indices in megaloblastosis and iron deficiency. Pathology 6: 107–117

Giorno R, Clifford J H, Beverly S, Rossing G 1980 Hematology reference values. American Journal of Clinical Pathology 74: 765–770

Hartsock R J, Smith E B, Petty C S 1965 Normal variations with aging on the amount of hemotopoietic tissue in bone marrow from the anterior iliac crest. American Journal of Clinical Pathology 43: 326–31

Kelly A, Munan L 1977 Haematologic profile of natural populations: red cell parameters. British Journal of Haematology 35: 153–160

McLennan W J, Andrews G R, Macleod C, Caird F I 1973 Anaemia in the elderly. Quarterly Journal of Medicine 42: 1–13

Okuno T 1972 Red cell size as measured by the Coulter model S. Journal of Clinical Pathology 25: 599–602

Whittingham S, Irwin J, Mackay I R, Marsh S, Cowling D C 1969 Autoantibodies in healthy subjects. Australian Annals of Medicine 18: 130–134

Williams W J 1983 In: Williams W J, Beutler E, Erslev A J, Lichtman M A (eds) Hematology, 3rd edn. McGraw-Hill, New York, p 47–53

Normal haematological values

INTRODUCTION

With the introduction of multiparameter semi-automated blood counters during the last decade, the interpretation of the blood count has undergone a change of kind rather than degree. That the indices and counts which were familiar from manual counting now appear and are rapid, precise and accurate is accepted and welcome. Less appreciated is the addition of new values, which are based on the capacity of the counters to measure new variables. Some of these variables are available before there are well-documented scales of normals, let alone well-understood bases for abnormal results. Since the automated blood count is generally the first step into a haematological evaluation, the clinician should make the most of the count. Therefore this chapter will show not only the normal values, but a brief explanation of the new variables: what is being measured, how it is reported and why it is of use.

Coagulation assays have not changed so dramatically in the routine laboratory, and the discussion of them will be briefer. However, important changes are likely in the next few years.

AUTOMATED BLOOD COUNTING

Red cells

1. The *red cell count* is measured directly. Red cells are defined by size rather than haemoglobin content, allowing artefactual high counts when cells of a similar size are present in substantial amounts — most commonly lymphocytes (Bessman, 1980). However, this artefact occurs rarely, and otherwise the count is reproducible within 1 per cent.

2. The *haemoglobin* is measured directly. It is artefactually elevated by severe hyperlipidaemia, but is otherwise reproducible within 2 per cent.

3. The *packed cell volume* (PCV) is no longer measured directly. The spun PCV measured the proportion of packed cells to the entire blood sample: this packed column included a small but ever-present amount of plasma trapped between the red cells. The greater the irregularity of red cell shape, the

greater the plasma trapping and the less accurate the PCV (Van Assendelft & England, 1982).

In contrast, the automated PCV is calculated as the product of red cell count (see above) and mean cell volume, MCV (see below). Thus the problem of plasma trapping no longer arises. However, since MCV is dependent to a small degree on red cell shape and deformability (see below), PCV will be artefactually increased in the same disorders that had an artefactually high PCV. The degree of artefact is much smaller in the automated PCV. This is probably the reason that the automated MCHC (see below) is of relatively little value. The automated PCV is reproducible within 3 per cent.

4. The *mean cell volume* (MCV) is directly measured in the automated counter. The scale for MCV is established for cells of an ideal shape and deformability: cells that are irregular register as slightly larger than they in fact are. It should be emphasised that there is no absolute reference standard for MCV (International Committee for Standardisation of Haematology, 1979, 1980, 1982). The duplicate error is about 1 fl.

5. The *mean cell haemoglobin* (MCH) is calculated as the ratio of haemoglobin to red cell count. Since haemoglobin varies little (see below), MCH varies essentially as does MCV and therefore has little independent value in interpreting the blood count.

6. The *mean cell haemoglobin concentration* (MCHC) is calculated as the ratio of haemoglobin to red cell count times MCV. Any artefact of any of the three directly-measured red cell variables will thus cause an abnormal MCHC: it is therefore an excellent indicator of machine error or specimen artefact. However, it varies little among normal or abnormal subjects; in particular, MCHC is not reliably low in iron deficiency (Gottfried, 1979). Therefore the automated MCHC is valuable for quality control and detection of artefact, but not for detection or classification of anaemic disorders. The duplicate error is 2 per cent.

7. *Red cell distribution width* (RDW) is calculated to be an index of the dispersion of red cell volume about the mean. While in most instruments this is calculated as a coefficient of variation, the ratio of standard deviation to mean of the distribution, in other instruments 'RDW' is simply the standard deviation. The latter measure is far less useful than the former. If only the standard deviation is used, the value will vary as MCV varies, and definition of normal becomes more difficult than necessary. If the coefficient of variation is used, normal values are the same whatever the MCV. However, even when the RDW is a coefficient of variation, the actual number reported for the same blood specimen varies substantially among machines, depending upon both program of the machine (Bessman, 1980) and manufacturer (Coulter Electronics, 1982; Technicon Corporation, 1983). This variability of reported number arises because the several manufacturers process the raw data of the curve differently to produce the data set that is analysed. In practice this means that the user should know what the normal values are for the equipment that is being used.

This is important because the RDW is potentially a valuable aid to the initial classification of red cell disorders, as shown below.

8. The *red cell volume distribution histogram* is an illustration of the distribution of red cell size in the blood sample. It is shown on the counter screen and/or printed. In normal subjects and in most abnormals the histogram is essentially unimodal and can be analysed with Gaussian statistics (Bessman, 1982). In certain abnormal circumstances, some of which are illustrated in this chapter, the red cell volume histogram is more complex: in such cases the histogram is often pathognomonic to the particular abnormality.

Classification of red cell disorders

Two classifications of red cell disorders have generally been used: the 'morphological', based on red cell indices (Wintrobe, 1981), and the 'physiological', based on reticulocyte count (Hillman & Finch, 1969). The morphological classification has the advantage of being precise and easy: the data are available in the automated blood count. However, red cell disorders are grouped without any apparent physiological basis: what is the similarity between iron deficiency, red cell fragmentation and thalassaemia, except for low MCV? In contrast, the physiological classification is based on clear distinctions of red cell production: increased versus decreased. Here, however, while the physiology of the disorders is highlighted, the reproducibility of the reticulocyte count is poor. The reticulocyte count is not part of the automated blood count. It must therefore be considered a secondary rather than a primary blood test.

In terms of a low or raised MCV, two large groups of disorders can be distinguished. *Small red blood cells* characterise iron deficiency, anaemia of chronic disorders, thalassaemia and hyperthyroidism. *Large red cells* are common to disorders with megaloblastic haemopoiesis (cobalamin and folate deficiency and some rare congenital disorders of pyrimidine and purine synthesis) and to a normoblastic group including alcoholism, hypothyroidism, hypoplastic anaemia, reticulocytosis, sideroblastic anaemia, neoplasia, drug therapy (particularly cytotoxics and anticolvulsants), liver disease and the preleukaemic syndrome. A normochromic anaemia (*normal-sized red cells*) often characterises renal failure, a variety of secondary anaemias and some haemolytic anaemias.

Use of the RDW along with the MCV allows a fuller classification of red cell disorders, and uses morphological criteria to make physiological distinctions. Table 2.1 lists the several categories that can be distinguished by MCV high, normal, and low, and RDW high or normal. As discussed earlier, MCHC is no longer a useful general classifier, and so the traditional terminology of normochromic and hypochromic is of little use. Instead, as shown in Table 2.2, the terms 'homogeneous' and 'heterogeneous', corresponding to normal or increased RDW, are more descriptive (Bessman et al, 1983).

Table 2.1 Automated classification of anaemias

MCV low		MCV normal		MCV high	
RDW normal (microcytic homogeneous)	RDW high (microcytic heterogeneous)	RDW normal (normocytic homogeneous)	RDW high (normocytic heterogeneous)	RDW normal (macrocytic homogeneous)	RDW high (macrocytic heterogeneous)
Heterozygous thalassaemia	Iron deficiency	Normal	Early iron, B_{12}, folate deficiency	Aplastic anaemia	B_{12} or folate deficiency
Chronic disease	HbH, thalassemia intermedia	Non-anaemic haemoglobinopathy	Anaemic haemoglobinopathy	Preleukaemia	Immune haemolytic anaemia
	RBC fragmentation★	Non-anaemic enzymopathy	Mixed deficiency		Cold agglutinins★
		Chronic disease			High-count CLL★
		Acute blood loss or haemolysis			
		CLL, CML			

★Indicates that the red cell distribution histogram is characteristically altered from the usual unimodal distribution.

The physiological significannce of RDW can be appreciated in this classification by noting that:

Disorders of *reduced cell proliferation* have *normal* RDW, whatever the MCV:
Microcytic homogencous: anacmia of chronic disease.
Normocytic homogeneous: anaemia of chronic disease.
Macrocytic homogeneous: aplastic anaemia.
Disorders of *nutrition* have *increased* RDW, whatever the MCV:
Microcytic heterogeneous: iron deficiency.
Normocytic heterogeneous: early iron, folate, or vitamin B_{12} deficiency.
Macrocytic heterogeneous: folate or vitamin B_{12} deficiency.

Haemolytic disorders (abnormal membrane, enzyme, or haemoglobin; or immune) have an RDW that is *increased in proportion to the degree of anaemia* that the haemolytic process causes, whatever the MCV.
Microcytic homogeneous: thalassaemia minor.
microcytic heterogeneous: thalassaemia major; haemoglobins H, or S with thalassaemia.
Normocytic homogeneous: sickle or haemoglobin C trait, mild G6PD deficiency.
Normocytic heterogeneous: sickle-cell anaemia.
Macrocytic homogeneous: rarely seen in haemolytic disorders.
Macrocytic heterogeneous: immune haemolytic anaemia, a minority of sickle-cell anaemia.

This is again illustrated in Figure 2.1.

Two important practical uses can be made. First, increased RDW despite normal MCV suggests either transfusion (Bessman et al, 1983) or early nutritional deficiency. While the first sign of iron deficiency is reduced iron stores, as shown by transferring saturation, ferritin, or bone marrow examination, the earliest evidence in the count is an increased RDW (Bessman et al, 1983); only later in the course of the disease do microcytosis and finally anaemia develop (Table 2.2). Second, low MCV with normal RDW suggests heterozygous thalassaemia. In contrast, low MCV with high RDW suggests iron deficiency, which does require further evaluation (Johnson et al, 1983; Kaye & Alter, 1982).

Finally, the red cell size distribution histogram should be examined routinely as part of the automated blood count. When the RDW is increased, usually the histogram remains a single, essentially symmetrical peak, but wider than normal. When the histogram has a different appearance, it is an important clue to specific disorders:

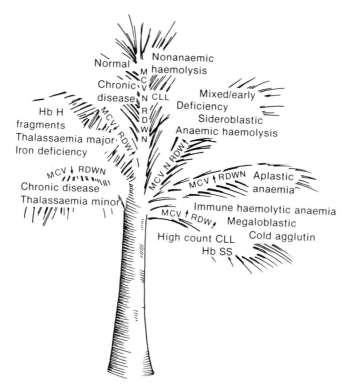

Fig. 2.1 Decision tree for evaluation of red cell disorders from automated blood count. Beginning with MCV and RDW, a small group of disorders can be distinguished as most likely, and subsequent tests can be directed at identifying which of the short list is responsible

Table 2.2   Progressive degrees of iron deficiency

	Iron stores	RDW	MCV	Haemoglobin
Hypoferremic	Low	Normal	Normal	Normal
Heterogenous	Low	High	Normal	Normal
Microcytic	Low	High	Low	Normal
Anaemic	Low	High	Low	Low

a. *Plateau to left of peak.* Red cell fragments will appear as smaller-than-normal cells, to the left of the peak of whole cells. Depending on their size, they may or may not be counted as red cells. Common causes include burns, traumatic cardiac valves, sickle-cell crisis, thrombotic thrombocytopenic purpura, and megaloblastic anaemia. An abnormal histogram is more quantitative than examination of the peripheral blood smear in detecting these fragments.

b. *Two red cell peaks,* both between 50 and 140 fl. This pattern indicates one population of red cells with a size disorder (either large or small) and a second population that reflects either transfused red cells or red cells produced after some specific therapy (e.g. treatment of iron deficiency). In this case the MCV will not accurately reflect the red cells, and the RDW will be dramatically increased.

c. *Two red cell peaks,* one above 140 fl. A peak of cells at about 165 fl indicates red cell agglutinins. Doublet (agglutinated) red cells are measured as one cell, but the measured volume, because of altered perceived red cell shape, is about 15 per cent less than double a single cell's volume. Therefore, the red cell count is reduced more than the MCV is increased, and the MCHC is artefactually high. This combination of histogram and high MCHC is pathognomonic for red cell agglutinins. Though it is a laboratory artefact, it may be the first clue to the underlying cause, whether idiopathic, pneumonia, or lymphocytic malignancy.

A peak of cells at about 200 fl suggests chronic lymphocytic leukaemia. Well-differentiated small lymphocytes may be this small. They are included as red cells even in normal blood, but in such low number as not to be important. When the lymphocytes exceed about $100 \times 10^9/l$, a second peak will be seen on the red cell histogram, the MCV will rise and MCHC will fall below normal.

Platelets

1. The *platelet count* is measured directly. As described for red cells, platelets are no longer defined by their morphological features, but rather by size (in the Coulter instrument, 2–20 fl). Thus any extraneous particle of this size will be counted as a platelet. When such extraneous particles (red cell or white cell fragments) are not present, the platelet count is reproducible within $10 \times 10^9/l$. This means that platelet counts below $10 \times 10^9/l$ cannot reliably be

distinguished from each other, and platelet counts up to $20 \times 10^9/l$ only marginally. Manual platelet counts are even less precise. In contrast, at higher platelet counts this level of duplicate error is not clinically important.

2. The *mean platelet volume* (MPV) is measured directly. It is taken from the distribution of platelet size. Any extraneous particles that affect the platelet count will also affect the MPV. The anticoagulant that is standard for the automated blood count is EDTA. This anticoagulant causes progressive disc-to-sphere platelet change; the shape change causes an increase of MPV of about 15 per cent during the first hour after anticoagulation (Salzman et al, 1969). MPV is then stable for the next 12 hours. Therefore, in evaluating whether MPV is normal or abnormal, the time in anticoagulant prior to measurement should be known. The duplicate error is 6 per cent.

Unlike many other variables, MPV has no single range of 'normal' size. Rather, in both the general run of hospitalised patients (Giles, 1981; Levin & Bessman, 1983) and in normal subjects (Bessman et al, 1981) there is an inverse relation between platelet size and platelet count even among subjects with a 'normal' platelet count. Instead of a single range of MPV, a nomogram thhat reflects this inverse relation should be used to judge whether an individual's MPV is normal or not. Figure 2.2 is appropriate for the Coulter instruments when calibrated as recommended by the manufacturer. A similar inverse non-linear relationship is seen with other instruments, though the absolute value for MPV will differ. The user should be provided with a nomogram that is appropriate to the instrument being used.

3. The *platelet volume distribution histogram* shows the distribution of platelet size. Ordinarily it is right-skewed enough to allow log-normal statistics for analysis. Certain artefacts are suggested by an abnormal histogram. If

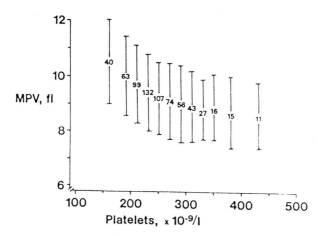

Fig. 2.2   Relation of platelet count and platelet volume in 683 normal subjects. Each group is shown as the mean (number) ± 2 *s.d.* (bar) of all subjects grouped by platelet counts of: 128–179, 180–199, 200–219, 220–239, 240–259, 260–279, 280–299–300–319, 320–339, 340–359, 361–403 and 406–462 × $10^9/l$. The number at mean position show how many subjects were in the group.

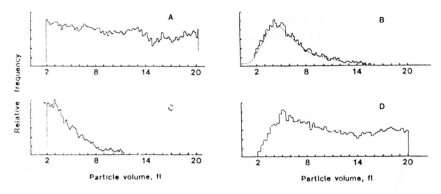

Fig. 2.3   Platelet volume distribution histograms: A, C, and D show contamination by non-platelet particles, while B shows the distribution of platelets alone. The platelet count and MPV from curve B will be accurate, while those from the others will not be

there is an exaggerated right tail whereby the histogram does not return to baseline by 20 fl, either small red cells (e.g. in iron deficiency) or platelet clumps (caused by EDTA) are probably present. Each of these artefacts is seen in about 0.1 per cent of blood specimens. If there is not a right-skewed histogram, but only an irregular pattern, and the platelet count is below $10 \times 10^9/l$, platelets are probably not being measured. Instead, the histogram shows electronic and cell-debris noise. This noise is always present, but is usually dwarfed by valid platelet signals. Appearance of the noise pattern is a sign that the platelet count is extremely low, lower than when there is an equal count that is accompanied by a normal-appearing histogram (Fig. 2.3).

4. The *platelet-crit* is the product of platelet count and MPV. Because of the non-linear inverse relation of platelet count and platelet size, platelet-crit has no single normal range. This index is not yet widely used in evaluation of the automated blood count.

5. The *platelet distribution width* (PDW) is a measure of the heterogeneity of platelet size. It varies directly but non-linearly with MPV (Bessman et al, 1982) but has not yet been widely used.

Classification of platelet disorders

Using the nomogram of normals shown in Figure 2.2, an individual's platelets now can be evaluated routinely for two morphological variables: MPV as well as platelet count:

MPV is higher than normal in subjects with heterozygous thalassaemia and those with chronic myelogenous leukaemia. In immune thrombocytopenic purpura, MPV is higher than normal only when platelet count is low; when platelet count is normal in well-compensated immune platelet destruction, MPV is the same as in normals with the same platelet count. MPV also is above normal after splenectomy.

MPV is lower than normal in subjects with aplastic anaemia, splenomegaly, megaloblastic anaemia, and in those receiving myelotoxic chemotherapy. In recovery from the latter two disorders, platelet size returns to normal (Bessman et al, 1982). It should be emphasised that these disorders of MPV can occur even while the platelet count is normal.

MPV is normal (for the platelet count) in subjects with diabetes, atherosclerosis and coronary heart disease. Recent reports of changes of MPV during acute myocardial infarction (Cameron et al, 1983; Martin et al, 1983) have not been confirmed (van der Lelie & Brakenhoff, 1983): any slight change in MPV is related to changes in platelet count, with MPV continuing to conform to the nomogram of normal values (Cameron et al, 1983).

Sequential changes of MPV

MPV will alter during changes in the development or recovery from bone marrow stimulation or suppression. During the course of recovery from immune thrombocytopenia, the MPV falls as platelet count rises, paralleling the nomogram of normal values (Fig. 2.4a). During marrow suppression by chemotherapy, MPV and platelet count both fall, progressively deviating from the nomogram even before the platelet count falls below normal. During the subsequent recovery, MPV rises before platelet count, as the first

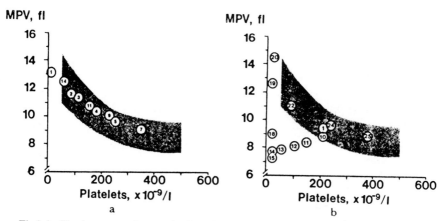

Fig 2.4   Platelet count and mean platelet volume, MPV, during recovery from nonseptic thrombocytopenia. The cross-hatched area is the nomogram of platelet count and mean platelet volume in normal persons and patients with immune thrombocytopenia purpura and platelet counts of 50–120 × 10⁹/l. The numbers indicate sequential days during the patient's course. a, Immune thrombocytopenia purpura. Mean platelet volume follows the inverse, nonlinear relation — during recovery and rising platelet counrts, days 1 to 7, mean platelet volume falls; during relapse, days 9 to 14, as platelet count falls, mean platelet volume rises. b, Recovery from chemotherapy, given on days 1 to 5. During the fall of platelet count, days 10 to 15, the mean platelet volume also falls, and so the relation of mean platelet volume and platelet count progressively diverges from the normal. During recovery, the mean platelet volume rises before the platelet count, days 18 to 20 and, then, as the platelet count rises, the mean platelet volume falls to enter the nomogram, days 20 to 25

peripheral-blood sign of platelet recovery. Then, as platelet count rises, MPV falls to follow the nomogram (Fig. 2.4b). Comparison of the course of MPV during other types of thrombocytopenia (e.g. sepsis) with the pure patterns of marrow suppression or peripheral platelet destruction (Fig. 2.4) allows a rough estimate of the relative contribution of these two causes of thrombocytopenia (Cameron et al, 1983).

White cells

1. The *white cell count* is measured directly. However, what cells are measured are not necessarily white cells by manual microscopy, but rather cells that fit the criteria of the individual machine, as described in the next section. The criteria have been adjusted to allow a satisfactory correlation between manual and automated results. The duplicate error is $0.3 \times 10^9/l$.

2. The *automated white cell differential* is now derived via several different methods. Each makes certain novel assumptions to define the several classes of leucocyte; each offers improved precision and speed over manual methods, but none completely replaces manual examination of a stained blood smear. Also, the new criteria for definition of cell types introduce new abnormalities that must be dealt with as there is increasing experience with these instruments.

The Coulter series uses nuclear size of nucleated cells as the criterion: a special lysing agent collapses the cell membrane upon the nucleus with most of the cytoplasm lysed away. This yields four relatively distinct peaks. Smallest are nucleated red cells, the peak of which becomes distinct at about 5 per cent of total white cell count. Next are lymphocytes, with a mode value of 60–80 fl. Third are 'mononuclear' cells, with modal values from 110 to 170 fl: cells in this category include atypical lymphocytes, monocytes, blasts, eosinophils, basophils and myelocytes. Finally, granulocytes appear generally above 200 fl. While there is some overlap, the lymphocyte and granulocyte percentages by this technique correlate with manual percentages with correlation coefficients above 0.98. However, the mononuclear percentage correlates rather less well with the percentage of any particular cell type on manual differential (correlation coefficient r = 0.84).

The Technicon series uses a combination of cell size and myeloperoxidase content to create a two-dimensional scattergram. Distinct subpopulations are seen for lymphocytes, monocytes, granulocytes, eosinophils and 'large unstained cells' which often are the category in which blasts appear. The correlation between the granulocyte, lymphocyte and eosinophil percentages in this instrument and manual percentages is above 0.95 for the former and probably nearly as good for the latter. In addition, hereditary and acquired myeloperoxidase deficiency can be detected from the characteristic pattern of the neutrophils. Nucleated red cells are not routinely detected.

The Ortho series uses a combination of forward and 90-degree light scatter to produce a scattergram of granulocytes, lymphocytes and monocytes. It is not yet precisely known how well these automated differentials compare with normal.

In contrast, the Hematrak pattern recognition system depends on an entirely different technology. The above three systems use flow cytometry: cells in suspension are analysed as they pass by a sensor single file. The criteria noted are chosen because they can be used with available sensors with flow cytometry. The Hematrak is automated image analysis: it scans a peripheral blood smear and identifies leucocytes by a set of image-analysis criteria that at least approximate manual criteria. With the Hematrak these criteria are more uniformly applied. All cell types recognised by manual microscopy are recognised by this technique. However, it is not so rapid as flow cytometry, and requires an instrument separate from the routine automated blood counter.

The advantages of the automated differential are its speed and reproducibility. However, as is described above, none of the automated techniques includes the band neutrophil as a separate type. Whether this lack is important remains to be determined. Current use of the automated differential is s a screening device: if it is completely normal, a manual differential is less likely to be done, or certainly less likely to be repeated after the initial differential. However, the automated differential does not detect either rare events or morphological variants. To detect such abnormalities, the peripheral blood smear must still be examined.

THE PERIPHERAL BLOOD SMEAR

Examination of the peripheral blood smear remains an important part of the haematological evaluation. The clinician should recognise that the peripheral smear will probably be examined after the automated blood count results are available. Therefore, time spent with the blood smear should be to glean additional information, not to attempt to duplicate the automated data. As a general principle, the automated blood counter is more efficient than manual examination to determine averages and count frequent events: red cell indices, cell counts, platelet size and lymphocyte and granulocyte percentage (if these are part of the automated count that is available). In contrast, the automated counter is at best unproved and often quite incapable of detecting rare events: nucleated red cells, immature granulocytes, red cell fragments.

Red cells

Rouleaux may be the first clue to a lymphoid or plasmacytic disorder. Agglutinins are similarly detected, but should be used to compare with the appearance of doublet red cells on the red cell histogram. Red cell fragments may be detected when they are as little as $1/2$ per cent of the cells, about the same level at which the red cell histogram becomes abnormal; thus the two techniques are complementary. Abnormalities of shape may indicate particular disorders, especially the sickling haemoglobinopathies, while teardrop cells suggest marrow infiltration by tumour or fibrosis. Target cells and burr cells are less specific abnormalities. The most common morphological abnormality reported is 'slight anisocytosis, slight poikilocytosis". Unfortunately, this abnormality is so non-specific as to make it unhelpful in discerning even whether there is a haematological disorder.

Polychromasia should be evaluated, with the clinician recognising that various degrees of polychromasia will indicate varying degrees of marrow stimulation. Basophilic stippling is another representation of residual RNA content; while most are associated with thalassaemias, basophilic stippling will occur in any type of erythroid stimulation. Nucleated red cells should be searched for carefully, since even if present, this indicates marked erythroid stimulation, loss of splenic function or marrow infiltration.

Platelets

The platelets should be examined to assure that they are about as numerous as indicated by the automated count (on a high-power field, each platelet seen will correspond to about $15 \times 10^9/l$). Marked clumping may cause an erroneous low platelet count. When there is marked thrombocytosis, the MPV usually is low, yet the relatively few largest platelets will stand out. When the platelet count and MPV are not given because of contaminant or artefact, it is especially important to look at the smear to find whether platelets are present, approximately how many and what appears to be the cause of the artefact. Red cell and white cell fragments are the particles most often confused by the counter for platelets (Armitage et al, 1978; Hanker & Giammara, 1983).

White cells

Check for infrequent cells: monocytes, eosinophils, basophils and for cells that normally are not present: myelocytes, plasma cells, blasts. Also, morphological abnormalities should be looked for. Pelger-Huet (congenital granulocyte hyposegmentation) and pseudo-Pelger-Huet (the same hyposegmentation, acquired with a myeloproliferative disorder) anomalies are uncommon but should be distinguished from increased bands. Hypersegmented neutrophils indicate either megaloblastic disease, renal failure or heat stroke. Toxic granulation is often seen, not always with a recognisable cause.

Finally, the clinician should recognise that only one experienced observer need look at the peripheral blood smear in all but a handful of cases. If a qualified technologist or consultant has interpreted the peripheral smear, little additional information will be gained by the second observer (Woo et al, 1981).

COAGULATION

Prothrombin and partial thromboplastin times

These are measures of portions of the humoral coagulation cascade. Normal values depend to a small degree upon the reagents and system used, but a typical set of normal values is shown in Table 2.3.

Table 2.3   Normal values of coagulation times for prothrombin and partial thromboplastim

	Normal time (seconds) ± 2 s.d.	Duplicate error (seconds)
Prothrombin Time	10.5 ± 1.5	1.0
Partial Thromboplastin Time	31.0 + 5.0	3.0

Both assays depend on inactivation of endogenous blood coagulation in the specimen tube; when the test is to be run, calcium (chelated by the anticoagulant) and a coagulation activator are added. The time required for observable coagulation is then measured. Most laboratories have converted from manual assays of coagulation to automated assays. Depending on the reagent added, portions of the coagulation cascade, such as are measured by the above tests, or single coagulation factors can be measured.

It is important to use a constant amount of plasma from the blood specimen. Severely anaemic patients will have more than usual plasma per volume of whole blood: a fixed amount of anticoagulant will chelate endogenous Ca^{++} less than normally. Therefore the blood will coagulate in an artefactually rapid manner under assay conditions and slight coagulation defects will be concealed. In contrast, polycythemic patients will have less than normal plasma per whole blood. Added Ca^{++} will be partially blocked by the collection tube's excess (for the plasma) anticoagulant, falsely lengthening the test coagulation time and suggesting a disorder.

Bleeding time

This is an *in vivo* assay of haemostatic competence, in which a standardised incision is made on skin under 40 mmHg pressure. Normal values are 3–6 minutes using the standard Mielke template. Duplicate error is 3 minutes, even with experienced technique. Even without a qualitative haemostatic defect, the bleeding time is prolonged proportional to the degree of thrombocytopenia. Correction of the bleeding time for thrombocyytopenia is done in some centers and may become more accepted with increasingly accurate platelet counts, but the bleeding time is difficult to interpret when the platelet count is under $50 \times 10^9/l$. A drawback is that discomfort and scar of the test may make multiple evaluations unacceptable to many patients.

Whole-blood clotting time

This is the time required for whole, unmodified blood to coagulate at room temperature *in vitro*. It is performed by repeated tilting of blood-filled tubes and measurement of the time for the blood to coagulate. The duplicate error of this method is quite high: when it is used to monitor anticoagulation, the potential for error is compounded if it is performed by more than one person. Sources of variation include differences in blood drawing (activation by tissue factors that is of little importance to the anticoagulated specimen is critical in this test), vigour in tube-tilting and diligence in serial observation.

Platelet aggregation

Platelets suspended in plasma will aggregate after exposure to ADP or other inducers, such as collagen, thrombin or epinephrine. The rate at which a turbid suspension of single platelets clears as platelet aggregates form and precipitate is recorded as a change in light transmission over time. Aspirin, uraemia, liver disease, alcoholism, myeloproliferative disorders and dys-proteinaemias will alter the response to aggregating agents. The several forms of von Willebrand's disease will diminish the aggregation response to ris-tocetin.

There is a substantial intra- and inter-laboratory variation in platelet aggregation studies. If the laboratory staff that perform aggregometry are personally not well experienced in the disorders under question, only gross abnormalities should be relied upon, while the subtle changes that are more often seen should be interpreted with great conservatism.

NORMAL VALUES

In apparently normal medical students, the range of values (mean ± 2 *s.d.*) for the automated blood count is shown in Table 2.4.

The data from a study of ambulatory, home-dwelling subjects suggest that there is no substantial difference in blood count values between normal students and normal septuagenarians (Kelly & Munan, 1977). Therefore it is incorrect to attribute anaemia or thrombocytopenia to 'old age' unless there is an underlying disease. However, since the bone marrow proliferative capacity progressively declines with age, there is progressively less marrow reserve (Lipschitz et al, 1981). It may therefore be expected that an elderly subject's marrow will compensate less well for a given degree of acute or chronic disease than will a young subject's, making the elderly more prone to the anaemia of chronic disease.

Similar studies show that the prothrombin and partial thromboplastin times do not vary with age among normals. This is not so thoroughly known for platelet aggregation or bleeding time.

Table 2.4 Range of values for the automated blood count

White cells, $\times 10^9$/l*	6.1 ± 2.3
Red cells, $\times 10^{12}$/l**	5.29 ± 0.75
Haemoglabin, g/dl**	16.2 ± 1.9
PCV, g/dl**	48.4 ± 5.8
MCV, fl***	90.3 ± 9.1
MCH, pg	30.6 ± 3.0
MCHC, %	33.6 ± 1.2
RDW, %	13.2 ± 1.6
Platelets, $\times 10^9$/l	288 ± 153
MPV, fl****	***
Lymphoctes, %	$36 + 14$
Neutrophils, %	60 ± 15

*These values for whites only; blacks, $5.4 \pm 2.7 \times 10^9$/l
**These values for males only; females, red cells 4.62 ± 0.70
   haemoglobin 14.0 ± 2.2
   PCV 41.6 ± 5.8
***Variation can be due to differences in machine setting.
****Depends on platelet count

INDICATIONS AND VALUE OF BONE MARROW EXAMINATION

Indications to examine the bone marrow fall into two general categories. If a primary bone marrow disorder is suspected, then the most important data are the distribution of cell types and the morphology of individual cells. Careful study of a satisfactory area of stained bone marrow aspirate is most useful in such cases, and may be supplemented by examination of a section from trephine biopsy. In contrast, if a systemic disorder — tumour, infection, or vasculitis — is suspected, the bone marrow is appropriately a tissue that can be examined to establish a diagnosis or document the disorder's extent. Examples are staging of lymphoma, culture for tuberculosis and identification of vasculitis. For these purposes a trephine biopsy, sometimes from multiple sites, is most useful.

The bone marrow examination should begin with a review of the specimen at low magnification to judge three variables. First, is the specimen satisfactory in quantity and quality? There should be spicular architecture, and the cells should be in a monolayer that allows study of individual cell morphology. Second, are there areas of homogeneity of cells? Normally marrow is a heterogenous mix of several cell types in a continuum of maturation. If there is a sheet or nodule of a single cell type, this may indicate a lymphoid nodule (normal) or leukaemia, lymphoma, myeloma, or metastatic solid tumour. Third, are megakaryocytes present? While other cell types are more easily identified at higher power, the megakaryocyte is relatively rare but distinctively large, making low-power scan the best to determine the approximate megakaryocyte number.

High-power examination of bone marrow is for three further purposes. First, what is the relative proportion of erythroid and myeloid cells? Often this is subjective, with a broad range of the 'normal' myeloid-to-erythroid ratio 2–4:1. A differential count of 500 or 1000 marrow cells allows more precise quantitation. Second, is erythroid and myeloid maturation normal? The maturation of nucleus and cytoplasm is examined and megaloblastic or other dysplastic changes are detected. Likewise, maturation arrest of erythroid and/or myeloid lines are detected. Third, are other cells present in abnormal numbers? Blast cells, plasmacytes, mast cells, lymphocytes and eosinophils are all present in normal marrow. However, an increase above 5 per cent in any of these cell types is clearly abnormal. Any tumour cell is abnormal. Finally, iron stores are determined by Prussian-blue stain. Sideroblasts are also best detected with this stain.

Most bone marrow examinations are to determine the presence or extent of haematological or non-haematological malignancy. Other frequent indications are as follows:

Thrombocytopenia

Decreased bone marrow megakaryocyte suggests a failure of adequate production as the cause of thrombocytopenia; increased megakaryocytes suggest peripheral platelet destruction. The distinction is clear only in rather advanced examples of either type of disorder. Probably the improved information available from MPV will somewhat reduce the number of cases in whom bone marrow examination is needed to distinguish these two causes.

Megaloblastic anaemia and iron deficiency anaemia

The bone marrow offers a pathognomonic picture in both disorders: megaloblastic nuclear-cytoplasmic dissociation, or absent stainable iron, and general or erythroid hyperplasia. However, with increased reliability of transferrin, iron, B_{12} and folate blood assays, as well as reliable cell indices, many such cases will be definitely diagnosed without the bone marrow. Whether this relatively risk-free but uncomfortable and costly procedure is essential in such proved cases will have to be determined in individual cases.

Aplasia of one or more cell lines

This is a qualitative rather than quantitative study. If there is a peripheral cytopenia, an increase in this cell line in the bone marrow suggest a peripheral destruction or ineffective haematopoiesis. In contrast, a decrease in this cell line suggests bone marrow failure, either primary or as a result of toxin or systemic disease.

REFERENCES

Armitage J D, Goeken J A, Feagler J R 1978 Spurious elevation of the platelet count in acute leukemia. Journal of the American Medical Association 239: 433–434
Bessman J D 1980 Evaluation of whole-blood automated particle counts and sizing. American Journal of Clinical Pathology 76: 289–293

Bessman J D 1982 Analysis and clinical application of red cell volume distribution. In: Van Assendelft O W, England J M (eds) Advances in hematologic methods: calibration and control. CRC Press, Boca Raton

Bessman J D, Williams L J, Gilmer P R 1981 Mean platelet volume: the inverse relation between platelet count and size in normal subjects and an artifact of small particles. American Journal of Clinical Pathology 76: 289–293

Bessman J D, Williams L J, Gilmer P R 1982 Platelet size in health and hematologic disease. American Journal of Clinical Pathology 78: 150–153

Bessman J D, Gilmer P R, Gardner F H 1983 Improved classification of anemia with MCV and RDW. American Journal of Clinical Pathology 30: 322–326

Cameron H A, Phillips R, Ibotson R M, Carson P H M 1983 Platelet size in myocardial infarction. British Medical Journal 287: 449

Cameron H A, Phillips R, Ibotson R M, Carson P H M 1983 Mean platelet volume in myocardial infarction. British Medical Journal 287: 1883

Coulter Electronics, 1982 Manual for S-Plus IV. Hialeah

Giles C 1981 The platelet count and mean platelet volume. British Journal of Haematology 48: 31–38

Gottfried E L 1979 Erythrocyte indexes with the electronic counter. New England Journal of Medicine 300: 1277

Hanker J S, Giammara B L 1983 Neutrophil pseudoplatelets: their discrimination by myeloperoxidase. Science 220: 415–417

Hillman R S, Finch C A 1969 The misused reticulocyte. British Journal of Haematology 17: 313–315

International Committee for Standardisation of Haematology: expert panel on cell counting: Berlin, 1979; Montebello, 1980; Leuven, 1982

Johnson C S, Tegos C, Beutler E 1983 Thalassemia minor: routine erythrocyte measurements and differentiation from iron deficiency. American Journal of Clinical Pathology 80: 31–36

Kaye F J, Alter B P 1982 Red cell size distribution analysis: a noninvasive evaluation of microcytosis. (abstract) Blood 60(Sup 1): 36a

Kelly A, Munan L 1977 Haematologic profile of natural populations: red cell parameters. British Journal of Haematology 35: 153–160

Levin J, Bessman J D 1983 The inverse relation between platelet volume and platelet number. Journal of Laboratory and Clinical Medicine 101: 295–307

Lipschitz D A, Mitchell C O, Thompson C 1981 The anemia of senescence. American Journal of Hematology 11: 47–54

Martin J F, Plumb J, Kilbey R S, Kishk Y T 1983 Changes in volume and density of platelets in myocardial infarction. British Medical Journal 287: 456

Salzman E W, Ashford T P, Chambers D A, Neri L L, Dempster A P 1969 Platelet volume: effect of temperature and agents affecting platelet aggregation. American Journal of Physiology 217: 1330–1336

Technicon Corporation, 1983 Manual for H-6000/601C. Tarrytown

Van Assendelft O W, England J M (eds) 1982 Advances in hematologic methods: calibration and control. CRC Press, Boca Raton

van der Lelie J, Brakenhoff J A C 1983 Mean platelet volume in myocardial infarction. British Medical Journal 287: 1471

Wintrobe M M 1981 Clinical hematology, 8th edn. Lea & Febiger, Philadelphia

Woo B, Jen P, Rosenthal D E, Bunn H F, Goldman L 1981 Anemic inpatients: Correlates of house officer performance. Archives of Internal Medicine 141: 1199–1202

Iron-deficiency anaemia

INTRODUCTION

Almost all the iron in the human body is complexed with protein. There are three major groups of iron metalloproteins: haem proteins that transport and store oxygen, enzymes involved in oxidising (redox) reactions, and specific iron transport and storage proteins (Wrigglesworth & Baum, 1980). Approximately three-quarters of the iron is functionally important. Sixty-two per cent is in the haemoglobin of circulating red cells, 8 per cent is found in muscle myoglobin and the rest in tissue enzymes. Most of the remaining 25 per cent constitutes a reserve that can be rapidly transferred to the functional compartments (Bothwell et al, 1979). Iron deficiency exists when total body iron is reduced, but this ranges in severity from diminished iron stores without loss of functional iron to absent stores with severe anaemia (Table 3.1).

IRON METABOLISM

Iron is rigorously conserved and reused by the human body. While there is a continuous exchange between storage sites and all functional compartments quantitative measurements of iron turnover are dominated by its role in

Table 3.1 Stages of iron deficiency

Stage	Synonyms	Iron stores	Anaemia
Iron storage depletion	Prelatent iron deficiency	Reduced	None
Iron-deficient erythropoiesis	Latent iron deficiency	Absent	None
	Iron deficiency without anaemia		
Iron-deficiency anaemia		Absent	Present

haemoglobin synthesis (Finch et al, 1970). Between 30 and 35 mg of iron pass through the plasma each day, most of it en route for the erythroid marrow where it is incorporated into the haemoglobin of developing red cells. This process can be measured readily by the introduction of a transferrin-bound radio-iron tag into the plasma (plasma iron turnover). About 80 per cent of such radio-iron is found in circulating red cells after 14 days in normal subjects (red cell utilisation, Hosain et al, 1967). The iron incorporated into red cells then remains in the circulation for about 120 days before the cells are engulfed by macrophages, principally in the spleen, and the iron is either returned to plasma immediately or incorporated into cellular stores for a variable period of time (Lynch et al, 1974).

Most measurements of internal iron transport have been made in younger individuals. However, Marx & Dinant (1982) carried out ferrokinetic studies in one man and six women aged between 61 and 80 years. Comparisons were made with seven men and three women between 19 and 50 years of age. The mean plasma iron turnover of the older subjects was somewhat higher than the younger controls (125 ± 47 μmol/l blood/24h vs 112 ± 27 μmol/l blood /24h) while red cell utilisation was a little less (82 per cent vs 85 per cent). Thus, non-erythroid iron turnover (iron destined for tissues other than the erythroid marrow) was significantly increased (29 vs 17 μmol/l blood/24h).

ABSORPTION

Iron homeostasis is maintained by matching variable absorption with an obligatory rate of excretion. Only three of the many factors known to affect iron absorption in experimental situations appear to be important under most physiological circumstances. They are: the amount of iron ingested, its bioavailability and the iron storage status of the individual being tested (Lynch & Morck, 1983). The average iron content of Western diets is about 6 mg/4.2 MJ (Wretlind, 1970). Recent dietary surveys carried out in the United States indicate that the average intake remains adequate in older people. This occurs even when caloric consumption falls because there is a concomitant rise in iron nutrient density from 6 to 8 mg/4.2 MJ (Lynch et al, 1982). Nevertheless, it is important to note that nutritional deficiencies may occur in certain disadvantaged groups. These include some nursing-home patients (Jansen & Harrill, 1977), those who have physical disabilities or live alone (Caird et al, 1975; Steen et al, 1977) and older people in whom dietary diversity is limited by poverty or strong food dislikes (Boykin, 1976).

Adequate nutrition depends as much on dietary iron availability as it does on overall intake (Bothwell et al, 1979). Haem iron in meat is absorbed as the intact porphyrin ring and is highly bioavailable in virtually all meals. However, haem iron represents only a small proportion of overall intake even in Western countries. All other forms of food iron (non-haem iron) are solubilised and enter a common luminal pool before being absorbed. Assimilation from this pool is markedly affected by meal composition. Meat and ascorbic acid appear to be the major dietary factors ensuring adequate absorption (Monsen et al, 1978). The bioavailability of food iron may thus be reduced in the elderly if food choices are limited. The second Health and Nutrition Survey carried out in the United States revealed a progressive fall in the proportion of dietary iron derived from meat with increasing age (Lynch et al, 1982). This trend could diminish iron bioavailability in two ways: the quantity of haem is less and the bioavailability of non-haem iron is reduced.

The physiological mechanisms responsible for iron assimilation may also be affected. Percentage absorption has been reported to fall (Bonnet et al, 1960; Freiman et al, 1963; Jacobs & Owen, 1969). Unfortunately, the earlier studies were not well controlled for iron storage status, making the interpretation of the findings difficult. However, Jacobs & Owen (1969) measured absorption from a standard meal in 8 men and 28 women, all of whom were healthy and considered iron replete on the basis of a normal haemoglobin level, a serum iron greater than 11.6 μmol/l (mean 20.9 μmol/l) and a percentage saturation over 18 per cent (mean 32 per cent). Their ages ranged from 21 to 78 years. Absorption of inorganic iron diminished with age while haem iron was unaffected. The authors suggested that this might be a consequence of an increasing incidence of gastric atrophy and hypochlorhydria, since hydrochloric acid facilitates the absorption of inorganic but not haem iron.

More recently Marx (1979) demonstrated that iron-replete young and old people absorb ferrous ammonium sulphate equally well, and that both groups respond appropriately to the stimulus of iron deficiency. Since hydrochloric acid is unimportant for the adequate absorption of both haem iron and soluble ferrous salts (Jacobs et al, 1964), the latter two studies taken together suggest that mucosal uptake and transport is unaltered by ageing but that hypochlorhydria limits the absorption of less soluble forms of food iron.

Approximately 80 per cent of the absorbed iron is found in circulating red cells after two weeks in iron-replete young individuals. Recent studies indicate that red cell incorporation of this iron is reduced in the elderly (Marx, 1979; Marx & Dinant, 1982). It appears that a greater proportion is retained as it passes through the liver.

EXCRETION

The body's ability to increase iron absorption is limited by dietary availability. Therefore, it is not surprising that iron deficiency occurs most often when requirements are augmented by rapid growth (early childhood) or accelerated loss (menstruation, pregnancy and lactation). In the elderly, obligatory physiological losses are minimal. They result from exfoliation of cells from the skin and gastrointestinal and urinary tracts as well as the excretion of small amounts of iron in sweat, bile and urine. Using radioisotopic methods, Finch (1959) reported a daily excretion rate of 0.61 ($\pm$ 0.08) mg and 0.64 ($\pm$ 0.05) mg in men aged 57–84 years and women aged 59–77 years respectively. Significantly higher values were obtained for menstruating women, 1.22 ($\pm$ 0.11) mg per day. Green et al (1968) used the same method to study three groups of younger men and obtained values between 0.90 and 1.02 mg per day.

STORAGE

The physiological factors discussed above protect the elderly against iron deficiency, a conclusion that is corroborated by direct and indirect measurements of iron stores. One-third of storage iron is found in the liver. Hepatic iron concentrations in unselected male victims of trauma or illnesses unlikely to affect iron metabolism rise after puberty and then remain unchanged even in old age. Women tend to have little liver iron until the menopause, after which the concentration rises to levels approaching those in men (Lynch et al, 1982).

Another important storage site is the bone marrow. Stainable iron in this organ also increases with age (Benzie, 1963). However, the most comprehensive data have been obtained indirectly by using serum ferritin measurements which correlate closely with body iron stores, 1 μg/l of ferritin in the plasma representing approximately 10 mg storage iron (Cook, 1982). Concentrations rise with increasing age (Fig. 3.1). In women the trend is most apparent after 50 years.

PREVALENCE OF IRON DEFICIENCY

Iron deficiency remains the most common cause of nutritional anaemia throughout the world. Prevalence rates are highest in developing countries.

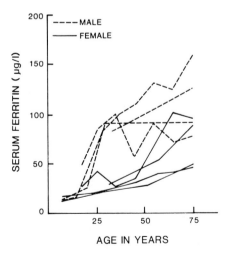

Fig. 3.1   The effect of age on serum ferritin concentration. Observations from four different studies (Cook et al, 1976; Valberg et al, 1976; Leyland et al, 1979; Casale et al, 1981). Reproduced with permission from the American Journal of Clinical Nutrition

While very little comprehensive information is available for the elderly, it appears that the same geographical variations in prevalence exist, but that the elderly are at lower risk than children and menstruating women. MacPhail et al (1981) reported that anaemia was present in 18.5 per cent of South African Indian women under the age of 45, as compared with only 6.9 per cent of those between 46 and 75 years. Mean serum ferritin concentrations for the two groups were 14.0 and 27.8 μ/l respectively. Similar conclusions were reached by Hershko et al (1979) who studied in a rural Israeli community with a high incidence of nutritional anaemia. Whereas 46 per cent of pregnant women and 20 per cent of children under the age of 6 had haemoglobins of less than 10 g/100 ml, this was the case in only 2 per cent of the 142 individuals aged 60–99 years.

Despite the availability of observations from several extensive epidemiological surveys, it is difficult to determine the true prevalence of iron deficiency among apparently healthy individuals living in Western countries. This is a result of the lack of a clear understanding of the factors that affect haemoglobin concentration in the elderly as well as the fact that anaemia has been equated with iron deficiency in many studies (Lynch et al, 1982). In a survey of the literature from Western countries, Bowering & Sanchez (1976) reported prevalence rates for anaemia (haemoglobin less than 11 or 12 g/dl) in elderly individuals not receiving medical care of 1.1–5.0 per cent for men, 1.5–16.0 per cent for women, and 4.0–4.4 per cent where the sexes were not separated. Three large-scale surveys from the United States and Canada demonstrated that the proportion of elderly individuals with haemoglobin concentrations below values considered to fall within the normal range for younger subjects varied widely in different ethnic and socioeconomic groups, but was highest in elderly men with low incomes (Ten-State Nutrition Survey, 1968–1970; Health and Nutrition Examination Survey United States, 1971–1974; Nutrition Canada, 1978). A similar age-related fall in mean haemoglobin levels is evident in four community studies carried out in the United Kingdom (Table 3.2).

While there appears to be little doubt that haemoglobin values decline in many older men, the validity of the assumption that this represents nutritional iron deficiency has been questioned recently (Lynch et al, 1982; Dallman et al, 1984). Dallman and his colleagues analysed the data from the Second National Health and Nutrition Examination Survey carried out in the United States, in a different way (Dallman et al, 1984). Reference ranges for haemoglobin were first derived from those subjects who had normal laboratory values for serum iron, iron-binding capacity, mean corpuscular volume and erythrocyte protoporphyrin. Using these standards, 4.4 per cent of elderly men had haemoglobin values below the 95 per cent reference range, compared with 5.7 per cent of the infants, 5.9 per cent of the teenage girls and 5.8 per cent of the young women. However, while the pattern of laboratory abnormalities suggested that iron deficiency was the predominant cause in

Table 3.2   Mean haemoglobin values and prevalence of anaemia in the elderly living at home

Study No.	Mean haemoglobin (g/dl)				Reference
	Men		Women		
	65–74*	75–90	65–74	75–90	
1	14.6 (7.2)+	14.1 (20.8)	13.7 (11.1)	13.0 (23.3)	Parsons et al, 1965
2	14.6 (1.9)	13.8 (31.0)	13.7 (7.5)	13.1 (21.4)	Hill, 1967
3	13.9 (8.8)	13.5 (17.0)	13.2 (9.4)	13.0 (14.7)	Myers et al, 1968
4	14.2 (4.0)	13.8 (12.0)	13.1 (15.0)	12.9 (25.0)	McLennan et al, 1973

* Age in years
\+ Numbers in parentheses indicate percentage anaemic (haemoglobin <12 for all women, and men in studies 3, 4, <12.5 for men in studies 1, 2).

infants, teenage girls and young women, the authors concluded that inflammatory disease was a more likely explanation in the elderly men.

It must be pointed out that few subjects met all the criteria for the diagnosis of anaemia associated with inflammation or neoplasms – 'the anaemia of chronic disease'. Moreover, Lipschitz et al (1981) found a relatively high prevalence of low haemoglobin values in a group of very carefully selected healthy elderly subjects. Neither iron deficiency nor inflammation appeared to be important factors, and modest reductions in neutrophil and platelet counts were also noted, suggesting that an overall decrease in haematopoiesis was present. While the specific reasons for lower haemoglobin values in apparently healthy older men require better definition, these observations lend support to the contention that iron-deficiency anaemia is unlikely to have a nutritional basis in the elderly living in industralised countries unless special circumstances pertain.

Documented iron-deficiency anaemia is considerably more common among individuals seeking medical care. Table 3.3 shows the results obtained in several surveys in which the incidence of anaemia in elderly hospital patients is reported. Between 6.4 and 41 per cent of patients were anaemic, and in 21–90 per cent of the anaemic individuals the cause was considered to be iron deficiency. Unfortunately, patient selection and criteria used for identifying both anaemia and iron deficiency vary considerably in the different surveys. In some studies the evaluation iron status was based on definitive information such as bone marrow examination or response to iron therapy, while in others serum iron and iron-binding capacity were used. Nevertheless, it is evident that while iron deficiency may not be prevalent in

Table 3.3   Prevalence of anaemia in hospital patients

Number surveyed	Criterion for anaemia (Hb g/dl)	Anaemia (%)	Iron deficient‡ (%)	Aetiology of iron deficiency	Reference
7941	<10.4	18.6	35	Blood loss in >50%	Monroe, 1951
156	<11.7	41	94	Blood loss in 78%	Bedford & Wollner, 1958
319	<11.9	37	21*	Blood loss in 50%	Lawson, 1960
1500	<120 male <11.5 female	33	26	Blood loss in 51%	Cooper et al, 1967
>400	<12.0	32	48*	ND	Davison, 1967
100	<11.7	33	60*	ND	Batata et al, 1967
2700	<10.0	6.4	67	Blood loss in 44%	Evans et al, 1968
500	<11.4	16	85	ND	Griffiths et al, 1970
1094	<11.0	21	45	Site of blood loss found in 24%	Bose et al, 1970
104	<11.0	15	30	Blood loss	Matzner et al, 1979
161	<12.0	41	42	Blood loss in 69%	Kalchthaler & Tan, 1980

ND Not defined
‡ Percentage of anaemic patients found to be iron-deficient
* Neoplasms causing blood loss excluded

the healthy elderly, it is a common cause of the more severe degrees of anaemia encountered in older hospital patients and that adequate evaluation of iron status is therefore essential.

AETIOLOGY

Inadequate intake

As discussed above, reduced physiological iron requirements protect the elderly against nutritional iron deficiency. Inadequate intake is a likely explanation for iron-deficiency anaemia only in populations where the overall prevalence of nutritional anaemia is very high or when poverty, living conditions or other factors limit food choices significantly.

Impaired absorption

Malabsorption of iron is unusual, even in the presence of extensive bowel disease, unless the stomach and upper small intestine are affected. The most common cause is gastric surgery (Bothwell et al, 1979). As many as 80 per cent of patients who have undergone gastric surgery may develop iron deficiency, although prevalence rates of 30–50 per cent have been reported in most series (Lloyd & Valberg, 1977). Robertson & Kirkham (1979) found 15 (57.7 per cent) of 26 patients aged between 58 and 94 years who had had an operation on the stomach between 5 and 40 years earlier to be anaemic.

Iron deficiency is considerably more likely when resection is combined with gastrojejunostomy (Lloyd & Valberg, 1977; Magnusson, 1976) and results as much from the loss of the reservoir function of the stomach and diversion of the gastric contents away from the proximal duodenum which is capable of maximal absorption as from loss of hydrochloric acid secretion. Despite impaired food iron absorption, the absorption of soluble iron salts remains adequate (Smith & Mallett, 1957).

Chronic blood loss

Chronic blood loss is the most important cause of iron deficiency in the elderly. Since epistaxis, haemoptysis, haematuria or uterine haemorrhage usually brings the patient to the doctor long before anaemia occurs, bleeding from the gastrointestinal tract is the most frequent reason. The major causes are listed in Table 3.4. Non-steroidal anti-inflammatory drugs, particularly

Table 3.4 Major sources of gastrointestinal blood loss in the elderly

Drugs
  Nonsteroidal anti-inflammatory drugs
    Aspirin
    Indomethacin
  Anticoagulants

Peptic ulcer disease
  Gastric
  Duodenal

Tumours
  Polyps
  Cancer of the stomach
  Cancer of the colon

Miscellaneous
  Hiatus hernia
    Oesophagitis
    Hernial pouch
  Vascular malformations
  Ischaemic colitis
  Haemorrhoids
  Diverticulosis

aspirin combinations, are frequently used by older people and are a common cause of chronic blood loss (McLennan et al, 1973, Steinheber, 1976; Raufmann & Dobbins, 1980; Beveridge et al, 1965). The importance of peptic ulcer disease is frequently overlooked, since most patients with this disorder present in the third to fifth decades of life. Nevertheless, clinical and autopsy surveys have demonstrated that these lesions are prevalent in the elderly (Narayanan & Steinheber, 1976) and that they are one of the most commonly encountered reasons for chronic blood loss (Kasper et al, 1965).

Tumours are a well-recognised source of bleeding. Colonic carcinoma is the most common malignancy, with a prevalence rate of about 3 per cent after the age of 70 years (Steinheber, 1976). Hiatus hernia is frequently present in the elderly, but should not be accepted as a cause of gastrointestinal blood loss unless associated oesophagitis or mucosal bleeding has been demonstrated by endoscopy. Similarly, diverticulosis is often found but may not necessarily provide a satisfactory explanation for chronic blood loss unless the latter is documented by colonoscopy.

Vascular malformations have recently been shown by angiographic and endoscopic techniques to be a prominent cause of chronic bleeding in older individuals (Boley et al, 1977) and may be responsible for that mistakenly attributed to diverticular disease (Raufmann & Dobbins, 1980). The frequency of degenerative vascular disease also increases with age, and ischaemic colitis with predominantly mucosal involvement may cause bleeding despite a minimum of other symptoms (Raufmann & Dobbins, 1980). Finally it should be remembered that haemorrhoids are not a common cause of rectal bleeding which appears for the first time in older patients. Care should also be taken not to accept this explanation without further investigation (Steinheber, 1976).

The elderly patient with iron deficiency merits a careful search for gastrointestinal blood loss (Croker & Beynon, 1981), although the extent of investigation for a precise anatomical diagnosis depends on the clinical setting. Improved instrumentation has made evaluation of the gastrointestinal tract possible even in elderly patients. Gibbins et al (1974) found that endoscopy was well tolerated in 114 patients aged between 65 and 89 years.

EFFECTS OF IRON DEFICIENCY

Related to anaemia

Anaemia is the most common clinically apparent consequence of iron deficiency, and there is a significant association between its severity and the degree of pallor (Davison et al, 1969). On the contrary, symptoms related to tissue hypoxia may not appear until the haemoglobin level falls below 8 g/dl because compensatory mechanisms improve the efficiency of oxygen delivery (Elwood et al, 1969). The two most important adaptations are a rise in cardiac output and improved oxygen release to the tissues as a result of increased red cell 2–3 diphosphoglyceric acid (2–3 DPG) concentration (Brannon et al, 1945; Andersen & Barkve, 1970; Torrance et al, 1970; Varat et al, 1972; Davies et al, 1973). Healthy young people can even perform strenuous exercise in the presence of mild anaemia (Schoene et al, 1983), although severe anaemia does limit the capacity for physical work (Sproule et al, 1960; Andersen & Barkve, 1970; Viteri & Torun, 1974; Gardner et al, 1977).

The functional consequences of mild anaemia are more evident in the elderly because adaptive mechanisms may be compromised and tissue perfusion less adequate. Cardiac output is often limited by coronary vascular disease. There is also a gradual fall in 2–3 DPG levels with age (Brewer, 1974). Furthermore, even minimal decreases in tissue oxygenation can provoke symptoms, the heart and brain being the organs most often affected (Hyams, 1978). Both congestive heart failure and left ventricular failure are seen. Angina is rare. Dizziness is common and confusion may occur.

Unrelated to anaemia

Mucosal and epithelioid

Atrophic glossitis and angular stomatitis have been regarded as prominent symptoms of iron-deficiency anaemia, particularly in older individuals (Beveridge et al, 1965). However, it is not clear whether these changes are attributable purely to iron lack or are the result of concomitant deficiencies of other essential nutrients such as pyridoxine (Jacobs & Cavill, 1968).

The reported association between iron deficiency and post-cricoid oesophageal webs (Paterson–Kelly or Plummer Vinson syndrome) has attracted considerable attention over the years (Beutler & Fairbanks, 1980). The disorder is more often seen in women over 40 years of age (Chisholm et al, 1971a), and carcinoma eventually develops in 4–16 per cent of patients (Chisholm et al, 1971a; Chisholm, 1974). Most surveys emanate from Europe and the United Kingdom, and the syndrome seems to be rare in the United States as well as in the developing countries where iron deficiency is most prevalent (Bothwell et al, 1979). Furthermore, some investigators have disputed the validity of the apparent association (Elwood et al, 1964; Nosher et al, 1975), and the possibility that other factors play a role is strengthened by the finding of a relationship with auto-immune disorders (Chisholm et al, 1971b; Blendis, 1964; Jacobs & Kilpatrick, 1964; Javett, 1972). Koilonychia, once considered a common clinical sign of severe iron deficiency, is rarely seen now and may have resulted from an associated or combined deficiency of zinc (Bothwell et al, 1979) or possibly methionine and cysteine (Jalili & Al-Kassab, 1959).

Muscular

Skeletal muscle performance is abnormal in iron deficiency (Finch et al,

1976; Koziol et al, 1978; MacLanē et al, 1981) and compounds the effects of anaemia on exercise tolerance. The functional impairment results from decreased activity of iron-containing enzymes. Some studies suggest that depletion of alpha-glycerophosphate dehydrogenase plays a primary role (Finch et al, 1979). Myocardial function is not affected (Llewellyn-Jones, 1965). While these findings may have significance for people undertaking severe exercise their importance in the relatively sedentary is less apparent (Charlton et al, 1977).

Behavioural and neurological

Severe iron deficiency is associated with a number of neurological abnormalities, although the pathogenetic mechanisms remain obscure. Perversions of appetite such as pica and pagophagia are well described (Crosby, 1971; Reynolds et al, 1968; Crosby, 1976; Bothwell et al, 1979). Paraesthesias, headaches and optic papillitis may occur (Fairbanks et al, 1971). Most descriptions of these disorders have been in younger people particularly young women. More recent studies have demonstrated intellectual and behavioural impairment in children (Pollitt & Leibel, 1976). The latter are poorly understood, and it is not known whether they occur only during the developmental period.

Infectious

Reduced granulocyte (Prasad 1979; Yetgin et al, 1979) and lymphocyte function (Hoffbrand et al, 1974; Narasinga Rao, 1978) as measured *in vitro* has been reported, as has impaired cell mediated immunity (Joynson et al, 1972; McDougal et al, 1975; Srikantia et al, 1976), although the clinical significance of these observations in terms of an increased risk of infection has not been established.

CLINICAL FEATURES

Iron-deficiency anaemia is rarely an isolated disorder in the elderly. The most prominent symptoms and signs may be related to the underlying disease process in many clinical situations. Skin pallor is a consistent feature and correlates closely with the haemoglobin concentration. Unfortunately, it is often overlooked in older people. Cardiovascular and cerebral symptoms frequently predominate in old age. Tachycardia, breathlessness and peripheral oedema are common, while dizziness, apathy and confusion may result from impaired oxygen delivery to the brain. The contribution of anaemia to these symptoms can be underestimated unless the blood is examined (DeNicola & Casale, 1983). Symptoms unrelated to anaemia such as glossitis, chelosis and angular stomatitis are less specific, while painful dysphagia in association with the Paterson–Kelly syndrome is a rare occurrence.

LABORATORY EVALUATION

Blood picture

The haemoglobin or packed cell volume (PCV) estimate is the basis of diagnosis, but mild anaemia may be difficult to detect with certainty because of a significant overlap in the frequency distribution curves of haemoglobin or PCV in anaemic and normal individuals (Garby et al, 1969; Cook et al, 1971). The use of the haemoglobin alone is further complicated in the elderly by the changes discussed above that appear to be associated with ageing. The peripheral blood cells of severely iron-deficient individuals typically show hypochromia and microcytosis with variable degrees of aniso- and poikilocytosis, but mild iron deficiency may not be recognised on morphological grounds alone in 50 per cent of patients (Fairbanks, 1971).

The advent of electronic counters has revolutionised the accuracy and sensitivity of red cell indices. A reduced mean corpuscular volume (MCV) and mean corpuscular haemoglobin are the most reliable parameters of iron deficiency, but decreased values are not specific, being equally characteristic of other disorders in which haemoglobin synthesis is impaired, such as thalassaemia and anaemia of chronic disorders. Moreover, the degree of change depends on the duration of iron-deficient erythropoiesis and on the quantitative discrepancy between iron supply and marrow demand (Bothwell et al, 1979). If erythropoiesis is sufficiently suppressed or iron deficiency of recent onset, values may fall within the normal range and further evaluation depends on specific biochemical tests that measure the size of body iron stores and the adequacy of iron supply to the developing red blood cells. Raper et al (1977) studied 69 patients aged between 65 and 100 years. An MCV between 71 and 82 fl failed to distinguish between iron deficiency and the anaemia of chronic disease, while eight patients with values below 70 had no marrow iron stores.

The white blood cells are usually normal but sometimes show hypersegmentation. Platelet numbers are normal, or increased in patients who are bleeding.

Evaluation of iron stores

Serum ferritin

Iron is stored in the liver, spleen, bone marrow and skeletal muscle in the form of ferritin or haemosiderin. Sensitive immunoradiometric assays have demonstrated that small quantities of the protein shell of ferritin are present in the plasma. Furthermore, the serum ferritin concentration is directly proportional to the size of body iron stores (Addison et al, 1972; Jacobs et al, 1972; Walters et al, 1973; Cook et al, 1974; Bezwoda et al, 1979). In young healthy adults, storage iron in milligrams can be calculated by multiplying the serum ferritin value in micrograms per litre by 10 (Cook, 1982). Mean serum ferritin concentrations measured in healthy men and women aged between 20 and 50 years who had no evidence of iron deficiency were 94 and 34 $\mu g/l$ respectively (Cook et al, 1974). Mean values reported for men and women aged 65 or older lie between 41 and 171 $\mu g/l$ (Table 3.5).

A serum ferritin below 12 $\mu g/l$ in an anaemic patient is diagnostic of iron deficiency. Cook (1982) reviewed 154 cases of uncomplicated iron deficiency drawn from the literature and found serum ferritin concentrations to be above this level in only 2.6 per cent of subjects. Unfortunately, serum ferritin values are less valuable in many clinical situations where infections, other inflammatory disorders, neoplasms, liver disease or chronic renal disease coexist. The usual relationship between iron stores and serum ferritin is disturbed, and ferritin levels tend to be higher and more variable. It is often necessary to resort to bone marrow examination for an accurate evaluation of iron stores.

Interpretation of serum ferritin concentrations in elderly individuals is also less well established. For the most part, the higher values reported in apparently healthy individuals probably reflect larger iron stores. However, Loria et al (1979) found that 10 of 55 subjects who had a haemoglobin response to iron therapy had normal or high serum ferritin values, suggesting that it may be less sensitive as a measure of iron deficiency in this population. The presence of concurrent but undetected inflammatory or neoplastic disorders could provide an alternative explanation for these observations. More detailed studies are needed to determine whether the relationship between serum ferritin and iron stores is altered in old age.

Table 3.5   Serum ferritin values in the elderly

Number of observations	Age (years)	Mean serum ferritin ($\mu g/l$)	Reference
Men			
165	>45	124	Cook et al, 1976
104	65–90	92	Valberg et al, 1976
31	60–69	73	Leyland et al, 1979
14	70–80	78	Leyland et al, 1979
28	60–96	171	Loria et al, 1979
31	73	166	Qvist et al, 1980
40	>71	128	Casale et al, 1981a
Women			
215	>45	89	Cook et al, 1976
98	65–87	52	Valberg et al, 1976
32	60–69	41	Leyland et al, 1979
25	70–80	48	Leyland et al, 1979
46	60–96	149	Loria et al, 1979
23	73	161	Qvist et al, 1980
48	>71	86	Casale et al, 1981a

Bone marrow

Once iron deficiency is established, the bone marrow usually demonstrates erythroid hypoplasia with normoblastic maturation. Haemoglobinisation is uneven in many developing red cells. The cytoplasm is reduced and cell borders are ragged. Haemosiderin granules are not seen in the reticuloen-dothelial cells, and there is marked reduction in sideroblast iron (Gale et al, 1963; Bainton & Finch, 1964; Baumgartner-Staubli & Beck, 1977). In anaemic patients the finding of significant quantities of bone marrow iron excludes the diagnosis of iron deficiency, with two exceptions. Soon after severe haemorrhage, iron mobilisation from the larger particles may be too slow to meet the demands of the erythroid marrow, leading to persistence of stainable iron despite an inadequate supply to red cell precursors (Stevens et al, 1953). Following iron dextran administration, stainable iron may be found in macrophages for some months despite the continued presence of iron deficiency (Olsson & Weinfeld, 1972).

Evaluation of iron supply

Serum iron and iron-binding capacity

Once iron stores are exhausted, the rate of delivery of iron to the plasma is exceeded by the requirements of the bone marrow, and the plasma iron concentration falls. On the other hand, the total iron-binding capacity (TIBC) rises before iron stores are totally depleted, and there is an inverse relationship between storage iron status and TIBC over a wide range of values (Weinfeld, 1964; Ballas, 1979). Used together as the percentage saturation of transferrin, the two assays provide the most reliable evidence of the adequacy of the iron supply to the bone marrow. When the saturation falls below 15 per cent, delivery of iron to the bone marrow is inadequate to support normal erythropoiesis (Bainton & Finch, 1964; Hillman & Hender-son, 1969).

The circadian rhythm in the plasma iron with higher concentrations in the morning is maintained in old age (Casale et al, 1981b). However, there are a number of reports indicating that the serum iron concentration is lower and total iron binding capacity higher in elderly patients (McFarlane et al, 1967; Powell et al, 1968; Powell & Thomas, 1969; Lloyd, 1971). Iron deficiency is a likely explanation in most of these patients, since more definitive tests of storage iron status such as serum ferritin or bone marrow examination were not carried out.

In one study (Cape & Zirk, 1975) percentage saturation was compared with the presence or absence of bone marrow iron in 34 women over 66 years of age. Eight of 13 individuals with no iron in the marrow had transferrin saturations below 16 per cent. The level was greater than 21 per cent in only one case. On the other hand, only two patients with demonstrable marrow iron had levels below 16 per cent. Similar although less clear-cut results were obtained by Mitchell & Pegrum (1971). Although these reports are based on small numbers of observations, they suggest that the percentage saturation of transferrin should be interpreted no differently in the elderly than it is in younger people.

Free erythrocyte protoporphyrin (FEP)

Protoporphyrin IX accumulates in the developing red cells when haem synthesis is impaired. Consequently, FEP is raised in iron deficiency as well as in conditions affecting the production of haem, such as lead poisoning, chronic inflammatory disease and erythropoietic porphyria. If these other disorders can be excluded, it is a sensitive indicator of an inadequate iron supply (Langer et al, 1972), providing the same information as the transferrin saturation. However values are more stable because the FEP content of each red cell remains fixed for the duration of its lifespan (Langer et al, 1972; Thomas et al, 1977). The advent of rapid simple techniques for measuring FEP on capillary blood have made the assay particularly attractive for evaluating children and for survey work (Blumberg et al, 1977). However, its validity has not been established in the elderly.

DIAGNOSIS

Iron deficiency is a common cause of anaemia in elderly hospital patients. Diagnosis depends on the evaluation of appropriate laboratory investigations. The optimal choice of tests will be determined by the clinical setting. For the out-patient, a blood count together with the red cell indices, serum ferritin, and transferrin saturation may be sufficient to make the diagnosis. However, in hospitalised patients with complicated illnesses, bone marrow examination is often still the best method. Once the presence of iron deficiency has been established, it is essential that the cause be identified, although the vigour with which further investigation is pursued will depend on clinical circumstances.

TREATMENT

Oral iron therapy

Iron deficiency can be corrected in the majority of patients by the administration of a simple ferrous salt. Ferrous sulphate tablets containing approximately 60 mg iron, is usually the least expensive preparation and is customarily given two to three times a day. Other ferrous salts, such as the gluconate, fumarate and lactate, are equally well absorbed (Brise & Hallberg, 1962). Since food reduces the absorption of inorganic iron by 20–60 per cent (Brise, 1962), treatment is more rapidly effective when the iron is given between meals.

Despite the simplicity of oral iron therapy, failure to respond is not uncommon. Some patients do not take their iron because of gastrointestinal side-effects that occur in 25 per cent of individuals (Solvell, 1970). Reducing the dose of iron may diminish nausea and epigastric discomfort, but has little effect on the frequency of abdominal distension, constipation and diarrhoea. Many unsuccessful attempts have been made to improve the therapeutic response to iron while at the same time reducing side-effects. Large quantities of ascorbic acid improve the absorption of ferrous sulphate by 30–40 per cent but side-effects are more common and there is no therapeutic advantage over an equivalent increase in iron dose. Since rapid correction of chronic iron deficiency is rarely necessary, reduction in iron dose or administration of iron with meals are the most practical approaches to reducing the severity of side-effects.

Forgetfulness may be an additional problem in older people. Compliance can be improved by decreasing the number of tablets (Parkin et al, 1976). Although there is no therapeutic advantage to the more expensive slow-release iron preparations over regularly administered ferrous sulphate (Elwood & Williams, 1970), this has been used as an argument for prescribing the former (Hyams, 1978; Fulcher & Hyland, 1981).

It is important to monitor the response to iron therapy, and an average rise in haemoglobin concentration of 0.5 g/dl per week, similar to that observed in younger age groups, has been reported in elderly patients (Fulcher & Hyland, 1981). Treatment should be continued for three to six months beyond the time required to correct the haemoglobin deficit in an effort to replenish iron stores. If available, the serum ferritin concentration is a useful means of monitoring the accumulation of storage iron (Cook, 1982).

An inadequate response to oral iron is most often due to failure to take the medication. If this can be excluded, other possibilities include inaccurate diagnosis or failure to recognise other important contributory factors such as continuing blood loss, renal impairment, infection or an underlying neoplasm. Malabsorption of elemental iron is rare and can be excluded by administering 100 mg ferrous sulphate in the fasting state and measuring the serum iron concentration one and two hours later. Failure of the value to rise above 17.9 μmol/l is presumptive evidence of impaired absorption (Bothwell et al, 1979).

Parenteral iron therapy

Parenteral iron therapy should be reserved for the rare patient who has proven malabsorption, a condition such as hereditary telangiectasia in which the rate of bleeding may mandate an iron requirement that cannot be met by the oral route, or severe side-effects that are not alleviated by modifying the iron dose or employing a delayed-release preparation. Iron dextran is used most frequently. Although it can be administered intramuscularly, intravenous injection is preferable. If there is no reaction to a small intravenous test dose, the drug can be given by repeated slow injections of 250 to 500 mg or by total dose infusion. If the latter method is used, the total iron requirement is calculated and the appropriate quantity of iron dextran diluted in normal saline to a concentration not exceeding 5 per cent. It is infused over four to six hours (Bothwell et al, 1979). Elderly patients appear to tolerate this method of administration satisfactorily (Wright, 1967; Andrews et al, 1967). The most important side-effect is anaphylaxis and, although infrequent, it necessitates the availability of equipment for resuscitation during therapy. Arthralgias sometimes occur, particularly in patients with rheumatoid arthritis (Lloyd & Williams, 1970).

Inappropriate iron therapy

The practice of prescribing iron for older patients who have anaemia without evaluating iron status or the possibility of blood loss should be discouraged. In a recent survey of prescription statistics in Sweden, Reizenstein et al (1979) reported that 83 per cent of patients over 75 years had been given iron without appropriate investigation. Furthermore, some elderly may already be taking large quantities of supplemental iron (Garry et al, 1982).

There are two important potential dangers. It has been demonstrated recently that idiopathic haemochromatosis is an autosomal recessive disorder and that a single gene for the disease may be present in 2–10 per cent of the population in Europe and the United States (Edwards et al, 1981). While there is at present no evidence that manifestations of the disease occur in individuals who carry only one gene, male heterozygotes accumulate 4 to 5 g of iron by the age of 40. Most of them appear to stabilise at this level. Nevertheless, it is possible that a high iron intake could lead to a progressive increase in body iron stores.

The second important danger of indiscriminate iron therapy lies in the failure to recognise occult gastrointestinal blood loss as the cause. This may significantly delay diagnosis in patients with potentially remediable disorders of the bowel.

REFERENCES

Addison G M, Beamish M R, Hales C N, Hodgkins M, Jacobs A, Llewellin P 1972 An immunoradiometric assay for ferritin in the serum of normal subjects and patients with iron deficiency and iron overload. Journal of Clinical Pathology 25: 326–329

Andersen H T, Barkve H 1970 Iron deficiency and muscular work performance. Scandinavian Journal of Clinical and Laboratory Investigation 25 (Suppl 144): 1–62

Andrews J, Fairley A, Barker R 1976 Total dose infusion of iron-dextran in the elderly. Scottish Medical Journal 12: 208–215

Bainton D F, Finch C A 1964 The diagnosis of iron deficiency anemia. American Journal of Medicine 37: 62–70

Ballas S K 1979 Normal serum iron and elevated total iron-binding capacity in iron-deficiency states. American Journal of Clinical Pathology 71: 401–403

Batata M, Spray G H, Bolton F G, Higgins G, Wollner L 1967 Blood and bone marrow changes in elderly patients, with special reference to folic acid, vitamin B_{12}, iron and ascorbic acid. British Medical Journal 2: 667–669

Baumgartner-Stauli R, Beck E A 1977 Sideroblast score: a sensitive indicator of iron deficiency and hypoproliferative anemia. Acta Haematologica 57: 24–31

Bedford P D, Wollner L 1958 Occult intestinal bleeding as a cause of anaemia in elderly people. Lancet 1: 1144–1147

Benzie R McD 1963 The influence of age upon the iron content of bone-marrow. Lancet 1: 1074–1075

Beutler E, Fairbanks V F 1980 The effects of iron deficiency. In: Jacobs A, Worwood M (eds). Iron in biochemistry and medicine, vol II. Academic Press, London, p 393–425

Beveridge B R, Bannerman R M, Evanson J M, Witts L J 1965 Hypochromic anaemia. A retrospective study and follow-up of 378 in-patients. Quarterly Journal of Medicine (New Series) 34: 145–161

Bezwoda W R, Bothwell T H, Torrance J D, MacPhail A P, Charlton R W, Kay G, Levin J 1979 The relationship between marrow iron stores, plasma ferritin concentration and iron absorption. Scandinavian Journal of Haematology 22: 113–120

Blendis L M, Sahay B M 1964 Paterson–Kelly syndrome. British Medical Journal 2: 311

Blumberg W E, Eisinger J, Lamola A A, Zuckerman D M 1977 Zinc protoporphyrin level in blood determined by a portable hematofluorometer: a screening device for lead poisoning. Journal of Laboratory and Clinical Medicine 89: 712–723

Boley S J, Sammartano R, Adams A, Di Biase A, Kleinhaus S, Sprayregen S 1977 On the nature and etiology of vascular ectasias of the colon. Gastroenterology 72: 650–660

Bonnet J D, Hagedorn A B, Owen C A 1960 A quantitative method for measuring the gastrointestinal absorption of iron. Blood 15: 36–44

Bose S K, Andrews J, Roberts P D 1970 Haematological problems in a geriatric unit with special reference to anaemia. Gerontologia Clinica (Basel) 12: 339–346

Bothwell T H, Charlton R W, Cook J D, Finch C A 1979 Iron metabolism in man. Blackwell, Oxford

Bowering J, Sanchez A M 1976 A conspectus of research on iron requirements of man. Journal of Nutrition 106: 985–1074

Boykin L S 1976 Iron deficiency anaemia in post-menopausal women. Journal of the American Geriatriatric Society 24: 588–589

Brannon E S, Merrill A J, Warren J V, Stead Jr E A 1945 The cardiac output in patients with chronic anemia as measured by the technique of right atrial catheterization. Journal of Clinical Investigation 24: 332–336

Brewer G J 1974 Red cell metabolism and function. In: Surgenor D M (ed), The red blood cell, 2nd end, vol 1. Academic Press, New York, p 473–508

Brise H 1962 Influence of meals on iron absorption in oral iron therapy Acta Medica Scandinavica 171 (Suppl 376): 39–46

Brise H, Hallberg L 1962 Absorbability of different iron compounds. Acta Medica Scandinavica 171 (Suppl 376): 23–38

Caird F I, Judge T G, MacLeod C 1975 Pointers to possible malnutrition in the elderly at home. Gerontologia Clinica 17: 47–54

Cape R D T, Zirk M H 1975 Assessment of iron stores in old people. Gerontologia Clinica 17: 101–106

Casale G, Bonora C, Migliavacca A, Zurita I E, de Nicola P 1981a Serum ferritin and ageing. Age and Ageing 10: 119–122

Casale G, Migliavacca A, Bonora C, Zurita I E, de Nicola P 1981b Circadian rhythm of plasma iron, total iron binding capacity and serum ferritin in arteriosclerotic aged patients. Age and Ageing 10: 115–118

Charlton R W et al 1977 Anaemia, iron deficiency and exercise: extended studies in human subjects. Clinical Science and Molecular Medicine 53: 537–541

Chisholm M 1974 The association between webs, iron and post-cricoid carcinoma. Postgraduate Medical Journal 50: 215–219

Chisholm M, Ardran G M, Callender S T, Wright R 1971a A follow-up study of patients with post-cricoid webs. Quarterly Journal of Medicine (New Series) 40: 409–420

Chisholm M, Ardran G M, Callender S T, Wright R 1971b Iron deficiency and autoimmunity in post-cricoid webs. Quarterly Journal of Medicine (New Series) 40: 421–433

Cook J D 1982 Clinical evaluation of iron deficiency. Seminars in Hematology 19: 6–18

Cook J D et al 1971 Nutritional deficiency and anemia in Latin America: a collaborative study. Blood 38: 591–603

Cook J D, Lipschitz D A, Miles L E M, Finch C A 1974 Serum ferritin as a measure of iron stores in normal subjects. American Journal of Clinical Nutrition 27: 681–687

Cook J D, Finch C A, Smith N 1976 Evaluation of the iron status of a population. Blood 48: 449–455

Cooper W M, Hieber R D, Chapman W L 1967 Anemia in the aged. Journal of the American Geriatrics Society 15: 568–574

Croker J R, Beynon G 1981 Gastro-intestinal bleeding — a major cause of iron deficiency in the elderly. Age and Ageing 10: 40–43

Crosby W H 1971 Food pica and iron deficiency. Archives of Internal Medicine 127: 960–961

Crosby W H 1976 Pica. Journal of the Amercian Medical Association 235: 2765

Dallman P R, Yip R, Johnson C 1984 Prevalence and causes of anemia in the United States, 1976–1980. American Journal of Clinical Nutrition 39: 437–445

Davies C T M, Chukweumeka A C, van Haaren J P M 1973 Iron-deficiency anaemia: its effect on maximum aerobic power and responses to exercise in African males aged 17–40 years. Clinical Science 44: 555–562

Davison W 1967 Anaemia in the elderly with special reference to iron deficiency. Gerontologia Clinica 9: 393–400

Davison A A, Ogston D Fullerton H W 1969 Evaluation of diagnostic significance of certain symptoms and physical signs in anaemic patients. British Medical Journal 3: 436–439

De Nicola P, Casale G 1983 Blood in the aged. In: Platt D (ed) Geriatrics 2. Springer, Berlin, p 252–292

Edwards C Q, Dadone M M, Skolnick M H, Kushner J D 1982 Hereditary haemochromatosis. Clinics in Haematology 11: 411–435

Elwood P C, Williams G A 1970 A comparative trial of slow-release and conventional iron preparations. Practitioner 204: 812–815

Elwood P C, Jacobs A, Pitman R G, Entwistle C C 1964 Epidemiology of the Paterson–Kelly syndrome. Lancet 2: 716–720

Elwood P C, Waters W E, Greene W J W, Sweetnam P, Wood M M 1969 Symptoms and circulating haemoglobin level. Journal of Chronic Diseases 21: 615–628

Evans D M D, Pathy M S, Sanerkin N G, Deeble T J 1968 Anaemia in geriatric patients. Gerontologia Clinica 10: 228–241

Fairbanks V F 1971 Is the peripheral blood film reliable for the diagnosis of iron deficiency anemia? American Journal of Clinical Pathology 55: 447–451

Fairbanks V F, Fahey J L, Beutler E 1971 Clinical disorders of iron metabolism. Grune & Stratton, New York

Finch C A 1959 Body iron exchange in man. Journal of Clinical Investigation 38: 392–396

Finch C A et al 1970 Ferrokinetics in man. Medicine 49: 17–53

Finch C A, Miller L R, Inamdar A R, Person R, Seiler K, Mackler B 1976 Iron deficiency in the rat. Physiological and biochemical studies of muscle dysfunction. Journal of Clinical Investigation 58: 447–453

Finch C A, Gollnick P D, Hlastala M P, Miller L R, Dillman E, Mackler B 1979 Lactic acidosis as a result of iron deficiency. Journal of Clinical Investigation 64: 129–137

Freiman H D, Tauber S A, Tulsky E G 1963 Iron absorption in the healthy aged. Geriatrics 18: 716–720

Fulcher R A, Hyland C M 1981 Effectiveness of once daily oral iron in the elderly. Age and Ageing 10: 44–46

Gale E, Torrance J, Bothwell T H 1963 The quantitative estimation of total iron stores in human bone marrow. Journal of Clinical Investigation 42: 1076–1082

Garby L, Irnell L, Werner I 1969 Iron deficiency in women of fertile age in a Swedish community. Estimation of prevalence based on response to iron supplementation. Acta Medica Scandinavica 185: 113–117

Gardner G W, Edgerton V R, Senewiratne B, Barnard R J, Ohira Y 1977 Physical work capacity and metabolic stress in subjects with iron deficiency anemia. American Journal of Clinical Nutrition 30: 910–917

Garry P J, Goodwin J S, Hunt W C, Hooper E M, Leonard A G 1982 Nutritional status in a healthy elderly population: dietary and supplemental intakes. American Journal of Clinical Nutrition 36: 319–331

Gibbins F J, Collins H J, Hall R G P, Dellipiani A W 1974 Endoscopy in the elderly. Age and Ageing 3: 240–244

Green R et al 1968 Body iron excretion in man. A collaborative study. American Journal of Medicine 45: 336–353

Griffiths H J L, Nicholson W J, O'Gorman P 1970 A haematological study of 500 elderly females. Gerontologia Clinica 12: 18–32

Harant Z, Goldberger J V 1975 Treatment of anemia in the aged: a common problem and challenge. Journal of the American Geriatric Society 23: 127–131

Health and Nutrition Examination Survey United States 1971–74 Dietary intake source data. Hyattsville, MD: DHEW publication no (PHS) 1979, 79–1221

Hershko C, Levy S, Matzner Y, Grossowicz N, Izak G 1979 Prevalence and causes of anemia in the elderly in Kiryat Shmoneh, Israel. Gerontology 25: 42–48

Hill R D 1976 The prevalence of anaemia in the over-65s in a rural practice. Practitioner 217: 963–967

Hillman R S, Henderson P A 1969 Control of marrow production by relative iron supply. Journal of Clinical Investigation 48: 454–460

Hoffbrand A V, Ganeshaguru K, Tattersall M H N, Tripp E 1974 Effect of iron deficiency on DNA synthesis. Clinical Science and Molecular Medicine 46: 12P

Hosain F, Marsaglia G, Finch C A 1967 Blood ferrokinetics in normal man. Journal of Clinical Investigation 46: 1–9

Hyams D E 1978 The blood. In: Brocklehurst J C (ed) Textbook of geriatric medicine and gerontology, 2d end. Churchill Livingstone, Edinburgh

Jacobs A, Kilpatrick G S 1964 The Paterson–Kelly syndrome. British Medical Journal 2: 79–82

Jacobs A, Cavill I 1968 The oral lesions of iron deficiency anaemia: pyridoxine and riboflavin status. British Journal of Haematology 14: 291–295

Jacobs A M, Owen G M 1969 The effect of age on iron absorption. Journal of Gerontology 24: 95–96

Jacobs A, Lawrie J H, Entwistle C C, Campbell H 1966 Gastric acid secretion in chronic iron-deficiency anaemia. Lancet 2: 190–192

Jacobs A, Miller F, Worwood M, Beamish M R, Wardrop C A 1972 Ferritin in the serum of normal subjects and patients with iron deficiency and iron overload. British Medical Journal 4: 206–208

Jacobs P, Bothwell T H, Charlton R W 1964 Role of hydrochloric acid in iron absorption. Journal of Applied Physiology 19: 187–188

Jalili M A, Al-Kassab S 1959 Koilonychia and cystine content of nails. Lancet 2: 108–110

Jansen C, Harrill I 1977 Intakes and serum levels of protein and iron for 70 elderly women. American Journal of Clinical Nutrition 30: 1414–1422

Javett S L 1972 Sideropenic dysphagia, Hashimoto's thyroiditis and chronic gastritis. South African Medical Journal 46: 1644–1645

Joynson D H M, Jacobs A, Walker D M, Dolby A E 1972 Defect of cell-mediated immunity in patients with iron-deficiency anaemia. Lancet 2: 1058–1059

Kalchthaler T, Tan M E 1980 Anemia in institutionalized elderly patients. Journal of the American Geriatriatrics Society 28: 108–113

Kasper C K, Whissell D Y E, Wallerstein R O 1965 Clinical aspects of iron deficiency. Journal of the American Medical Association 191: 359–363

Koziol B J, Ohira Y, Simpson D R, Edgerton V R 1978 Biochemical skeletal muscle and hematological profiles of moderate and severely iron deficient anemic adult rats. Journal of Nutrition 108: 1306–1314

Langer E E, Haining R G, Labbe R F, Jacobs P, Crosby E F, Finch C A 1972 Erythrocyte protoporphyrin. Blood 40: 112–128

Lawson I R 1960 Anaemia in a group of elderly patients. Gerontologia Clinica 2: 87–101

Leyland M J, Harris H, Brown P J 1979 Iron status in a general practice and its relationship to morbidity. British Journal of Nutrition 41: 291–295

Lipschitz D A, Mitchell C O, Thompson C 1981 The anemia of senescence. American Journal of Hematology 11: 47–54

Llewellyn-Jones D 1965 Severe anaemia in pregnancy. Australian and New Zealand Journal of Obstetrics and Gynaecology 5: 191–197

Lloyd D A, Valberg L S 1977 Serum ferritin and body iron status after gastric operations. American Journal of Digestive Diseases 22: 598–604

Lloyd E L 1971 Serum iron levels and haematological status in the elderly. Gerontologia Clinica 246–255

Lloyd K N, Williams P 1970 Reactions to total dose infusion of iron dextran in rheumatoid arthritis. British Medical Journal 2: 323–325

Loria A, Hershko C, Konijn A M 1979 Serum ferritin in an elderly population. Journal of
    Gerontology 34: 521–524
Lynch S R, Morck T A 1983 Iron deficiency anemia. In: Lindenbaum J (ed) Nutrition in
    hematology. Churchill Livingstone, New York, p 143–165
Lynch S R, Lipschitz D A, Bothwell T H, Charlton R W 1974 Iron and the reticuloendothelial
    system. In: Jacobs A, Worwood M (eds) Iron in biochemistry and medicine. Academic Press,
    London, p 563–587
Lynch S R, Finch C A, Monsen E R, Cook J D 1982 Iron status of elderly Americans.
    American Journal of Clinical Nutrition 36: 1032–1045
MacDougall L G, Anderson R, McNab G M, Katz J 1975 The immune response in iron
    deficient children: impaired cellular defence mechanisms with altered humoral components.
    Journal of Pediatrics 86: 833–843
McFarlane D B, Pinkerton P H, Dagg J H, Goldberg A 1967 Incidence of iron deficiency with
    and without anemia in women in general practice. British Journal of Haematology 13: 790–796
McLane J A, Fell R D, McKay R H, Winder W W, Brown E B, Holloszy J O 1981
    Physiological and biochemical effects of iron deficiency on rat skeletal muscle. American
    Journal of Physiology 241: C47–C54
McLennan W J, Andrews G R, MacLeod C, Caird F I 1973 Anaemia in the elderly. Quarterly
    Journal of Medicine (New Series) 42: 1–13
MacPhail A P, Bothwell T H, Torrance J D, Derman D P, Bezwoda W R, Charlton R W,
    Mayet F G H 1981 Iron nutrition in Indian women at different ages. South African Medical
    Journal 59: 939–942
Magnusson B E O 1976 Iron absorption after antrectomy with gastroduodenostomy.
    Scandinavian Journal of Haematology 26 (Suppl): 1–111
Marx J J M 1979 Normal iron absorption and decreased red cell iron uptake in the aged. Blood
    53: 204–211
Marx J J M, Dinant H J 1982 Ferrokinetics and red cell iron uptake in old age: evidence for
    increased liver iron retention? Series Haematologica 67: 161–168
Matzner Y, Levy S, Grossowicz N, Izak G, Hershko C 1979 Prevalence and causes of anemia in
    elderly hospitalized patients. Gerontology 25: 113–119
Mitchell T R, Pegrum G D 1971 The diagnosis of mild iron deficiency in the elderly.
    Gerontologia Clinica 13: 296–306
Monroe R T 1951 Diseases in old age. A clinical and pathological study of 7941 individuals over
    61 years of age. Harvard University Press, Cambridge, Mass, p 253–262
Monsen E R, Hallberg L, Layrisse M, Hegsted D M, Cook J D, Mertz W, Finch C A 1978
    Estimation of available dietary iron. American Journal of Clinical Nutrition 31: 134–141
Myers A M, Saunders C R G, Chalmers D G 1968 The haemoglobin level of fit elderly people.
    Lancet 2: 261–263
Narasinga Rao B S 1978 Studies on iron deficiency anemia. Indian Journal of Medical Research
    68 (Suppl): 58–69
Narayanan M, Steinheber F U 1976 The changing face of peptic ulcer in the elderly. Medical
    Clinics of North America 60: 1159–1172
National Center for Health Statistics 1982 Hematological and nutritional biochemistry reference
    data for persons 6 months – 74 years of age: United States, 1976–80. U S Department of
    Health and Human Services Publication No. (PHS): 83–1682 Hyattsville, MD
Nosher J L, Campbell W L, Seaman W B 1975 The clinical significance of cervical esophageal
    and hypopharyngeal webs. Radiology 117: 45–47
Nutrition Canada. National survey. Information Canada, Ottawa, KIA OS9. Canada, 1978
Olsson K S, Weiinfeld A 1972 Availability of iron dextran for haemoglobin synthesis. Acta
    Medica Scandinavica 192: 543–549
Parkin D M, Henney C R, Quirk J, Crooks J 1976 Deviation from prescribed drug treatment
    after discharge from hospital. British Medical Journal 2: 686–688
Parsons P L, Withey J L, Kilpatrick G S 1965 The prevalence of anaemia in the elderly. The
    Practitioner 195: 656–660
Pollitt E, Leibel R L 1976 Iron deficiency and behavior. Pediatrics 88: 372–381
Powell D E B, Thomas J H 1969 The iron-binding capacity of serum in elderly hospital
    patients. Gerontologia Clinica 11: 36–47
Powell D E B, Thomas J H, Mills P 1968 Serum iron in elderly hospital patients. Gerontologia
    Clinica 10: 21–29
Prasad J S 1979 Leucocyte function in iron-deficiency anemia. American Journal of Clinical
    Nutrition 32: 550–552

Qvist I, Norden A, Olofsson T 1980 Serum ferritin in the elderly. Scandivanian Journal of Clinical and Laboratory Investigation 40: 609–613

Raper C G L, Rosen C, Choudhury M 1977 Automated red cell indices and marrow iron reserves in geriatric patients. Journal of Clinical Pathology 30: 353–355

Raufmann J P, Dobbins W O 1980 Evaluation of chronic gastrointestinal blood loss. In: Fiddian-Green R G, Turcotte J G (eds) Gastrointestinal hemorrhage. Grune & Stratton, New York, p 23–38

Reizenstein P, Ljunggren G, Smedby B, Agenas I, Penchansky M 1979 Overprescribing iron tablets to elderly people in Sweden. British Medical Journal 2: 962–963

Reynolds R D, Binder H J, Miller M B, Chang W W Y, Horan S 1968 Pagophagia and iron deficiency anemia. Annals of Internal Medicine 69: 435–440

Robertson D, Kirkham B 1979 Screening for nutritional deficiencies in the elderly following gastric surgery. Age and Ageing 8: 216–221

Schoene R B, Escourrou P, Robertson H T, Nilson K L, Parsons J R, Smith N J 1983 Iron repletion decreases maximal exercise lactate concentrations in female athletes with minimal iron deficiency anemia. Journal of Laboratory and Clinical Medicine 102: 306–312

Smith M D, Mallett B 1957 Iron absorption before and after partial gastrectomy. Clinical Science 16: 23–34

Solvell L 1970 Oral iron therapy – side effects. In: Hallberg L, Harwerth H-G, Vannotti A (eds) Iron deficiency. Pathogenesis. Clinical aspects. Therapy. Academic Press, London, p 573-583

Sproule B J, Mitchell J H, Miller W F 1960 Cardiopulmonary physiological responses to heavy exercise in patients with anemia. Journal of Clinical Investigation 39: 378–388

Srikantia S G, Prasad J S, Bhaskaram C, Krishnamachari K A V R 1976 Anemia and immune response. Lancet 1: 1307–1309

Steen B, Isaksson B, Svanborg A 1977 Intake of energy and nutrients and meal habits in 70-year-old males and females in Gothenburg, Sweden. A population study. Acta Medica Scandinavica 61 (Suppl): 39–86

Steinheber F U 1976 Interpretation of gastrointestinal symptoms in the elderly. Medical Clinics of North America 60: 1141–1157

Stevens A R, Coleman D H, Finch C A 1953 Iron metabolism: clinical evaluation of iron stores. Annals of Internal Medicine 38: 199–205

Stone W D 1968 Gastric secretory response to iron therapy. Gut 9: 99–105

Ten-State Nutrition Survey 1968–70: V Dietary. DHEW publication No. (HSM) 72–8133. Atlanta, GA: US Department of Health, Education and Welfare Center for Disease Control, 1972

Thomas W J, Koenig H M, Lightsey Jr A L, Green R 1977 Free erythrocyte porphyrin: hemoglobin ratios, serum ferritin and transferrin saturation levels during treatment of infants with iron-deficiency anemia. Blood 49: 455–462

Torrance J, Jacobs P, Restrepo A, Eschbach J, Lenfant C, Finch C 1970 Intraerythrocytic adaptation to anemia. New England Journal of Medicine 283: 165–169

Valberg L S, Sorbie J, Ludwig J, Pelletier O 1976 Serum ferritin and the iron status of Canadians. Canadian Medical Association Journal 14: 417–421

Varat M A, Adolph R J, Fowler N O 1972 Cardiovascular effects of anemia. American Heart Journal 83: 415–426

Viteri F E, Torun B 1974 Anemia and physical work capacity. In: Garby L (ed) Clinics in haematology, vol 3 (3). Saunders, London, p 609–626

Walters G O, Miller F M, Worwood M 1973 Serum ferritin concentration and iron stores in normal subjects. Journal of Clinical Pathology 26: 770–772

Weinfeld A 1964 Storage iron in man. Acta Medica Scandinavica 427 (Suppl): 1–155

Wretlind A 1970 The supply of food iron. In: Blix G (ed) Occurrence, causes and prevention of nutritional anaemias. Symposia of the Swedish Nutrition Foundation VI. Almqvist & Wiskell, Stockholm, p 73–91

Wrigglesworth J M, Baum H 1980 The biochemical functions of iron. In: Jacobs A, Worwood M (eds) Iron in biochemistry and medicine, vol II, Academic Press, London, p 29–86

Wright W B 1967 Iron deficiency anaemia of the elderly treated by total dose infusion. Gerontologia Clinica 9: 107–115

Yetgin S, Altay C, Ciliv G, Laleli Y 1979 Myeloperoxidase activity and bactericidal function of PMN in iron deficiency. Acta Haematologica 61: 10–14

Macrocytosis and megaloblastic anaemia

INTRODUCTION

The size of red blood cells is measured accurately and reproducably by modern automated blood counters. The result is termed the mean corpuscular volume, abbreviated as MCV, and the unit is the femtolitre, abbreviated as fl. The larger and red cell, the more haemoglobin it will contain, and therefore changes in the size of red cells are mirrored by changes in the haemoglobin content of the red cell. This is termed the mean corpuscular haemoglobin, or MCH, expressed in picograms (pg). These two parameters move in parallel; if they do not, this generally suggests technical error in setting the blood counter.

A significant proportion of patients have red cells that are either smaller or larger than the norm, and this is an important manifestation of a disease process. An explanation of changes in red cell size should be sought at least in so far as the commoner disorders are concerned and steps taken to confirm or exclude these conditions.

The size of red blood cells differs little from person to person. Nevertheless, normal ranges that are quoted in laboratory reports show surprising variation. This is to some extent due to the manner in which automated blood counters are set. Generally the mean value for the MCV should be about 86–88 fl and the normal range between 80 to not more than 94 fl. Indeed, in the author's laboratory, healthy persons consistently fall into the 80–90 fl range. Minor increases above the normal range (up to 4 fl) are commonplace in clinical practice and it is not useful to investigate small increases. But a persistent increase of 5 fl or more above the normal range is more significant.

Macrocytosis may be associated with normoblastic haemopoiesis or with megaloblastic haemopoiesis, and a marrow smear is valuable in determining into which of these two broad categories a particular patient falls.

NORMOBLASTIC MACROCYTOSIS

Causation

Causes of normoblastic macrocytosis are shown in Table 4.1. Not infrequent-

Table 4.1   Conditions associated with macrocytosis

Physiological	New born, Pregnancy
Normoblastic	Young red cell population (reticulocyte increase)
	Alcoholism
	Hypothyroidism
	Drugs (cytotoxics such as melphalan, chlorambucil, azathioprine, antidepressants such as imipramine and related compounds, anticonvulsants)
	Neoplasia
	Leukaemic and preleukaemic syndromes including sideroblastic anaemia, deletion of part of chromosone 5
	Aplastic and hypoplastic anaemia
	Liver disease
	Chronic obstructive airway disease
	Down's syndrome
	Unexplained
Megaloblastic	Cobalamin deficiency
	Folate deficiency
	Orotic aciduria
	Lesch-Nyhan syndrome
	Drugs (cytosine arabinoside, 5-fluorouracil, methotrexate, pyrimethamine)

ly, considerable investigation fails to disclose a recognised explanation for an increase in the MCV. Tobacco smoking is associated with small increases in the MCV (1–3 fl) (as do oral contraceptive preparations in women of fertile age), but it is doubtful whether these have a large enough effect to produce a significant increase in MCV. A familial macrocytosis has been claimed in one family.

Alcoholism

Macrocytosis is the commonest abnormality in the blood count in subjects taking more than 80 g ethanol daily. This is contained in one third of a bottle of spirits, half a bottle of fortified wine such as sherry, a bottle of wine, or four pints of beer. Indeed, alcoholism should be the first diagnosis in an adult when the blood count shows macrocytosis with a normal haemoglobin level. About 85 per cent of alcoholics are macrocytic. Cessation of alcohol intake will reverse the process, so that when a new red cell population replaces the old one (about a hundred days later) the MCV becomes normal. A recent survey among executives of a large insurance company disclosed that 3 per cent were macrocytic. Recall of 17 of these subjects showed that 16 were taking excessive amounts of alcohol.

Hypothyroidism

Primary or secondary myxoedema of whatever causation is associated with significant increases in red cell size in almost all patients. Even those with a

MCV in the conventional normal range show a marked fall in MCV when they are receiving adequate replacement therapy. Thus the MCV may fall from 88 to 82 fl.

Leukaemia and preleukaemia

This is a relatively common cause of macrocytosis in the elderly. Whereas the diagnosis of overt acute leukaemia with an excess of blast cells in peripheral blood and marrow is self-evident, more chronic forms and preleukaemic syndromes are less obvious. Unexplained anaemia, a low neutrophil count with poor granulation in the stained blood film and a monocytosis all suggest a chronic myelomonocyte leukaemia.

Drugs

The association between antidepressant drugs and macrocytosis is not well recorded, but the author has seen many examples of macrocytosis where long-term antidepressant drugs appeared to be the only possible factor. Treatment for neoplastic disease is one of the commonest causes of macrocytosis in hospital practice.

Young red cell population

Reticulocytosis for whatever reason will give an increase in the MCV. This can be due to a large bleed, e.g. malaena, or to a chronic haemolytic state, either congenital or due to therapy, for example with sulphasalazine, dapsone or methyldopa.

WHY INVESTIGATE?

It is of course simple to prescribe cobalamin injections and folate tablets to a patient who, one suspects, may have a megaloblastic anaemia — and, indeed, unnecessry investigation is to be deplored, not least in the elderly. However, deficiencies of cobalamin and folate may not be primary events but secondary to other disorders (Table 4.2) which also require management. Further, patients with normoblastic macrocytosis (Table 4.1) will not benefit from such therapy but will continue to deteriorate. Thus it is in both the patient's and doctor's interest to withhold 'blunderbuss' therapy until material has been collected for diagnosis. It is not necessary to delay therapy until a firm diagnosis is reached.

Procedure

History

A careful history is of great value. Patients with megaloblastic anaemia

Table 4.2 Causes of megaloblastic anaemia in the elderly

Cobalamin deficiency	Pernicious anaemia
	Postgastrectomy
	Anatomical abnormality of small gut
	Nutritional in Hindu vegetarians
Folate deficiency	Nutritional
	Coeliac disease
	Chronic haemolytic states
	Chronic myelofibrosis
	Anticonvulsant drugs
	Tropical sprue
	Drugs
Combined deficiency	Nutritional
	Tropical sprue

complain of tiredness, lethargy, sore tongue, paraesthesiae. There may be a family history of pernicious anaemia, or thyroid disease. Has the patient undergone abdominal surgery such as a gastrectomy? What drugs is he or she taking? How much alochol? Is the diet adequate?

Examination

A smooth tongue is found in most untreated patients with pernicious anaemia. Smoothness may be apparent only on the edges, but often on the whole tongue. A small, thin subject may indicate coeliac disease even in the elderly. Patients with anatomical abnormalities of the small bowel tend to have prominent abdominal symptoms such as a noisy tummy, colic and even bulky stools. Megaloblastic anaemia with a large spleen may suggest folate deficiency in myelofibrosis.

Blood count

Not all patients whose marrows show megaloblastosis are macrocytic. Thus among 75 patients with a megaloblastic marrow, three patients had a normal MCV (Chanarin, 1979). In these the red cell count was above 4.3 million/μl. However, severe megaloblastic anaemia can occur with a normal MCV when the patient has a concurrent disorder associated with small red cells. Occasionally this is a thalassaemia trait when the MCV in the uncomplicated state ranges from 60–70 fl in ß-thalasaemia and from 70–80 fl in $\propto$-thalassaemia. The increase in MCV that occurs when these patients become megaloblastic brings the MCV into conventional normal range of 80–92 fl. The blood film is very abnormal with many red cell fragments.

More usually macrocytosis is the only finding in early cases of megaloblastic anaemia, with perhaps some increase in those neutrophil polymorphs having 5 or more nuclear segments. In more severe cases oval macrocytosis develops with variation in cells size (anisocytosis) and a fall in the white cell and platelet counts. In severe cases the diagnosis of megaloblastosis can be made from the blood and even circulating megaloblasts may be seen.

Marrow

A marrow aspiration is often necessary, particularly in investigating non-anaemic patients. Thus if the patient is not taking alcohol or any medication, if the thyroid function tests are normal and cobalamin and folate levels are indecisive, it is very helpful to know whether there is megaloblastic change in the marrow or not. This is usually done in a hospital environment, although apsiration of the marrow is a minor procedure.

A diagnosis of megaloblastic haemopoiesis can be made only by examination of the blood and marrow and not by any other way.

Diagnosis of cobalamin deficiency

Two criteria are required to establish a diagnosis of cobalamin deficiency: (a) evidence of low stores of vitamin B_{12} usually taken as a low serum vitamin B_{12} level, and (b) evidence of failure of intestinal absorption of vitamin B_{12}.

The only exceptions to this generalisation are patients with nutritional cobalamin deficiency. These are strict vegetarians who take no eggs, cheese or meat but usually some milk. Since cobalamins are absent from vegetables, cobalamin is present in a vegetarian diet only as a result of microbial contamination of foodstuffs. These patients can be deficient in vitamin B_{12} but still absorb vitamin B_{12} normally.

There are considerable problems in performing cobalamin absorption tests in the elderly, since the standard test requires an accurate 24-hour urine collection. Incomplete collection may give an incorrectly low result. However, the measurement of plasma radioactivity after an oral dose of $[^{57}Co]$-vitamin B_{12} is a very reliable and satisfactory adjunct to the standard urinary excretion test. Plasma radioactivity is counted in a blood sample collected 8–12 hours after the oral dose, and the plasma activity is a reliable index of cobalamin absorption.

Where whole-body counting is available, this is a totally reliable means of assessing absorption, the subject being scanned before and half an hour after swallowing the oral labelled dose of cobalamin and, again, about one week later when unabsorbed radioactivity will have been excreted.

Finally, two isotopes of vitamin B_{12}, one free and the second bound to an intrinsic-factor preparation, may be given together. Normally in a subject who has normal amounts of gastric intrinsic factor the free cobalamin will be absorbed as well as the intrinsic-factor-bound cobalamin. Normally both isotopes will therefore be excreted into the urine after absorption in approximately equal amounts. If the patient lacks his or her own intrinsic factor (pernicious anaemia, gastric atrophy, gastrectomy), only the vitamin B_{12}

attached to intrinsic factor will be absorbed and appear in the urine. The advantage of this approach is that only a specimen of urine is required and not a complete collection. The difficulty is that exchange of the two forms of B_{12} on intrinsic factor occurs *in vivo*, so that the result may become blurred.

The haematological response to cobalamin therapy is a useful confirmation of a correct diagnosis and this should not be obscured by unnecessarily giving folic acid to patients who are likely to have uncomplicated vitamin B_{12} deficiency.

Diagnosis of folate deficiency

The decisive investigation for folate deficiency is the red cell folate concentration. Folate enters red cells during erythropoiesis in marrow, and there are no further fluxes of folate in mature red cells. In this sense red cells are a tissue and the level of folate in red cells (145–450 ng/ml packed red cells) is some twenty or more times greater than in serum. Changes in red cell folate occur only with entry into the circulation of new red cells of different folate content, so that changes are slow. A reduced red cell folate content implies long-standing folate deficiency.

Serum folate is more labile and can fall in days in a subject not eating normally. A low serum folate should be regarded as indicating a negative folate balance but not necessarily folate deficiency. Traces of haemolysis in a sample will elevate the folate content of a serum sample and vitiate the result.

Clinically a patient with megaloblastic anaemia who has a normal serum cobalmin level or who absorbs vitamin B_{12} normally, irrespective of the serum vitamin B_{12} level, has folate deficiency. Persistent megaloblastosis after cobalamin therapy also indicates folate deficiency.

PERNICIOUS ANAEMIA

Definition

Pernicious anaemia is a disorder characterised by megaloblastic haemopoiesis and/or a neuropathy due to vitamin B_{12} deficiency, the result of severe atrophic gastritis.

Frequency

In northern Europe and in populations of North European descent, the frequency of pernicious anaemia (PA) is 110–180 per 100 000 of the population. Above the aage of 60 the frequency approaches 1 per cent. It was 2.5 per cent in Glasgow for persons over the age of 65 and 3.7 per cent in North-West England for persons over the age of 75 (Chanarin, 1979). Where there is a family history of PA, the age of presentation is younger. The female-to-male ratio is consistently 10:7.

Causation

There are three threads to be woven together in the pathogenesis of PA: (a) its familial incidence, (b) the presence of severe atrophic gastritis, (c) an auto-immune association.

In the UK a family history of PA is present in 19 per cent of patients, and in Denmark this was the case in 30 per-cent. The mean age of diagnosis was 51 years in those with a family history, as compared to 66 years in the absence of such a history. Identical twins both usually show evidence of PA at about the same time. A study of relatives of patients with PA by Callender & Denborough (1957) showed that a quarter had achlorhydria and a third of these (8 per cent of the total) had low serum cobalamin levels and impaired cobalamin absorption. There is an association between blood group A on the one hand, and PA and gastric cancer on the other. There is, however, no clear link with the HLA system.

It is now more than a hundred years since Fenwick (1870) demonstrated gastric atrophy and loss of pepsinogen in the stomach in PA. Absence of acid from the gastric juice is common to all patients, as is the virtual absence of the intrinsic factor. Both are products of the gastric parietal cell. Gastric atrophy involves the proximal two-thirds of the stomach. There is gross or total loss of secreting cells and replacement by mucus-secreting cells which may be of intestinal type. There is lymphocytic and plasma cell infiltration. This appearance, however, is not unique to PA. It also occurs in simple atrophic gastritis in patients who are normal haematologically and who do not, after more than twenty years of follow-up, develop PA.

The third thread is the immune component. Two gastric antibodies have been associated with PA: the parietal-cell antibody and the intrinsic-factor antibody.

Sera from between 80 and 90 per cent of PA patients have antibodies reacting with the gastric parietal cell demonstrated by an immunofluorescent method. A similar antibody is present in 5–10 per cent of sera from healthy subjects. The frequency of parietal-cell antibodies in sera from elderly women reaches 16 per cent. Gastric biopsy shows evidence of gastritis in almost all patients with parietal-cell antibody in serum. Infusion of parietal-cell antibody into rats results in the development of mild atrophic changes, a marked fall in acid and in intrinsic factor secretion (Tanaka & Glass, 1970). This antibody may well play an important role in the development of gastric atrophy.

Intrinsic-factor antibody is present in sera of 57 per cent of patients with PA, and it is rare to find this antibody in patients without this disease. When taken by mouth, intrinsic-factor antibody will prevent cobalamin absorption by combining with intrinsic factor and so preventing the binding of cobalamin to intrinsic factor.

Not only are these antibodies present in sera but they are also present in gastric juice and are produced by plasma calls in the gastric mucosa. Thus the gastric juice may contain intrinsic-factor antibody of an IgA type, whereas that in serum is an IgG immunoglobulin. In some patients the antibody is present only in gastric juice and is not detectable in serum. Combining the data on the frequency of the antibody from these two sites, intrinsic-factor antibodies are detectable in about 76 percent of patients.

A further form of immunity against intrinsic factor is cell-mediated immunity detectable by either migration-inhibition tests or by leucocyte transformation. It is present in 86% of patients (Chanarin & James, 1974). when results with all these tests were combined — that is, either humoral antibody in serum, in gastric secretion, immune complexes in gastric secretion or cell-mediated immunity to intrinsic factor — evidence of immunity was present in 24 out of 25 patients with PA.

Current views are that lymphocytes carry all the information they require to make all antibodies but are prevented from doing so by suppressor T-lymphocytes. For reasons that are not clear, in these disorders the B-lymphocytes escape from suppressor-cell control and produce 'auto-antibodies' against parietal cells, intrinsic factor and, quite commonly, against thyroid, parathyroid, adrenal and islets of Langerhans. The tendency to do this is familial; otherwise healthy relatives have a high frequency of these antibodies and some have the corresponding disorders. What comes first in the development of atrophic gastritis is not clear. There is always a strong tendency to regeneration in gastric mucosa and this is prevented by parietal-cell antibody. It may be that the antibody initiates the atrophic process. Steroids, by destroying lymphocytes, reverse the process and allow the atrophic mucosa to regenerate (Ardeman & Chanarin, 1965). Atrophy will substantially reduce the volume of gastric secretion and the amount of intrinsic factor available.

The appearance of intrinsic-factor antibody will neutralise the remaining amounts of intrinsic factor and so reduce a just adequate cobalamin absorption to an inadequate one. There is thus a negative cobalamin balance and a slow development of cobalamin deficiency. Cessation of vitamin B_{12} absorption (as after total gastrectomy) will lead to deficiency after five years, and lesser degrees of negative balance will require a correspondingly longer period before leading to manifest deficiency.

Clinical features

Patients with pernicious anaemia complain of tiredness, lethargy and loss of drive and of interest. A quarter have a sore mouth or some tongue and one-third symmetrical paraesthesia in feet and/or hands. There is some weight loss and loss of appetite. Far less common are difficulties with gait, urinary difficulty, impotence, visual difficulties and, rarely, hallucinations and even psychiatric problems.

Examination usually shows a smooth tongue and, in more anaemic patients, pallor with somewhat icteric sclera. Neurological examination may show loss of vibration sense, of passive movement and sometimes other evidence of lateral and posterior cord involvement.

Diagnosis

The changes in blood and marrow have been mentioned. All patients have a low serum vitamin B_{12} level and fail to absorb vitamin B_{12} unless additional intrinsic factor is supplied.

Gastric juice shows a histamine-fast achlorhydria and gastric biopsy severe atrophic gastritis. Endoscopy is also valuable in excluding a carcinoma of the stomach. There is normally a full haematological response to cobalamin alone.

Not uncommonly, the investigations do not conform to the expected pattern. Some of these deviations are discussed.

Vitamin B_{12} absorption test does not return into the normal range when the test is repeated with intrinsic factor. The common cause of low values in the urinary excretion test (Schilling test) is lost urine. Thus the test must be accompanied by a plasma sample. If both results are low, this indicates a low absorption result, but if plasma radioactivity is normal but urine excretion is low, it indicates lost urine. A poor result in the intrinsic-factor supplemented test occurs when the patient has substantial intrinsic-factor antibody in the gastric juice.

Long-term cobalamin deficiency also impairs ileal function with depressed cobalamin uptake. This only corrects after several months of cobalamin therapy. Thus if all investigations point to PA, a poor response to added intrinsic factor in the absorption test is still compatible with the diagnosis.

All tests point to PA but the cobalamin absorption result is normal. This can be due to the presence of another isotope in urine — for example, technetium. As this has a very short half-life, the urine sample should be recounted after a few days. In other cases $[^{57}Co]B_{12}$ may be contaminted with ^{57}Co that is not cyanocobalamin. Repeat the absorption test with $[^{57}Co]B_{12}$ from a different batch. If the absorption is still normal, the diagnosis cannot be PA.

There is a low serum cobalamin, impaired cobalamin absorption improved by intrinsic factor but a normal blood picture. Rarely PA with neuropathy can present with normoblastic haemopoiesis. In the absence of neuropathy the diagnosis is simple atrophic gastritis and not PA (see below).

The patient appears to have PA but does not benefit clinically or haematologically from adequate cobalamin therapy. A response can be completely abrogated by the presence of a co-existing disorder such as renal failure, infection e.g. pyelonephritis, anaemia of chronic disorders, uncontrolled thyroid disease or gastric or other neoplasm. These should be searched for before it is decided that the diagnosis is wrong. Even in the absence of response, if the patient has PA, cobalamin will restore normoblastic haemopoiesis.

Treatment

It is customary to attempt to restore cobalamin stores by giving about six injections of 1 mg (1000 μg) of hydroxocobalamin initially. Hydroxocobalamin is retained much better than cyancobalamin. Thus about 70–80 per cent of a 1 mg dose of hydroxocobalamin is retained as compared to less than 30 per cent of a comparable dose of cyanocobalamin. There is no evidence whatsoever that the cyano-moiety of cyanocobalamin is harmful.

Maintenance should aim at supplying about 5 μg cobalamin daily, and this is achieved with 250 μg hydroxocobalamin monthly, continued for the remainder of the patient's life. After about three to six months, a few patients show iron deficiency as evidenced by a fall of the MCV below 80 fl. A short course of oral iron is indicated.

The return of normal blood values depends on the initial severity of the anaemia. Patients with severe anaemia have a very substantially reduced red cell survival and these patients show the most rapid restoration of a normal MCV (25–35 days). Mildly anaemic patients have red cells with an essentially normal survival, and restoration of a normal MCV takes up to 80 days.

Neuropathy is arrested and all patients recover normal urinary continence etc. Paraesthesias may take four to six months to disappear. Impaired vision, if due to optic atrphy, does not recover, but where it is due to retinal haemorrhage in the region of the macula, recovery is rapid.

Many patients show evidence of myxoedema within a few years of diagnosis of PA and this is a reason for follow-up in the first instance. Of 5217 patients with PA, 1.8 per cent had Graves' disease and 2.4 per cent myxoedema. Nine per cent of patients with primary hypothyroidism also had PA (Chanarin, 1979).

The study of Zamcheck et al (1955) showed that ultimately 5.8 per cent of patients developed a gastric carcinoma. Two Scandinavian studies showed that the frequency of diagnosed pernicious anaemia among patients having gastric carcinoma at autopsy was 2.2 per cent (Elsborg & Mosbech, 1979) and 2.1 per cent (Ericksson et al, 1981).

GASTRIC ATROPHY AND SEVERE ATROPHIC GASTRITIS

Changes in the gastric mucosa which lead to the loss of secreting cells and eventually to their virtual disappearance from the gastric mucosa are common. Their frequency increase with age, and some degree of atrophic gastritis is present in over 80 per cent of gastric biopsy samples after the age of 60 years. A few patients have symptoms of non-ulcer dyspepsia, but the vast majority of such patients have no such symptoms. In about 10 per cent of elderly subjects the appearance of the gastric biopsy is indistinguishable from that in PA.

The subjects with severe atrophic gastritis generally have a histamine-fast achlorhydria. The production of intrinsic factor declines with the loss of parietal cells and is abnormally low in all patients with severe atrophic gastritis (Ardeman & Chanarin, 1965). Some five hundred intrinsic factor units are required for normal absorption of 1 μg of cobalamin. The normal daily secretion of intrinsic factor ranges from 50 000 to 100 000 units. Thus only about 1 per cent of the normal output is needed to maintain normal cobalamin absorption. Impaired cobalamin absorption thus indicates severe loss of intrinsic factor, other causes of malabsorption being excluded. Vitamin B_{12} absorption was impaired in 6 out of 64 patients with atrophic gastritis of moderate severity and in 78 out of 159 patients with severe atrophic gastritis as determined by biopsy. These figures represent pooled data from seven studies (Chanarin, 1979). Although the amount of cobalamin absorbed by patients with atrophic gastritis (0.22 μg of a 1.0 μg dose) was below normal, it was on average twice that absorbed in PA (0.10 μg) (Whiteside et al, 1964).

When malabsorption of cobalamin is found in severe atrophic gastritis, the absorption is improved by the addition of intrinsic factor, and this was so in 36 out of 42 patients tested (Chanarin, 1979).

The resemblance to PA is heightened when serum cobalamin levels are measured. In 34 out of 120 patients the serum vitamin B_{12} was below 150 pg/ml (Chanarin, 1979). However, the parallel between low cobalamin levels and impaired cobalamin absorption is not absolute. In fact, in almost half of those with reduced cobalamin levels, the absorption was normal.

Why are these patients not regarded as early cases of pernicious anaemia? There are two good reasons for regarding them as different. The first is that they are usually normal from the haematological and neurological point of view, that is, they show none of the clinical consequences of vitamin B_{12} deficiency. Second, of 116 patients followed up for 19–23 years only two developed pernicious anaemia, although 11 developed carcinoma of the stomach (Siurala et al, 1974). Another group of 363 patients followed up for 11–18 years shows 13 per cent developing carcinoma of the stomach, but PA was not mentioned (Cheli et al 1973). Thus the majority of patients with severe atrophic gastritis are probably in cobalamin balance, absorbing just the amount of cobalamin needed despite lowered plasma levels and diminished absorption. Parietal-cell antibodies in serum are not uncommon, but intrinsic-factor antibodies are rare.

Screening for cobalamin deficiency in the elderly must be done by a reliable blood count and looking for an increase in the MCV. Measurement of serum vitamin B_{12} levels and cobalamin absorption will uncover many patients with atrophic gastritis, very few of whom will have PA.

On the other hand, symptoms due to vitamin B_{12} deficiency can precede changes in the blood by quite a long period. Where symptoms of lethargy etc.

are present in a patient who has a low cobalamin level and malabsorbs cobalamin, it may be good clinical practice to treat with vitamin B_{12} and stop if the symptomns do not improve in the long term.

POSTGASTRECTOMY MEGALOBLASTIC ANAEMIA

Partial gastrectomy as a treatment for peptic ulceration has been replaced largely by other surgical procedures in cases where medical treatment has failed. Nevertheless, megaloblastic anaemia following partial gastrectomy is still encountered. Total gastrectomy is still performed in gastric carcinoma and such patients should be given cobalamin replacement therapy indefinitely starting immediately after surgery.

Incidence

If followed up for long enough, roughly half the patients who have had about three-quarters of the stomach removed develop anaemia. In the majority this is an iron-deficiency anaemia due to poor absorption of food iron. In about 5 per cent it is a megaloblastic anaemia, and even in these cases the diagnosis is usually complicated by iron deficiency.

Causation

Secretion of intrinsic factor is confined to the body of the stomach. Resection usually leaves the fundal portion of the stomach behind; loss of intrinsic factor follows atrophy in the gastric remnant. Cobalamin deficiency never appears in less than five years after partial gastrectomy but in others maybe delayed for fifteen years or longer.

Clinical features

Symptoms are those of weakness, tiredness, lack of energy and dyspnoea on exertion. Unpleasant epigastric fullness after meals with nausea may be present. Glossitis is common. In those who are folate-deficient, alcoholism is not uncommon.

Diagnosis

The blood may be similar to that described in PA. In many patients, however, there is an overlay of iron deficiency. On the one hand there may be microcytosis (low MCV) with an unusual degree of neutrophil hypersegmentation in the stained blood film. In others the MCV may be only modestly raised or may be normal. There may be a dimorphic picture in the blood film, that is, both hypochromic and macrocytic cells. The marrow may just show iron deficiency, or show early or more frankly megaloblastic features. The serum cobalamin level is low, but in those with folate deficiency it may be normal with low serum and red cell folate levels.

Treatment

Where there is any doubt in a patient with mixed deficiency, it is advisable to treat first with oral iron alone for at least six weeks, or longer if the blood continues to improve, and then re-assess the situation. The marrow appearance will then show more decisive megaloblastic change if this is present. In those who do not have true cobalamin deficiency, the serum vitamin B_{12} level rises slowly to a plateau over about six months. These patients do not need cobalamin treatment. In others the rise in serum vitamin B_{12} is transient or does not occur at all. If the marrow is megaloblastic, these patients require vitamin B_{12} in the same way as patients with PA.

In a small number of cases the features are those of a blind-loop syndrome. This applies to those who have undergone a Polya gastrectomy. There is no improvement in cobalamin absorption with intrinsic factor, but this may improve after one week on an antibiotic such as tetracycline.

In some patients the marrow remains megaloblastic after cobalamin therapy. These patients require folic acid. Megaloblastic anaemia in the presence of a normal serum cobalamin level or normal cobalamin absorption is due to folate deficiency and is treated with 5 mg folic acid daily given for about three months.

MEGALOBLASTIC ANAEMIA DUE TO AN ABNORMAL INTESTINAL BACTERIAL FLORA

The small gut is normally sterile and any organisms are transient, entering via food or by reflux at the ileocolic junction. Anatomical abnormalities of the small gut, however, lead to the establishment of a permanent bacterial flora consisting of enteric organisms, both aerobic and anaerobic. These disorders are surgically produced blind loops, strictures of the small gut, entero-entero-anastomoses, fistulae between gut segments, diverticulitis of the small gut, poorly functioning gastroenterostomy, impairment of gut motility (in scleroderma, Whipple's disease, post-vagotomy), gut resection and hypogammaglobulinaemia.

These micro-organisms have an avid appetite for vitamin B_{12} which they take up from the diet. A the same time they may release some folate which is absorbed by the host. Thus these disorders may be accompanied by megaloblastic anaemia due to vitamin B_{12} deficiency.

In addition to cobalamin deficiency, these patients have steatorrhoea. Among 186 patients the intestinal lesions were strictures in 5, anastomoses and fistulate in 55 and small intestinal diverticulosis in 80. The patients present with signs and symptoms of a megaloblastic anaemia, but abdominal symptoms tend to be prominent. These include borborygmi, colic and bulky, smelly stools. Serum vitamin B_{12} is low, serum and red cell folate normal or even raised, the patients malabsorb vitamin B_{12} even with intrinsic factor, but this improves after a week on an antibiotic such as tetracycline.

In addition to therapy with vitamin B_{12}, dietary management involving reduction in fats is required.

Small gut resection occupies a special place. Cobalamin is absorbed in the ileum, and when above 600 mm or more are removed, malabsorption of vitamin B_{12} follows (Thompson & Wrathell, 1977).

NUTRITIONAL VITAMIN B_{12} DEFICIENCY

The normal origin of cobalamin in nature is bacterial synthesis, and mammals acquire cobalamin from synthesis by bacteria in the foregut of ruminants, by consumption of insects found on the surface of fruits by monkeys or fruit bats or, in the case of carnivores, by eating meat. Cobalamin is absent from plants, and a diet of clean food of vegetable origin contains cobalamin only as a result of contamination by bacteria.

Although only small numbers of dietary faddists are strictly vegetarian in habit, the bulk of vegetarians are Hindu Indians, and nutritional megaloblastic anaemia is commonly encountered in such communities. There is a high incidence of both $\propto$-and ß-thalassaemia trait among Indians, and because of this a minority of such patients may present with a megaloblastic anaemia with a normal MCV. The majority present in the usual way with lethargy, tiredness, sore mouth and a macrocytic blood picture. The anaemia can occur at any age and is equally common in both sexes.

Proof of the diagnosis depends on a haematological response to oral cobalamin (not parenteral cobalamin). The dose of Cobalamin should equal that present in a mixed diet, namely about 5 μg vitamin B_{12} daily. The haematological response is not as striking as that obtained with a large injection of vitamin B_{12} with a lower and later reticulocyte peak (days 10–12 instead of days 5–7). However, the response should be complete unless there is accompanying iron or folate deficiency. Those patients, unlike those with PA, absorb vitamin B_{12} normally.

NUTRITIONAL FOLATE DEFICIENCY

In the elderly, folate deficiency can arise from an inadequate intake of folate. Unlike cobalamin, folate is labile and deteriorates in stored, cooked or processed food and in food exposed to light. Inadequate amounts of poor-quality food, particularly if accompanied by alcoholism, may give rise to an inadequate folate intake. Mentally disturbed patients are more likely to have folate deficiency.

In the UK, Varadi 8 Elwis (1964) found that 14 per cent of elderly patients admitted to hospital had reduced red cell folate levels, and Elwood et al (1971) found that 8.1 per cent had low red cell folate values.

A review of folate nutrition in the elderly in North America (Rosenberg et al 1982) concluded that among Americans (not in institutions) there was no significant folate problem. On the other hand, surveys of various groups reported that among urban low-income groups the proportion of subjects with low red cell folates was 60 per cent (Baker et al 1979), 31 per cent (Bailey et al, 1982), 13 per cent (quoted by Rosenberg et al, 1982) 5 to 6 per cent (quoted by Rosenberg et al, 1982; Hoppner & Lampi, 1980). Poor urban populations were most at risk. These variable statistics raise questions about the reliability of these assay procedures and about what is a normal folate intake.

A recent survey in the UK indicated that daily intake ranged from 129 to 300 μg per day (Chanarin, 1975). In Sweden the daily folate intake was 103–239 μg in elderly males and 49–180 in elderly women (Jägerstad & Westesson, 1979). In Canada it averaged 151 μg per day in elderly men and 130 μg daily in elderly women (Nutrition Canada, 1977). In elderly Florida residents, daily folate intakes ranged from 184 to 250 μg per day (Rosenberg et al, 1982).

Unfortunately, recommended folate intakes are all put at an unrealistically high level. Thus both the WHO and United States recommend a daily intake of 400 μg folate. On this basis, a large proportion of the population would be receiving an inadequate intake. A more realistic value would be an intake of 150–200 μg daily for an adult.

Megaloblastic anaemia due to folate deficiency can only be diagnosed after other causes discussed in this chapter have been excluded while at the same time a dietary assessment shows a poor folate intake. Treatment is by oral folate, 5 mg daily.

COELIAC DISEASE

In coeliac disease sensitivity to gluten, present in dietary wheat products, provokes a reaction in the small gut leading to atrophy of the villi on the surface of the small gut. Loss of the villus absorbing surface in turn results in intestinal malabsorption. The proximal gut is affected to a much greater extent than distal gut, since the proximal gut is the first to make contact with dietary gluten. It is probable that the disease starts shortly after the weaned infant makes contact with gluten. Nevertheless, the diagnosis may not be made until late in adult life.

The elderly patients seen by the author in whom coeliac disease was diagnosed for the first time all have in common a megaloblastic anaemia and all were short in stature, kyphotic and grossly underweight. The cause of the megaloblastic anaemia in all uncomplicated coeliac patients is folate deficiency and only folate (and, in some, iron) is required for a response. Thus they show low serum and red cell folate levels, and jejunal biopsy shows villus atrophy. There is steatorrhoea.

The blood picture may be complicated by splenic atrophy common in coeliacs. Thus in addition to the changes described, the blood film may show target cells, Howell-Jolly bodies, red cell fragments and erythroblasts.

Coeliac patients do not require cobalamin. Nevertheless, laboratory testing shows that one-third have a low serum cobalamin level and one-third (not necessarily the same third) have impaired cobalamin absorption. These defects disappear on a gluten-free diet. Therapy with cobalamin alone produces no response at all.

Clinically, considerable benefit is obtained even by elderly patients with newly-diagnosed coeliac disease when they are put on a gluten-free diet. Response of the blood is hastened by treatment with folic acid 5 mg daily. Many patients will run out of iron shortly after folate therapy has started. This will be seen as a fall in the MCV below the lower limit of the normal range of 80 fl. Folate therapy should only be continued for about three to four months, but the gluten-free diet is maintained indefinitely. Some patients may have problems related to malabsorption of vitamin D and calcium and require appropriate therapy.

TROPICAL SPRUE

This is a disorder of intestinal malabsorption of unknown causation present in very high numbers among the indigenous population of India, the Far and Middle East, the Caribbean, Natal in South Africa and perhaps Zimbabwe. It also effects European migrants to those countries, and evidence of the disease may persist many years later. In chronic cases the only evidence of the disease may be cobalamin malabsorption and megaloblastic anaemia due to vitamin B_{12} deficiency. In others steatorrhoea is also present.

It is always necessary to determine whether a patient with megaloblastic anaemia has lived for any length of time in an area where tropical sprue is endemic. If the anaemia does not correspond to any recognised pattern, then chronic tropical sprue should be considered as a possible diagnosis. Confirmation requires intestinal absorption studies for fat, xylose, vitamin B_{12}, as well as a jejunal biopsy, and tests for the presence of *Gardia lamblia*. Patients may have deficiency of both vitamin B_{12} and folate, and, apart from correcting the nutritional deficiency, the absorption of cobalamin should be retested after a wide-spectrum antibiotic such as tetracycline which itself is valuable in therapy. The subject has been reviewed recently by Tomkins (1981).

ANTICONVULSANTS

Megaloblastic anaemia in association with administration of anticonvulsant drugs can occur at any age and is a relatively uncommon cause of megaloblastic anaemia in the elderly. Far more common is macrocytosis in the absence of megaloblastic marrow changes. This occurs in at least half the patients taking these drugs, and the increase in MCV is fairly modest in degree. It is not affected by treatment with folic acid. The range of MCV in 108 patients receiving diphenylhydantain and primidone was 74 to 105 fl, whereas it was normal in 18 untreated epileptics (Chanarin, 1979).

Megaloblastosis in the marrow in the absence of anaemia is probably not uncommon and, like the effect of alcohol, may be unrelated to folate status. In two studies involving marrow samples from 194 patients, megaloblastic changes were reported to be present in 34 per cent (Chanarin, 1979). Wickramasinghe et al (1975) carried out deoxyuridine suppression tests in 11 such patients with megaloblastic marrow changes. This test assesses the ability of marrow cells to synthesise thymidine from a precursor, deoxyuridine. It is always abnormal in megaloblastic anaemia due to cobalamin and folate deficiency. Only two out of 11 patients whose marrows were megaloblastic gave abnormal results, and the test was normal in the other nine patients. The implication was that the megaloblastic change was unrelated to folate or cobalamin metabolism.

In 47 patients with overt megaloblastic anaemia due to anticonvulsants, 12 were taking diphenylhydantain, 20 diphenylhydantain and phenobarbital, 11 diphenylhydantain and primidone and 12 primidone alone. Rarely other barbiturates (phenobarbital, amylobarbitone, quinalbarbitone and phenylmethylbarbituric acid) alone have been involved.

The megaloblastic anaemia may be mild or very severe, and there are no laboratory or clinical features that enable one to distinguish it from other causes other than that it has occurred in a patient taking anticonvulsant drugs. Serum folate and red cell folate levels are low and, in addition, the serum cobalamin level may be low. Hence in an elderly subject one must exclude pernicious anaemia as an alternative diagnosis. When the absorption of labelled cobalamin is normal, this does not present a problem, but in some the absorption of cobalamin is depressed temporarily and recovers only after folate therapy. Where available, the deoxyuridine suppression test may be helpful since, if the megaloblastic anaemia is due to cobalamin deficiency, an abnormal test will be partially corrected by adding cobalamin to the incubation mixture *in vitro*.

Treatment is by oral folic acid at conventional doses (5 to 10 mg daily for three months) and the anticonvulsant drugs are continued unchanged. Folate therapy is accompanied by improvement in energy, alertness, speed of thought and action in epileptics. It has also been claimed that, in the long term (that is, after six months) there is an increase in fit frequency etc., but this remains controversial.

The mode of action of anticonvulsants is rather complex. Firstly, it has an effect on cell division by interfering with the incorporation of thymidine into DNA. This effect is dose-related and can occur at therapeutic concentrations of diphenylhydantoin. Cells that are unable to complete cell division die. Increased cell turnover increases the requirement for folic acid. This, too is probably the explanation for the depression of immunoglobulin levels noted in treated epileptics. Secondly, there have been many studies on the effect of anticonvulsants on the intestinal absorption of folic acid. About half report an impairment and half do not. If there is impaired absorption (transient impairment of cobalamin absorption has been mentioned), it could be the result of defective renewal of enterocytes through the defect in DNA synthesis. Thirdly, many anticonvulsant drugs are enzyme inducers, and such a mechanism, it is suggested, may increase the rate of catabolism of folate and hence increase folate requirements. Administration of diphenylhydantoin is accompanied by a fall in the serum folate level. Kelly et al (1979) showed that in mice diphenylhydantoin caused an increased urinary excretion of folate breakdown products. Thus all these three factors lead to folate deficiency and, if the dietary intake is only marginal, may lead to a folate-deficient megaloblastic anaemia.

CO-TRIMOXAZOLE

This drug combination consists of trimethoprim and sulphamethoxazole. Trimethoprim is a folate antagonist binding to the enzyme, dihydrofolate reductase. Dihydrofolate reductase is an important enzyme which restores two hydrogens to folate which are utilised in thymidine synthesis. The end product is the active tetrahydrofolate. Trimethoprim binds strongly to bacterial dihydrofolate reductases but only weakly to the mammalian enzyme. Under some circumstances it can have quite a profound effect in humans and this is when the patient has accompanying folate or cobalamin deficiency. When this is the case, it can lead to marrow arrest.

Less dramatic effects may occur in elderly subjects given long-term prophylactic co-trimoxazole for chronic urinary tract or pulmonary infections. There may be a slow steady rise in the MCV with a gradual onset of anaemia. This is reversed by folic acid.

It is as well to ensure that a patient who may benefit from long-term prophylactic co-trimoxazole has normal serum cobalamin and normal red cell folate levels at the start.

CHRONIC HAEMOLYTIC STATES

There are a group of disorders characterised by an increased requirement for folic acid. When this requirement exceeds the dietary intake, a negative folate balance ensues and in time may lead to a folate-deficient megaloblastic anaemia. In the elderly there are at least two important disorders, chronic haemolytic states and chronic myelofibrosis which can be complicated by folate deficiency.

Chronic haemolytic states that have an increased folate requirement include hereditary spherocytosis (not treated by splenectomy), haemoglobinopathies such as sickle-cell anaemia, haemoglobin H disease and auto-immune haemolytic anaemias including that due to Aldomet (methyldopa) given to treat hypertension and that complicating chronic lymphocytic leukaemia.

Clinically when such patients develop a megaloblastic anaemia, they present with the signs and symptoms of severe anaemia and often jaundice. The sudden onset of anaemia in a patient known to have a red cell disorder of the type listed should suggest marrow failure due to folate deficiency. In severe cases, anaemia is accompanied by neutropenia and thrombocytopenia. Marrow is essential and shows florid megaloblastic change.

Treatment is with oral folic acid. In some patients with haemolytic anaemia complicating chronic lymphocytic leukaemia and a marrow packed with lymphocytes, high-dose steroids and even cytotoxic therapy may be needed. Transfusion will be necessary in these more severe cases.

It is reasonable to continue folate therapy indefinitely in such patients with chronic haemolytic states since these have a permanently increased folate requirement. Cobalamin absorption must be shown to be normal in these patients. Five milligrams of folate daily, or on alternative days, are adequate. Patients with auto-immune haemolytic anaemia will require high-dose steroid therapy and other appropriate management.

CHRONIC MYELOFIBROSIS

This chronic disorder in characterised by massive splenomegaly and a leuco-erythroblastic blood picture. The red blood cells may show a characteristic 'teardrop' deformity. Marrow trephine confirms an increase in marrow reticulin and sometimes even excess collagen which can become calcified (myelosclerosis). Attempts at marrow aspiration, however, are usually unsuccessful — so-called dry tap.

Generally, the course of this disease is at some time complicated by folate deficiency. Thus of 49 patients 16 had severe megaloblastic anaemia and 17 recognisable megaloblastic changes without significant anaemia (Hoffbrand et al 1968). In patients with severe involvement, the development of severe folate deficiency, if unrecognised, leads to repeated blood transfusions to maintain a falling haemoglobin level. Neutropenia may also be a feature. Others have an unexplained fall in the platelet count. This marrow failure is progressive and, if not recognised and treated, could prove fatal.

The diagnosis of megaloblastic marrow failure in chronic myelofibrosis requires a high degree of clinical awareness. In some patients the diagnosis can be confirmed by finding that circulating normoblasts are replaced by megaloblasts. In others, a buffy coat preparation is helpful. Where this is not decisive, attempts at marrow aspiration should be made. Even when fragments are not forthcoming, strong suction with a 20 ml syringe and withdrawal of the marrow needle while maintaining a negative pressure will yield sufficient fluid to spread one or two films which, when stained, confirm megaloblastosis.

Serum and red cell folates are low but the serum vitamin B_{12} level very high, as is the case in many patients with myeloproliferative disorders. Treatment is with oral folic acid and this should be continued indefinitely. Again the absorption of cobalamin should be shown to be normal.

BLOOD TRANSFUSION IN SEVERELY ANAEMIC MEGALOBLASTIC PATIENTS

It is not uncommon to encounter elderly patients with severe megaloblastic anaemia and red cell counts below 1.5 million/μl who are in congestive cardiac failure. In the majority the anaemia is the major factor in precipitating cardiac failure and hence there is a strong temptation to transfuse several units of blood. However, in such patients there is a considerable risk in overloading the circulation and great care has to be taken. It has been suggested that transfusion should not exceed 250 ml of packed red cells given very slowly over 4–6 hours. It should be accompanied by the administration of a rapidly acting diuretic such as frusemide, 40 mg.

Circulatory overload is indicated by a rise in jugular venous pressure, restlessness, the patient's head feeling full, a dry cough and moist sounds in the lung bases. Should this occur the transfusion is stopped, the patient propped up in bed and a further dose of diuretic given. If there is no response, a venesection should be carried out. Circulatory overload can lead to a fatal outcome after twelve or more hours with pulmonary oedema.

If it is possible to postpone transfusion in order to see if a response cannot be obtained to combined vitamin B_{12} and folate therapy (after laboratory samples have been taken) this should be done and the patient re-assessed at frequent intervals.

Although much has been made of a fall in serum potassium levels (which is maximum, if it occurs at all, two to three days after treatment is given), this is rarely of sufficient significance to warrant potassium supplements. The fall in serum potassium is greatest in elderly severely anaemic patients and perhaps these may need a supplement.

RFERENCES

Ardeman S, Chanarin I 1965 Steroids and addisonian pernicious anemia. New England Journal of Medicine 273: 1352–1358
Ardeman S, Chanarin I 1966 Intrinsic factor secretion in gastric atrophy. Gut 7: 99–101
Bailey L B et al 1982 Folacin and iron status and hematological findings in Black and Spanish–American adolescents from urban low-income households. American Journal of Clinical Nutrition 35: 1023–1032
Baker H, Frank 0, Thind I S, Jaslow S P, Louria D P 1979 Vitamin profile in elderly persons living at home or in nursing homes, versus profile in healthy young subjects. Journal of the American Geriatrics Society 27: 444–450
Callender S T, Denborough M A 1957 A family study of pernicious anaemia. British Journal of Haematology 3: 88–106
Chanarin I 1975 The folate content of foodstuffs and the availability of different folate analogues for absorption. In: Getting the most out of food. Van den Bergh & Jurgens, London, p 41
Chanarin I 1979 The megaloblastic anaemias, 2nd edn. Blackwell, Oxford
Chanarin I, James D 1974 Humoral and cell-mediated intrinsic-factor antibody in pernicious anaemia. Lancet 1: 1078–1080
Cheli R, Santi L, Ciancameria G, Canciani G 1973 A clinical and statistical follow-up of atrophic gastritis. Digestive Diseases 18: 1061–1065

Elsborg L, Mosbech J 1979 Pernicious anaemia as a risk factor in gastric cancer. Acta Medica Scandinavica 206: 315–318

Elwood P C, Shinton N K, Wilson C I D, Sweetnam P, Frazer AC 1971 Haemoglobin, vitamin B_{12} and folate levels in the elderly. British Journal of Haematology 21: 557–563

Ericksson S, Clase L, Moquist-Olsson I 1981 Pernicious anemia as a risk factor in gastric cancer. Acta Medica Scandinavica 210: 481–484

Fenwick S 1870 On atrophy of the stomach. Lancet ii: 78–80.

Hoffbrand A V, Chanarin I, Kremenchuzky S, Szur L, Waters A M, Mollin D L 1968 Megaloblastic anaemia in myelosclerosis. Quarterly Journal of Medicine NS 37: 493–516

Hoppner K, Lampi B 1980 Folate levels in human liver from autospies in Canada. American Journal of Clinical Nutrition 33: 862–846

Jägerstad M, Westesson A-K 1979 Folate. In: Bergström B, Nordin A, Akesson B, Abdulla M, Jägerstad M (eds) Nutrition and old age. Universities Forlaget, Oslo, ch 24, p 196

Kelly D, Weir D, Reed B, Scott J 1979 Effect of anticonvulsant drugs on the rate of folate catabolism in mice. Journal of Clinical Investigation 64: 1049–1096

Nutrition Canada 1977 Food consumption patterns report. Department of National Health and Welfare, Ottawa

Rosenberg I H, Bowman B B, Cooper B A, Halsted C H, Lindenbaum J 1982 Folate nutrition in the elderly. American Journal of Clinical Nutrition 36: 1060–1066

Siurala M, Lehtola J, Ihamäki T 1974 Atrophic gastristis and its sequelae, results of 19–23 years' follow-up examinations. Scandinavian Journal of Gastroenterostamy 9: 441–446

Tanaka A, Glass G-B J 1970 Effect of prolonged administration of parietal cell antibodies from patients with atrophic gastritis and pernicious anemia on the parietal cell mass and hydrochloric acid output in rats. Gastroenterlogy 58: 482–494

Thompson W G, Wrathell 1977 The relation between ileal resection and vitamin B_{12} absorption. Canadian Journal of Surgery 20: 461–464

Tomkins A 1981 Tropical malabsorption: recent concepts in pathogenesis and nutritional significance. Clinical Science 60: 131–137

Varadi S, Elwis A, 1964 Megaloblastic anaemia due to dietary deficiency i: 1162.

Whiteside M G, Mollin D L, Coghill N F, Williams A W, Andersen B 1964 The absorption of radioactive vitamin B_{12} and the secretion of hydrochloric acid in patients with atrophic gastritis. Gut 5: 385–399

Wickramasinghe S N, Williams G, Saunders, J Durston J H 1975 Megaloblastic erythropoiesis and macrocytosis in patients on anticonvulsants. British Medical Journal iv: 136–137

Zamcheck N, Grable E, Ley A, Norman L 1955 Occurrence of gastric cancer among patients with pernicious anemia at the Boston City Hospital. New England Journal of Medicine 252: 1103–1110

Normocytic Anaemia and Anaemias of General Disease

INTRODUCTION

Recent work on the haemopoietic system and the effects of ageing suggests that there is no real difference in the type of blood disease which may occur in the elderly from that which occurs in the younger population. The natural history may vary but the basic pathology is much the same and response to therapy in the main is also the same. Some of the newer therapeutic man-eouvres such as bone marrow transplantation have been considered unsuit-able for the elderly, but this reflects their inability to withstand the rigours of the procedure, and a greater liability to graft versus host disease, rather than any real change in the haemopoietic system. In any case, the biological process of ageing is only one factor which may affect the natural course of disease in old age. Other factors include the presence of infections or other chronic disorders and the general state of nutrition. Despite the well-known effect of oestrogens on the haemoglobin level, the female haemoglobin level remains slightly lower than that in the male even after the menopause and into old age.

Many surveys in elderly people have been undertaken to determine the incidence and severity of anaemia, but they are not strictly comparable, since different values were used for the diagnosis of anaemia (Elwood, 1971; Milne & Williamson, 1972; Davidson, 1967; Evans et al, 1968; Department of Health and Social Security, 1970 and 1972; Kilpatrick, 1961; Morgan, 1967; MacLennon et al 1973). Even when the values recommended by the World Health Organisation are adopted (1968), and anaemia is defined as a Hb of less than 13.0 g/dl in males and less than 11.9 g/dl in females, there are wide differences in the reported incidences of anaemia which may vary from over 40 per cent to as low as 5 per cent. The general conclusions, however, are that the incidence increases rapidly after the age of 60, that it carries with it an increasing mortality in the elderly and that it is more common in females than males.

Normocytic anaema is that anaemia which occurs with a lowered haemog-lobin level but in which the other indices are normal i.e. MCV remains normal (76–96 fl) and MCH 27–32 pg (see Table 5.1). There are

Table 5.1   Normocytic normochromic anaemia (MCV 76–96fl, MCH 27–32pg)

Hypoproliferative
  1. Anaemia of chronic disorders
      Infection
         Tuberculosis
         Bacterial endocarditis
         Bronchiectasis
         Lung abscess
         Brucellosis
         Pyelonephritis
         Osteomyelitis
         Fungal infections
         Actinomyeces
      Malignancy
         Lymphoma
         Carcinoma
      Collagen Diseases
         Rheumatoid arthritis
         Giant cell ateritis
         Polyarteritis nodosa
         Systemic lupus erythematosus
      Liver disease
         Acute
         Chronic
  2. Impaired erythropoietin secretion
      Endocrine disorders
         Hypothyroidism
         Hypopituitarism
         Addison's disease
      Renal disease
  3. Primary marrow failure
      Aplastic anaemia
      Pure red cell aplasia

some anaemias which may occur in primary form as normocytic, e.g. aplastic anaemia, and others which occur as a manifestation of some other underlying disease (see Table 5.2). Those disorders which are not covered elsewhere in this book will be discussed.

ANAEMIA OF CHRONIC DISORDERS

This is the most common of all anaemias in the elderly. The precise mechanism is still uncertain. Cartwright & Lee (1971) describe it as 'that anaemia usually mild in degree and not progressive in severity which is characterised by decreased plasma iron, decreased total iron-binding capacity of the plasma, decreased saturation of transferrin with iron, decreased marrow sideroblasts and normal or increased reticuloendothelial iron'. This type of anaemia may be associated not only with chronic infection but with malignancy, collagen diseases e.g. rheumatoid arthritis, and after certain injuries both to soft tissue and bone. The anaemia does not occur immediately following the onset of the illness but gradually develops over a period of weeks. The haemoglobin level is only slightly or moderately depressed and may remain so

Table 5.2 Pathogenesis of aplastic anaemia

Stem cell failure	2. Irradiation
1. Drugs and chemicals	X-rays and neutrons
Antibiotics	3. Infections
Chloramphenicol	Viruses
Sulphonamides	Hepatitis
Analgesics	Infectious mononucleosis
Phenylbutazone	Parvovirus
Oxyphenbutazone	Rubella
Anticonvulsants	Influenza
Phenytoin	Mumps
Methoin	Bacteria
Troxidone	Tuberculosis
Heavy metals	Brucellosis
Gold salts	4. Immunological disturbances antibodies to CFUE
Organic chemicals	Antibodies to erythropoietin
Antithyroid drugs	5 Idiopathic
Potassium perchlorate	Damage of micro-environment of marrow
Thiouricil	Evidence from experimental animals
Carbimazole	
Oral hypoglycaemic drugs	
~Tolbutamide	
Chlorpropamide	
Benzene derivatives	

for long periods of time. It is usually normocytic and normochromic in type but occasionally there is a mild element of hypochromia with a slightly reduced MCH and MCHC. It is only rarely that the degree of hypochromia can be compared with that seen in iron deficiency. The peripheral blood film therefore is unremarkable and the reticulocyte count is less than 2 per cent. Examination of the bone marrow shows an increase in the myeloid to-erythroid ratio, but there may also be a reactive increase in the number of granulocytes present, making it difficult to decide whether there is an absolute decrease in red cell precursors (although this is said to occur). There may be an increase in the proportion of basophilic normoblasts with abnormally large and immature nuclei with a proportionate reduction in more mature blasts and reticulocytes (Cartwright & Wintrobe 1952). In some instances, particularly those involving inflammation of the liver and bile ducts, there is plasmacytosis. Trephine biopsy usually shows diffuse hypoplasia (Begmann & Rasletter, 1972). The anaemia develops over a period of three or four weeks with a progressive fall in haemoglobin levels and it then levels out to around 9 or 10 g/dl with a packed cell volume (PCV) of 0.30–0.40 (Hardisty & Wetherall 1983). The eventual degree of anaemia is related to the severity and duration of the underlying disorder.

Pathogenesis

One of the main mechanisms of the cause of anaemia seems to be impaired utilisation of iron for incorporation into haemoglobin, and ferrokinetic studies indicate that either oral or parenteral iron therapy results in iron deposi-tion into the iron stores and utilisation of such iron only when the cause of the anaemia has been appropriately treated. Impaired utilisation in this manner appears to result from impaired release of reticuloendothelial iron to the developing erythroblasts within the bone marrow. The abnormality in iron metabolism is reflected by a reduced serum iron, reduced transferrin levels and reduced transferrin saturation, but the marrow iron stores are in fact increased. This in turn is reflected by a rise in the serum ferritin levels unless of course there is associated iron deficiency. (Zucker et al, 1976; Lipshitz et al 1974, Walsh and Frederickson 1977 and Birgegard et al 1978). There are several indications of an increase both in ferritin synthesis by the liver and spleen and retention of iron released from effete red cells by these organs (Herscshko et al, 1974; Torrence et al, 1978; Fillet et al, 1974). Other mechanisms contributing to the anaemia include shortened red cell survival and impaired erythropoietin response. The shortened red cell survival is associated with an increase in reticuloendothelial activity and the consequent increase in phagocytic activity results in slight haemolysis. Such haemolysis would normally be easily compensated for by normal marrow activity, but there appears to be an inadequate erythropoietin response to the anaemia and both serum and urinary erythropoietin levels are less than would be expected for the degree of the anaemia (Wallner et al, 1977).

Clinical features

The clinical features are predominantly those of the underlying disease, although on occasions anaemia may be a presenting feature.

A blood count usually reveals a normocytic normochromic anaemia, although occasionally it may be slightly hypochromic. There is reduced plasma iron and reduced total iron-binding capacity. Transferrin is reduced less than the plasma iron, so that the degree of saturation falls to below 30 per cent but not below 15 or 16 per cent as in iron deficiency. An iron stain carried out on a bone-marrow smear shows increased deposits of iron but marrow sideroblasts are decreased in numbers. Plasma copper and free erythrocyte protoporphyrin are also increased, but these levels are not mea-sured in routine practice. The bone marrow changes are described above and are none-diagnostic.

Treatment

The treatment is that of the primary condition. Iron therapy is useless and parenteral iron only adds to the reticuloendothelial load. In some instances, corticosteroids appear to release iron from the reticuloendothelial system, but in many cases they are contra-indicated. Cartwright & Lee (1971) suggested that it would be of great interest to treat patients with a continuous infusion of saturated transferrin and erythropoietin, which should restore both the quality and quantity of erythropoiiesis to normal.

Malignant disease

In many patients with malignant disease, the anaemia of chronic disorders is apparent and it is by far the commonest type of anaemia seen in malignancy. It may be associated with all forms of malignancy, including lymphoma, and the aetiological mechanisms are described above. In some instances it is obscured by other causes of anaemia such as blood loss, haemolysis or folate deficiency, but often it is a presenting feature and may be apparent even when the site and nature of the neoplasm is unknown. If dissemination of the tumour occurs, then other types of anaemia such as microangiopathic haemolytic anaemia or leucoerythroblastic anaemia may result. Occasionally bone marrow fibrosis occurs, as in Hodgkin's disease. The clinical features are those of the underlying neoplasm, but blood and bone marrow examination reveals features of the resulting anaemia. Bone pain is often associated with a rise in alkaline phosphatase levels and in certain tumours, such as prostatic carcinoma, there may be specific markers such as a rise in tartrate-resistant acid phosphase levels. Carcinoma cells should be looked for in the bone marrow smear and trephine biopsy, but even when they are present it is often difficult to determine the tissue of origin.

Other types of anaemia that may be associated with malignancy, such as sideroblastic anaemia and megaloblastic anaemia, are discussed elsewhere.

Infection

Nearly all bacterial infections, both acute and chronic, are complicated by some degree of anaemia which is of the normochromic normocyytic type. Haemolytic anaemia may occur in some infections such as *Clostridium welchi*, but this is much less common. In the acute infections the anaemia is complicated by a neutrophil leucocytosis with a shift to the left indicated by an increase in the numbers of neutrophils and sometimes of metamyelocytes or myelocytes in the peripheral blood. In some instances the neutrophil response is inadequate and in such cases an underlying cause, for example a haematological disorder or other debilitating condition such as alcoholism, should be looked for. In some of these patients a frank neutropenia is present, but this is much less common.

In chronic bacterial infections, the ESR tends to be very high, and in patients presenting with a high ESR and a low-grade anaemia, chronic infections should be sought for, e.g. chronic pyelonephritis, brucellosis and tuberculosis. In tuberculosis the degree of anaemia parallels closely the degree of disease activity, and appropriate therapy usually corrects the anaemia. Persistence after adequate treatment should raise the suspicion of other underlying covert diseases such as sideroblastic anaemia. Spiro chaetal infections are a much less common cause of this type of anaemia, and most of them are associated with a polymorphonuclear leucocytosis and sometimes an eosinophilia. Occasionally there is intravascular haemolysis and thrombocytopaenia.

Viral infections are an extremely uncommon cause of anaemia, with the possible exception of the hepatitis virus which may cause haemolytic or aplastic anaemia, and this relationship will be discussed later. Protozoal infections are outside the scope of this discussion.

Rheumatoid Arthritis

Many patients with rheumatoid arthritis present with a haemoglobin level of around 11 g/dl for women and 12.6 g/dl for men (Bennett, 1977), and it is estimated that around 50 per cent of all patients with rheumatoid arthritis suffer from anaemia. The red cell count is reduced in parallel with the haemoglobin level, but the MCH is only slightly reduced and the MCV is either low or remains within the normal range. Iron deficiency is occasionally associated with this picture and is best diagnosed by measurement of serum ferritin levels (Bentley & Williams, 1974). It has been suggested that there is an abnormality in iron metabolism with the retention of endogenous iron from senescent red cells in the reticuloendothelial system. There is a failure to release this iron, but it may be released following the administration of corticosteroids (Owen & Lawson, 1966). Other workers, however, have failed to confirm this finding (Williams et al, 1974). Increased amounts of storage iron has been found in the spleen, liver and lymph nodes, but the most interesting finding is that of high concentrations of ferritin in the synovial tissues (Bennett et al, 1974).

While there is no evidence of erythropoietin deficiency, there is nevertheless an inappropriate increase in erythropoietin levels for the degree of anaemia (Ward et al, 1969). It should be mentioned, for the sake of completeness, that megaloblastic anaemia is also recognised with increasing frequency in rheumatoid arthritis. It is usually due to folate deficiency consequent upon increased demands for folate consequent upon increased demands for folate and impaired nutrition, and may be corrected by simple folate supplements. Vitamin B_{12} deficiency is much less common and, when present, other causes such as pernicious anaemia should be looked for (Chanarin, 1979).

Some patients may be truly iron-deficient, particularly if receiving salicylate therapy, and a trial of oral iron therapy is advisable, especially in those patients in whom the serum ferritin level is reduced, but it is not recommended in all patients. Parenteral iron therapy, on the other hand, significantly improves the haemoglobin level in the vast majority of patients (Richmond et al, 1958). Two to three grams of intra-muscular iron appear to be about the correct dose, and its efficacy may be due to its ability to overcome the avidity of the reticuloendothelial system for iron.

If the disease itself can be brought under control, then there is usually a further dramatic improvement in haemoglobin levels. Corticosteroid therapy is often very effective in this respect and may reflect a reduction in the activity of the reticuloendothelial system with a consequent reduction in iron sequestration. This results in a greater amount of iron for red cell utilisation and improved marrow iron stores. It is of course customary to withhold corticosteroids and attempt to control the disease by other means before resorting to this form of therapy.

Felty's Syndrome

Felty first described the syndrome, which was later named after him, in 1924 (Felty, 1924). The clinical features described by Felty consisted of neutropaenia, pigmentation of exposed surfaces and lymphadenopathy, in association with splenomegaly and rheumatoid arthritis. There seems to be no direct correlation between the size of the spleen and the degree of neutropenia, and most patients with rheumatoid arthritis have some degree of splenomegaly, although it might not be clinically detectable. Leucopenia is the result of a reduction in both neutrophils and lympocytes. The platelet count may also be reduced but seldom falls below 100×10^9, per litre. Bacterial infections are frequently found and may be severe, but such infections are not necessarily confined to those patients with detectable splenomegaly.

Although this syndrome superfically resembles hypersplenism, there is no evidence of haemolytic anaemia and the cause of the splenomegaly is unknown. It is not associated with bone marrow hyperplasia as in true hypersplenism but in most cases there is some degree of maturation arrest of the granulocyte series. It seems likely that the cause of neutropaenia is overactivity of the spleen possibly in association with neutrophil antibodies. There is some evidence of reduced granulocyte colony formation in the bone marrow (Greenberg and Schrier 1973, Abdou et al 1978). Factors suggesting that there may be contributory immunological mechanisms to the neutropenia, include a positive ANF in many cases, high rhumatoid factor levels and raised immunoglobulin levels.

Splenectomy is sometimes undertaken, but it should only be performed in those cases where neutropenia is associated with recurrent and severe infections. There is no clear evidence that the operation reduces the incidence or the severity of infections, even though the neutrophil count rises in about 60 per cent of cases (Barnes et al, 1971; Seinknicht et al, 1977). Splenectomy may occasionally be undertaken because of thrombocytopenia, but this is not usually a clinical problem.

Steroid therapy in large dose, e.g. prednisolone 50 or 60 mg daily, will also restore the neutrophil count to normal, but once it is reduced to safe maintenance levels the neutrophils tend to fall again. Small rises in the neutrophil count may be obtained by lithium therapy (Gupta et al, 1975) but the rise is not sustained and the leucocytosis obtained is seldom maintained once the drug is withdrawn.

Systemic Lupus Erythematosus (SLE)

This is a collagen disease in which severe disturbances in the immune system result in disease of many other systems of the body. About 75 per cent of patients develop anaemia of chronic disorders (Budman & Steinberg, 1977; Harvey et al, 1954; Dubois & Tufanelli, 1964) which may be associated with auto-immune haemolytic anaemia and a positive Coombs test or with blood loss from administration of non-steroid anti-inflammatory agents or as a result of thrombocytopenia. Treatment is by corticosteroid therapy or other immunosuppressive agents.

Polymylgia rheumatica — temporal arteritis syndrome

Patients with this syndrome may present with a high ESR, normocytic normochromic anaemia and other symptoms such as weight loss, night sweats, fever and in temporal arteritis, temporal headaches which may be associated with visual loss. Such symptoms may suggest severe underlying disease in the form of disseminated malignancy, and careful investigation should be performed to exclude such a disorder. In polymyalgia rheumatica there is usually a dramatic response to small doses of prednisolone (5–10 mg daily) but temporal arteritis may require larger doses of 60–100 mg per day. The diagnosis of temporal arteritis may be confirmed by a temporal artery biopsy, but treatment should not be delayed in view of the risk of blindness. Some elderly patients present with a normochromic normocytic anaemia and a high ESR for which no cause can be found. In such patients a diagnosis of polymyalgia rheumatica should be entertained since the condition may be a variant of this disorder. If so, it would respond dramatically to small doses of prednisolone.

Scleroderma (progressive systemic sclerosis)

About one-third of patients develop normocytic normochromic anaemia, but it may be complicated by iron deficiency as a result of bleeding telangiectases or very occasionally haemolytic anaemia (Holt & Wright, 1967; Fundenberg & Wintrobe, 1955).

Ankylosing spondilitis

Anaemia of chronic disorders is found in about one-quarter of such patients and is usually mild in nature (Polley & Slocumb, 1947). Previous radiotherapy may result in some degree of marrow hypoplasia with a tenfold increase in the risk of developing leukaemia in subsequent years.

Dermatomyositis and Reiter's disease

In these disorders there are no specific abnormalities, although very occasionally normochromic anaemia may be found in association with an elevated ESR.

Chronic liver disease

Haematological findings associated with *acute* liver disease will be discussed later and consist mainly of the rare occurrence of haemolytic anaemia or hypoplastic anaemia.

Many years ago Wintrobe (1936) studied the incidence of various types of anaemia in *chronic* liver disease and found a macrocytic picture in 32.6 per cent, normocytic in 30.3 per cent, no anaemia in 22.7 per cent and microcytic anaemia in 14.4 per cent of patients.

Macrocytic anaemia may be due to folate deficiency, to accompanying alcoholism, or even coincident pernicious anaemia, but is usually unassociated with any vitamin deficiency and seems to be derived from macronormoblasts in the bone marrow. The macrocytes are much more uniform than is the case in megaloblastic anaemias of similar severity. The volume of these macrocytes is not significantly increased above normal but they are thinner, with an increased diameter over the normal erythrocyte. These cells are known as leptocytes (Binghan, 1961; Werre et al, 1970) of which there appear to be two types, one with and one without targeting. Targeting is due to the effects of serum factors and normal cells, when introduced into the circulation of patients with circulating leptocytes, take up excessive cholesterol and assume the same characteristics, including resistance to saline. In severe hepatocellular disease these changes may be marked, and some cells take on the appearance of acanthocytes seen in $\propto$-ß lipoproteinaemia; such cells carry a poor prognosis, and patients who exhibit them usually, die within a month or two.

Very commonly, particularly in association with chronic hepatitis or cirrhosis, there is a moderate anaemia in which the haemoglobin level rarely falls below 10 g/dl. In these uncomplicated cases the red cells are normocytic, normochromic.

Whether the red blood cells in the peripheral blood are normocytic or mildly macrocytic, the bone marrow is found to be hypoplastic and erythroblasts macronormoblatic (Nunally & Levine, 1961). The macronormoblasts have large nuclei, the chromatin network is more open and contains blocks or wedges of chromatin rather than the dense 'ink spot' nuclei of most late normoblasts. Giant metamyelocytes do occur, but some plasmacytosis is occasionally present. Megaloblastic changes are seen only in the presence of folate deficiency.

The changes of true iron deficiency in both the peripheral blood and bone marrow are seen occasionally as a result of blood loss, e.g. bleeding from oesophageal varices which may be complicated by a haemorrhagic diathesis as a result of liver disease.

The anaemia of liver disease is associated with a shortened red cell survival (Chaplin & Mollison, 1953; Cooksley et al, 1973). Red cells from patients with liver disease have shortened survival when transfused into normal recipients, but normal cells transfused into patients with liver disease also have a shortened survival, so it would appear that there is both an extracorpuscular and intracorpuscular haemolytic factor. The role of the spleen is uncertain and there is no direct correlation between the size of the spleen and haemolysis (Cooksley et al, 1973). Splenectomy is only rarely of benefit, and red cell survival is usually unaffected. The possibility that damage might be caused to the red cells during their passage through the liver has been suggested (Dacie, 1967) but Cooksley et al (1973) concluded that this was not primarily responsible for the haemolysis and that the liver only phagocytised effete red cells that were presented to it. Ferrokinetic studies have indicated that the bone marrow is unable to compensate for the increased red cell destruction in a normal manner. Erythropoiesis is in fact increased, but not to a sufficient degree to prevent a mild degree of anaemia. There is no evidence of ineffective erythropoiesis (Kimber et al, 1965).

Shortened red cell survival may also occur in acute liver disease, but apart from occasional aplasia already referred to, any shortening of the red cell survival is so well compensated for, that anaemia rarely results.

Occasionally, severe haemolytic anaemia may occur in patients with chronic liver disease as a result of superimposed acute episodes. One of these is known as Zieve's syndrome and was first described in 1958. The condition occurs after an acute bout of alcohol ingestion and is associated with severe haemolytic anaemia consequent upon hyperlipidaemia and hypercholesterolaemia. It may also be accompanied by malaise, vomiting and fever, with pain in the upper abdomen or lower chest. Severe haemolytic anaemia may also follow an attack of acute viral hepatitis or be consequent upon a Coombs positive haemolytic anaemia in association with chronic active hepatitis.

It should be remembered that heavy alcohol ingestion may produce megaloblastic or sideroblastic changes which may be superimposed upon the original anaemia of chronic liver disease.

IMPAIRED ERYTHROPOIETIN SECRETION

Chronic renal failure

All patients with chronic renal failure suffer from some degree of anaemia (Anagnostou & Fried, 1979). The anaemia is roughly proportional to the degree of renal failure, although there are some exceptions, for example patients with polycystic disease often suffer from less anaemia than might be expected, and those patients with the haemolytic-uraemia syndrome and microangiopathic haemolytic anaemia have a greater degree of anaemia than would be predicted by the level of renal failure.

Aetiology

The anaemia appears to be multifactorial, with a decrease in red cell survival (Brain, 1979) which seems to relate to the degree of uraemia, impaired erythropoiesis and haemodilution. Metabolic abnormalities occur in the erythrocytes in the presence of a raised blood urea, but these changes are reversible.

The bone marrow response is adequate for the degree of anaemia and this in turn appears to be due to an inappropriately low level of erythropoietin, in the production of which the kidneys play a vital role. It is, however, difficult to be certain of the significance of apparently low levels of erythropoietin, since, with the sensitivity of present techniques of erythropoietin assay, it is impossible to detect significant levels in normal plasma and it has been shown that erythrocyte 2, 3-DPG is increased in patients with chronic renal failure, as is the intracellular pH. These factors result in a reduced oxygen affinity of the red cell with increased uptake by the tissues and therefore reduced requirements for increased erythropoietin secretion. Uraemic serum itself has also been shown to reduce the iron uptake by red cells *in-vitro*.

Haemodilution has a very variable effect, but undoubtedly in some patients it does make the anaemia appear worse than it really is. And added factor in other patients is blood loss, which tends to take place from the gastrointestinal tract as a result of gastric erosions or peptic ulceration or as a result of a haemostatic defect.

Clinical features

There is a normocytic normochromic anaemia, but occasionally burr cells are present. They are caused by the change that occurs in the membrane lipids of the red cell, but other abnormal forms include poikilocytes, triangular and helmet cells. If gastrointestinal haemorrhages occur, then hypochromic cells may also be seen. The morphology of the leucocytes and platelets is normal, but the reticulocyte count is very variable and may be either reduced, normal or increased. Microangiopathic haemolytic anaemia may be present, but this is outside the scope of this chapter and will not be discussed further.

The marrow changes are relatively unimportant. The expected increase in erythropoietic activity is not present, and erythropoietic activity may in fact be reduced in some patients.

Treatment

The treatment is basically that of chronic renal failure. There is no specific therapy apart from long-term administration of erythropoietin, but this is not commercially available in sufficient quantities. Other preparations, including androgenic steroids and cobalt, have proved to be ineffective. Blood transfusions are not usually required, but in any case should be kept to a minimum since there is a danger of depressing the erythropoietic activity in the patient's own bone marrow and of inducing iron overload. Other risks include blood-transfusion-induced hepatitis.

ENDOCRINE DISORDERS

Hypothyroidism

Up to 50 per cent of patients with hypothyroidism may show some degree of anaemia, but it is only of slight degree (Horton et al, 1976)

Aetiology

The total red cell mass is said to be reduced in hypothyroidism (Muldowney et al, 1957), but the changes may be masked to some extent by parallel decreases in plasma volume. Both morphological examination of the bone marrow and ferrokinetic studies indicate that erythropoiesis is reduced, and this has been thought to be due to the reduced oxygen consumption by the tissues (Fisher & Gross, 1977) and as a result of reduced metabolic demands. This is thought to have an indirect effect on erythropoietin secretion with reduced erythropoietin levels (Hollander et al, 1967; Fisher & Gross, 1977; Dass et al, 1975), but erythropoiesis does not seem to be stimulated by thyroxine (Fisher et al, 1964). As already mentioned, however, the difficulty in making such assertions is that erythropoietin levels cannot be detected in normal plasma and therefore a reduction in levels cannot be substantiated. Moreover, there is some recent evidence to suggest that thyroid hormone has a direct stimulatory effect on erythroid colony growth in the presence of erythropoietin (Adamson et al 1978).

Clinical features

The anaemia is mild, the MCV is often increased and the blood film may also show occasional irregular contracted red cell (Wardrop & Hutchinson, 1969). The bone marrow shows evidence of erythroid hypoplasia, and ferrokinetics indicate a reduced iron clearance from the plasma and reduced iron utilisation for red cell formation. There is a high incidence of chronic atrophic gastritis and associated iron deficiency or vitamin B_{12} deficiency in patients with hypothyroidism, and such deficiences may modify the clinical picture. It is not proposed to discuss these features here, but the possibility of their occurrence in hypothyroid states should be remembered.

Therapy

Thyroxine therapy results in a slow but sure return of all parameters to normal, but concomitant iron or vitamin B^{12} deficiency will require appropriate replacement.

Addison's disease

Anaemia in association with Addison's disease was first described by Addison himself in 1849. The anaemia is mild in nature and is of the normocytic normochromic type. Other changes in the peripheral blood include leucopenia with a relative lymphocytosis and eosinophilia. Addison's disease may be associated with pernicious anaemia (Irvine et al, 1965) and in this case the anaemia may be macrocytic with megaloblastic bone marrow changes. In these cases there are often organ-specific antibodies against both the adrenal gland and the gastric parietal mucosa (Irvine et al, 1965; Gaudie et al, 1966). The serum iron level is normal, but erythrocyte utilisation of iron is slightly reduced. The plasma volume is also reduced, thus masking the degree of anaemia.

The mechanism of the anaemia is obscure, but adrenalectomy regularly results in hypoplasia of the erythrocyte precursors in the bone marrow (Gordon et al, 1951). It seems likely that cortisol has a controlling influence on the rate of erythropoiesis indirectly, since its administration results in an increase in oxygen consumption with subsequent stimulation in erythropoietin production (Peschle et al, 1975).

Therapy with adrenocorticosteroids results in gradual correction of the anaemia.

Hypopituitarism

A mild normochromic anaemia is a common feature in patients suffering from hypopituitarism (Sheenan, 1939; Summers, 1952) and may be a presenting feature. As in Addison's disease, there is often a leucopenia with a mild eosinophilia. The mechanism of the anaemia is the same as that described for hypothyroidism (see above), but it is also possible that growth hormone has an erythropoietic effect which is not related to oxygen consumption (Bozzini et al, 1970).

The diagnosis may be made clinically on the basis of other associated features such as loss of body hair and depigmentation of the areolate. Therapy with replacement endocrine hormones is effective in correcting the anaemia.

REFERENCES

Abdou N I, Naponeja, Balentine L, Abdou N L 1978 Suppressor cell mediated neutropenia in Felty's syndrome. Journal of Clinical Investigation 61: 738–741
Adamson J W, Popovic W J, Brown J E 1978 Modulation of *invitro* erythropoiesis: normal interactions and erythroid colony growth. In: Differentiation of normal and neoplastic hematopoietic cells. Clarkson B, Marks P A, Till J F (eds) Cold Spring Harbor, p 235 vol A.
Anagnostov A, Fried W 1979 Anemia of renal disease in hematological problems. In: Jepson J H Renal disease (ed). Adison-Wesley, Menlo Park, California

Barnes C G, Turnbull A L, Vernon-Roberts B 1971 Felty's syndrome. A clinical and pathological survery of 21 patients and their response to treatment. Annals of the Rheumatic Diseases 30: 359–374

Begmann H, Rasletter J 1972 Atlas of clinical haematology, 2nd edn. p 140

Bennett R M 1977 Hematological changes in rheumatoid disease. Clinics in Rheumatic Diseases 3: 433–470

Bennett R M, Holt P J L, Lewis S M 1974 Role of reticuloendothelial system in the anaemia of rheumatoid arthritis. Annals of Rheumatic Diseases 33: 147–152

Bentley D P, Williams P 1974. Serum ferritin concentrations as an index of storage iron in rheumatoid arthritis. Journal of Clinical Pathology 27: 786–788

Bingham J 1961 The macrocytosis of hepatic disease, thin, thick and target macrocytosis. Canadian Medical Association Journal 85: 178–185

Birgegard G, Haoogren R, Kiland A, Strombers A, Venge P, Wide L 1978 Serum ferritin during infection, a longitudinal study. Scandinavian Journal of Haematology 21: 33

Bozzini C E, Kofoed J A, Niotti H F, Alippi R M, Barrionuevo J A 1970 Relationship of red cell mass and energy metabolism to lean body mass in hypophysectomized rats. Journal of Applied Physiology 29: 10–12

Brain M C 1979 Hemolysis in renal disease. In: Hematalogical problems in renal disease, Jepson J H (ed) Addison-Wesley, Menlo Park, California

Budman D R, Steinberg A D 1977 Hematological aspects of systemic lupus erythematosus. Current concepts. Annals of Internal Medicine 86: 220–230

Cartwright G E, Lee G R 1971 The anaemia of chronic disorders. British Journal of Haematology 21: 147–152

Cartwright G E, Wintrobe M N 1952 The anaemia of infection XVIII In: A review in advances in internal medicine Dock W, Snapper (eds), vol V. The Year Book Publishers, p 165–276

Chanarin I 1979 The magaloblastic anaemias, 2nd edn. Blackwell, Oxford

Chaplin H Jr, Mollinson P L 1953 Red cell life span in nephritis and in hepatic cirrhosis. Clinical Science 12: 351–360

Cooksley W G E, Powell L W, Haliday J W 1973 Reticuloendothelial phagocytic function in liver disease and its relation to haemolysis. British Journal of Haematology 25: 147–164

Dacie J V 1967 The haemolytic anaemias, congenital and acquired, 2nd edn, part 3. Churchill

Dass K C, Mucka D M, Sarkar T K, Dash P J Rasting G K 1975 Erythropoiesis and erythropoietin in hypo-and hyper-thyroidism. Journal of Clinics in Endocrinology 81: 1007–1017

Davidson W 1967 Anaemia in the elderly with special reference to iron deficiency. Gerontologia Clinica 9: 293–400

Department of Health and Social Security 1970 First report on nutrition in the elderly. A nutritional survey of the elderly; Reports on public health and medical subjects No 123. London, HMSO

Department of Health and Social Security 1972 Final report on nutrition on the elderly. A nutritional survey of the elderly; Reports on Health and Social subjects. London, HMSO

Dubois E L, Tufanelli D L 1964 Clinical manifestations of systemic lupus erythematous. Computer analysis of 520 cases. Journal of the American Medical Association 190: 104–111

Ellwood P C 1971 Epidemiological aspects of iron deficiency in the elderly. Gerontologia Clinical 13: 2–11

Evans D M D, Pathy M S, Sonerkin N G, Deeble T J 1968 Anaemia in geriatric patients. Gerontologia Clinical 1: 228–241

Felty A R 1924 Chronic arthritis in the adult associated with splenomegaly and leucopaenia. A report of 5 cases of an unusual clinical syndrome. Johns Hopkins Medical Journal 35: 16–22

Fillet G, Cook J D, Finch C A 1974 Storage iron kinetics VIII. A biological model for reticuloendothelial iron transport. Journal of Clinical Investigation 53: 1527–1531

Fisher J W, Gross D M 1977 Hormonal influences on erythropoiesis anterior, pituitary, adrenal corticol, thyroid, growth and other hormones. In: Kidney hormones II: erythropoietin Fisher J W (ed) Academic Press, New York, p 415

Fisher J W, Roh B L, Couch C, Nightingale W O 1964 Influence of cobolt sheep erythropoietin and several hormones on erythropoiesis in bone marrows of isolated prefused hind limbs of dogs. Blood 23: 87–98

Fudenberg H, Wintrope M N 1955 Scleroderma with symptomatic hemolytic anaemia. A case report. Annals of Internal Medicine 3: 210–202

Gaudie R B, Anderson J R, Gray K K, Whyte W G 1966 Auto-antibodies in Addison's disease. Lancet i: 1173–1176

Gordon S, Piliero S H, Landau D 1951 Relation of the adrenal to blood formation in the rat. Endocrinology 49: 497–511

Greenberg P L, Schrier S L 1973 Granulopoiesis in neutropaenic disorders. Blood 41: 753–760

Gupta R C, Robertson W A, Smyth C J 1975. Efficacy of Lithium in rheumatoid arthritis with granulocytopaenia (Felty's syndrome). Arthritis and Rheumatism 18: 179–184

Hardisty R M, Weatherall D J 1983 Blood and its disorders. Oxford, Blackwell

Harvey A N, Shulman L E, Jumelti P A, Conley C L Schoenrach E H 1954 Systemic lupus erythematosus. Review of the literature and clinical analysis of the 138 cases. Medicine (Baltimore) 33: 291–296

Herscshko C, Cook J D, Finch C A 1974 Storage iron kinetics VI. The effect of inflammation on iron exchange in the rat. British Journal of Haematology 28: 67

Hollander C S, Thompson R H, Barrett P V D, Berlin N I 1967 Repair of the anaemia and hyperlipidaemia of the hypothyroid dog. Endocrinology 81: 1007–10117

Holt J M, Wright R 1967 Anaemia due to blood loss from telangiectases of sclerodenma. British Medical Journal iii: 537–540

Horton L, Coburn R J, England J M, Himsworth R L 1976 The haematology of hypothyroidism. Quarterly Journal of Medicine (New Series) 45: 101–106

Irvine W J, Davies S H, Tietelbaum S, Delamore I W, Wynn Williams A 1965 The clinical and pathological significance of gastric parietal cell antibody. Annals of the New York Academy of Science, 242 Part II: 657–691

Kilpatrick G S 1961 Prevalence of anaemia in the general population. British Medical Journal ii: 1736–1738

Kimber C, Deller D J, Ibotttson R N, Lander H 1965 The mechanism of anaemia in chronic liver disease. Quarterly Journal of Medicine (N.S.) 34: 33–64

Lipshitz D A, Cook J D, Finch C A 1974 A clinical evaluation of serum ferritin. New England Journal of Medicine 290: 1213–1218

MacLennon W J, Andrews G R, MacLoud C, Caird F I 1973 Anaemia in the elderly. Quarterly Journal of Medicine 42: 1–13

Milne J S, Williamson J 1972 Haemoglobin, haematocrit reading, leucocyte count and blood grouping in a random sample of older people. Geriatrics 27: 118–126

Morgan R H 1967 Anaemia in elderly housebound patients. British Medical Journal iv: 171

Muldowney F P, Crooks J, Wayne E J 1957 The total red cell mass thyrotoxicosis and myxoedema. Clinical Science 16: 309–314

Nunally R M, Levine I 1961 Macronormoblastic hyperplasia of the bone marrow in hepatic sclerosis. American Journal of Medicine 30: 972-976

Owen E T, Lawson A A H 1966 Nature of anaemia in rheumatoid arthritis vi. Metabolism of endogenous iron. Annals of Rheumatic Diseases 25: 547–552

Peschle C, Marmount A M, Marone G, Genovese A, Sasso G F, Konderelli M 1975 The cellular basis for the defect in haemopoiesis in flexed tailed mice iii. Restriction of the defect to erthropoietic progenitors capable of transit colony formation in vitro. British Journal of Haematology 30: 411–417

Polley H F, Slocumb C H 1947 Rheumatoid Spondylitis. A study of 1035 cases. Annals of Rhumatic Diseases 6: 95–105

Richmond J, Roy L M H, Gardner D L, Alexander W R M, Daffy J J 1958.. Nature of anaemia in rheumatoid arthritis IV. Effects of intravenous administration and saccarated oxide of iron. Annals of Rhematic Diseases 17: 406–415

Sienknicht C W, Vrowitz M B, Pruzanski W, Stein H B 1977 Felty's syndrome. Clinical and serological analysis of 34 cases. Annals of Rheumatic Diseases 36: 500–505

Sheehan H L 1939 Simmons disease due to post partum necrosis of the anterior pituitary. Quarterly Journal of Medicine 8: 277–309

Summers E K 1952 The anaemia of hypopituitarism. British Medical Journal i: 787–790

Torrence J D, Charlton R W, Simon M O, Lynch S R, Bothwell T H 1978 The mechanism of endotoxin-induced hypoferraemia. Scandinavian Journal of Haematology 21: 403–410

Wallner S F, Kurnick J E, Vautrin R M, White J M J, Chapman R G, Ward H B 1977 Levels of erythropoietin in patients with the anaemias of chronic disease and liver failure. American Journal of Hematology 3: 37

Ward H P, Gordon P, Pickett J C 1969 Serum levels of erythropoietin in rheumatoid arthritis. Journal of Laboratory and Clinical Medicine 74: 93–97

Wardrop C, Hutchinson H E 1969 Red cell shape in hypothyroidism Lancet ii: 1243–1245

Walsh J R Frederickson M 1977 Serum ferritin. The erythrocyte protoporphyrin and urinary iron excretion in patients with iron disorders. American Journal of the Medical Sciences 273: 293–300

Werre J M, Helleman P W, Verloop M C, De Gier J 1970 Causes of macroplasia of erythrocyte in diseases of the liver and biliary tract with special reference to leptocytosis. British Journal of Haematology 19: 223–235

W.H.O. 1968. Nutritional anaemias. Report of a WHO scientific group. WHO Technical Report Series No 405. Geneva

Williams P, Cavill I, Kanakakorn K 1974 Iron kinetics and the anaemia of rheumatoid arthritis. Rheumatology and Rehabilitation 13: 17–20

Wintrobe M N 1936 The relation of disease of the liver to anaemia, type of anaemia to histopathological changes in liver, spleen and bone marrow. Archives of Internal Medicine vol: 289–306

Zucker S, Lysik R N, Freidman S 1976 Diminished bone marrow responsiveness to erythropoietin in myelophthistic anaemia. Cancer 37: 1308–1312

Cytopenias due to bone marrow failure; hypersplenism

INTRODUCTION

Blood cytopenia, involving one or more of the main haemopoietic cell lines, is a relatively common finding in the elderly patient, and can be due to a wide variety of causes, both intrinsic and extrinsic to the marrow (Table 6.1). A description of cytopenias due to peripheral immunological destruction of blood cells in dealt will in Chapter 15. It must be recognised, however, that

Table 6.1 The causes of pancytopenia in the elderly

Bone marrow infiltrations
  Acute leukaemia
  Oligoblastic leukaemia and preleukaemia ('myelodysplastic syndromes')
  Carcinomatosis
  Myeloma, lymphoma*, hairy-cell leukaemia*
  Myelofibrosis, osteomyelosclerosis, myeloid metaplasia

Hypersplenism
  Portal hypertension, splenic vein thrombosis etc (congestive splenomegaly)
  Felty's syndrome*
  Lymphoma*, leukaemia
  Chronic infections: malaria, kalaazar, tuberculosis, sarcoidosis
  Tropical and non-tropical idiopathic splenomegaly; 'primary splenic pancytopenia'

Immune cytopenias*
  Systemic lupus erythematosus, diffuse eosinophilic fasciitis etc.
  Drug reactions

Bone marrow aplasias and dysplasias
  Aplastic anaemia
  Paroxysmal nocturnal haemoglobinuria
  Refractory dyserythropoietic anaemias

Metabolic, endocrine and infective causes
  Megaloblastic anaemia (B_{12} and folate deficiency)
  Malnutrition, alcoholism
  Septicaemia (often with disseminated intravascular coagulation)
  Miliary tuberculosis, brucellosis, sarcoidosis
  Hypopituitarism, hypothyroidism

*Some diseases may produce pancytopenia by more than one mechanism: for example in Felty's syndrome, in addition to hypersplenism, there may be humoral and/or lymphocytotoxic auto-antibodies directed against specific blood cells. Reduced marrow production of granulocytes has also been demonstrated in this disorder. Lymphomata infilitrate the marrow, and may also cause secondary hypersplenism.

processes which produce cytopenia mainly by destruction of cells in the blood may also sometimes attack haemopoietic precursor cells in the marrow.

BONE MARROW FAILURE

Today this term is often used loosely to describe an intrinsic functional disturbance of the marrow, irrespective of its cellularity, i.e. including both quantities and qualitative abnormalities. Strictly speaking, such reversible causes as megaloblastic anaemia should be included, and they certainly enter into the differential diagnosis of pancytopenia. The term 'aplastic anaemia' (AA) is best reserved for cases in which there is simple fatty atrophy of the haemopoietic tissue, not associated with marrow infiltration or fibrosis (although, in the elderly, cases in the latter category are much more numerous).

However, pancytopenia due to chronic marrow failure may also be associated with a morphologically cellular or hypercellular marrow ('dysplastic anaemia') and these cases are especially likely to be encountered in the elderly. Even in pancytopenic patients with predominantly hypocellular marrows, it is ofen possible to identify islands of active haemopoiesis ('hot pockets'), and some clinicians have urged that there is no clear cut division between such cases and pancytopenic patients with hyperplastic marrows. However, the natural history of the latter group is different from those with true aplasia: for example, eventual termination in leukaemia is more likely. Moreover, drug-induced marrow failure is characteristically associated with hypocellularity rather than hypercellularity.

APLASTIC ANAEMIA

The incidence of AA is one of the order of 6–13 per million per year in Europe, but is significantly higher in Asia and South America (Bottiger, 1979; Aoki et al, 1980). An incidence of 0.9–2.4/1000 hospital admissions was reported from one Paris clinic in the 1960s (Bernard & Najean, 1965), but the disease seems slowly to be increasing in frequency. As defined above, this is a haematological syndrome due to a number of different causes, all having in common a quantitative defect in haemopoietic stem cells, of which the cardinal morphological sequalae are blood pancytopenia and fatty atrophy of marrow tissue. Functional evidence of a hypoproliferative marrow is provided, in most cases, by reticulocytopenia, a prolonged plasma iron clearance time and reduced incorporation of iron into red cells.

In pathophysiological terms, aplastic anaemia is a group of diseases rather than a single entity. Clinical and experimental evidence suggests that there is a drastic reduction in the normal stem cell population in the marrow, leading to deficiencies in the maturing ('transit') cell population. Bone marrow culture shows that the ability of the patient's marrow to produce granulocytic and erythroid colonies (CFU-GM and BFU-E) is much reduced (Chapter 2).

However, evidence from animal experiments suggests that mice can survive for long periods with stem cell populations reduced to 1 per cent of the normal level (Morley et al, 1975). It is possible that, in some cases, there is also a disturbance in the proliferative behaviour of the stem cell or its earliest descendants, or in maturation (Schofield, 1979). There is certainly morphological evidence of abnormal residual haemopoiesis in the marrows of aplastic patients.

Another possibility is that the specialised stromal environment ('haemopoietic inductive environment') is damaged and is unable to support normal haemopoiesis. X-irradiation is known to injure the marrow sinusoidal vasculature as well as stem cells; it has been postulated that auto-immune processes might produce the same effects. The fact that bone marrow transplantation cures a high proportion of younger patients with AA does not necessarily prove that the basic lesion is simply a deficiency of stem cells, since vascular and other stromal cells such as macrophages and fat cells are transferred with the graft.

It should be noted that, theoretically, an aetiological agent acting at a later stage than the stem cell could produce AA if it were to damage all the major committed cell lines simultaneously. However, such an agent would have to act continuously, since normal stem cells would make good the deficiency in the short term. In practice, damage to the marrow's transit compartment is more likely to be associated with an isolated cytopenia such as red cell aplasia.

Aetiology

The aetiology of AA is summarised in Table 6.2. Although the precise cellular mechanisms in AA are not completely understood, epidemiological studies suggest that many cases in the adult are associated with exposure to environmental agents. Earlier reports of 50 per cent cases of AA as 'idiopathic' may be an overestimate. Congenital disorders of the bone marrow (e.g. Fanconi's anaemia) are recognised, and may not present clinically until early adult life, but these account for only a small proportion of the total. Moreover there is little evidence that gradual senescence of undamaged

Table 6.2   Aetiology of aplastic anaemia (after Benestad, 1974)

I Ionising radiation Cytotoxic chemicals	} dose-dependent

II Chemicals, drugs
  Conditional
  Immunological
	} largely dose-independent

III Viral cytotoxicity
  Direct
  Immunological	

IV Auto-immune cytotoxicity	
V Hereditary defect	

haemopoietic cells ('stem cell exhaustion') accounts for aplastic anaemia. AA is relatively more common in the elderly, however; in one study from Europe, 80 per cent of the cases diagnosed were over the age of 50. (Bottiger, 1979), possibly reflecting more frequent exposure to drugs at this age. The age distribution in the Far East does not seem to follow this pattern.

There are broadly three ways in which drugs and chemicals might produce marrow damage: a dose-related effect, an idiosyncratic effect and provocation of an abnormal immunological response (hypersensitivity). The last two mechanisms are likely to be genetically determined. Idiosyncratic (or 'conditional') mechanisms imply that either the target cells or drug metabolism are abnormal: bone marrow cells are thus rendered unusually sensitive to the toxin. Although such conditional reactions are unexpected, increasing doses will often give more marked effects. In immunological reactions, on the other hand, dose and time relationships are erratic: marrow damage usually appears after second or later exposure to the drug (Benestad, 1979).

AA due to physical and chemical agents

Certain physical and chemical agents will produce aplastic anaemia in all individuals if used in sufficiently high doses: X-irradiation and alkylating agents, such as the nitrogen mustards, are good examples. A dose-related myelotoxic effect can also be demonstrated with benzene in animals. In humans, heavy exposure to benzene produces a variety of abnormal marrow and blood pictures, often culminating in aplasia, or even leukaemia, but clinical evidence suggest that some individuals react idiosyncratically to small doses of benzenne, and possibly other organic solvents, especially if exposure is repeated (Saita, 1973). These predictable, largely dose-related effects of known myelosuppressive agents account for only a few cases of chronic aplastic anaemia, since, except after massive exposure, sufficient stem cells survive to ensure recovery of apparently normal haemopoiesis after a period of days or a few weeks. However, such individuals may be unusually susceptible to further doses of X-irradiation or cytotoxic drugs, and this is particularly true of the elderly. There is also an increased risk of late leukaemia after such episodes.

AA due to idiosyncratic responses to drugs

Many cases of AA encountered in clinical practice today are, unfortunately, examples of iatrogenic disease. Bone marrow damage here represents an unusual response to a drug which, in the vast majority, is innocuous or only very slightly myelosuppressive. A good example is chloramphenicol, which produces a reversible reticulocytopenia and toxic changes in erythroblasts in most individuals, but devastating aplastic anaemia in a tiny minority. Examples of this type of reaction are unpredictable and may occur after exposure to only small amounts of the drug: for instance, cases have been described after the use of chloramphenicol eye-drops (Fraunfelden et al, 1982), The first effect is a result of temporary inhibition of protein synthesis by mitochondria, analogous to the action of the antibiotic on bacteria. The second, however, represents an irreversible change in the haemopoietic stem cell, leading to defective replication and maturation (Yunis, 1973). Many other commonly used drugs are believed, occasionally, to produce AA, but the majority of cases seem to be associated with a relatively small group of substances.

Obviously, the importance of a particular drug as a cause of AA depends not only on the incidence of bone marrow damage following its use (estimated at 1:30 000 in the case of chloramphenicol and as rarely as 1:100 000 with butazones) but also on the frequency with which that drug is used within the community. For example, because of its potentially dangerous side-effect, chloramphenicol is now avoided when alternative antibiotics are available. This drug, conspicuous in earlier lists of drugs causing AA, did not appear in a recent study from Sweden (Arneborn & Palmblad, 1982). These workers found that sulphonamides, antithyroid drugs and antihistaminics were most frequently encountered in cases of marrow depression.

The position occupied by sulphonamides in this list seems to relate to their widespread use in the community rather than to a particularly high risk in the individual patient. It must not be forgotten that sulphonamides may be present in 'composite' preparations; for example, several cases of fatal agranulocytosis have recently been described after use of proprietary malarial prophylactics containing sulphonamides (Arneborn & Palmblad, 1982). In our own clinic, gold, phenylbutazone and, rarely, phneytoins are also encountered as apparent causes of chronic marrow depression.

AA due to infective agents

AA is an occasional complication of infections such as tuberculosis, atypical mycobacteria, dengue, brucellosis and viral hepatitis; recently infection with the papova virus has been linked to transient erythroid depression in children. There are rare reports of aplasia following other common virus infections, including infections mononucleosis, rubella, mumps and even influenza (Curzon et al, 1983). A very small number of cases in which aplasia was linked to fungal or parasitic infections have been described (Aymard et al, 1980). In general the association of marrow aplasia with bacterial infections (apart from *M. tuberculosis*) is ill-defined; the best-documented clinical association with infection is that involving viral hepatitis. Such studies as have been done suggest that type A hepatitis is more likely to be incriminated than type B.

Various clinical forms of acute viral hepatitis have been noted in association with marrow hypoplasia, ranging from subclinical cases to severe disease with subacute hepatic necrosis (Camitta, 1979; Aymard et al, 1980). Some studies have shown that in many cases of acute AA there is biochemical evidence of disturbance of liver function, even when no clear history of hepatitis is obtained. Possibly such damage impairs metabolism and detox-ification of drugs or other chemicals and increases the myelotoxic effect of these substances. However, impaired liver function per se does not seem to predispose to bone marrow depression, since AA is not increased in patients with chronic liver failure. Virus infection may produce blood deficiencies by a direct cytotoxic effect on marrow cells, but chronic hypoplasia is more likely to follow an auto-immune process leading to cell destruction.

AA as an auto-immune disease

There is currently much interest in the immunological abnormalities found in some cases of AA, and their possible relationship to its pathoegenesis. AA is, however, rarely found in the setting of well-defined auto immune syndromes such as systemic lupus erythematosus and Sjogren's syndrome (although it has been described as a complication of diffuse eosinophilic fasciitis) (Hoff-man et al, 1979); on the other hand, isolated cytopenias due to immune destruction are relatively common in such patients (Cline & Golde, 1978).

Both humoral and cell-mediated inhibitors of haemopoietic cells have been described in AA, though in some cases these seem to represent allantibodies (due to blood transfusion) rather than auto-antibodies. Nevertheless, there is evidence that T-lymphocytes derived from the marrows, and even occasional-ly the blood, of untreated aplastic patients can inhibit haemopoiesis in healthy marrows (Ascensao et al, 1976). Some of the most compelling evi-dence favouring an immunological basis for some cases of AA derives from the field of bone marrow transplantation. Thus, intensive immunosuppres-sive therapy, given to prepare the patient for a marrow graft, has occasionally resulted in regrowth of the patient's own marrow. In the case of identical twin transplants, when, theoretically, no immunosuppressive conditioning should be required, successful engraftment has been achieved without such therapy in only some 50 per cent of the reported cases. The inference is that an abnormal immunological process must be abrogated before normal haemopoiesis can occur. A disturbance in the ratio of suppressor to 'helper' lymphocytes has been postulated. As explained above, such processes might be triggered by drug exposure or virus infection. Whether this type of AA is more common in the elderly, when the incidence of other types of auto-immune disease is increased, is unknown. However, chronic red cell aplasia, one haematological syndrome in which marrow cells are known to be injured by auto-antibodies, is usually found in older patients. The reader is referred to the excellent account of this subject by Camitta et al, 1982.

Clinical picture

The onset of AA can be dramatic and rapidly fatal, or insidious; the latter picture is more likely to be encountered in the elderly. Symptoms in a new case of AA relate, usually, to a haemorrhagic tendency or to the effects of chronic anaemia, or a combination of the two. In one series, evidence of bleeding, such as skin purpura, or retinal haemorrhages, was found in 84 per cent of newly diagnosed cases (Williams et al, 1973). Infection is seldom the presenting episode in AA, though it may dominate the picture later. Since the main leucocyte deficiency is of granulocytes, with relatively normal numbers of T-and B-lymphocytes, at least in the early stages, viral infections are less common than bacterial.

Physical examination reveals, usually, only evidence of anaemia and a haemorrhagic tendency. Lymphadenopathy is almost never found except in response to local infection. Although some clinical studies suggest that slight splenomegaly is occasionally found in AA, its presence should arouse suspicion of an underlying disorder such as lymphoma or leukaemia.

Blood and bone marrow examination

AA is by definition a pancytopenic disorder. Most patients have pancytopenia at diagnosis, though the major cell lines are often affected asymmetrically. Over 80 per cent of patients have haemoglobin levels of below 12 g/dl, total granulocyte counts of less than $1500/\mu l$ and platelet counts of less than $100\,000/\mu l$ at diagnosis. A minority do not show this diagnostic triad at presentation, but the counts usually fall into an abnormally low range within two months (Heimpel, 1979). Normal granulocyte counts at diagnosis are seen more frequently than normal haemoglobin levels or platelet counts. Lymphocyte counts are often normal, but there is evidence that B-lymphocyte populations decline during chronic aplasia; hypogammaglobulinaemia may also occur (Mir et al 1977).

The absolute reticulocyte count (of greater value than the conventional reticulocyte count) is an important adjunct to assessment of bone marrow function. Two-thirds of patients have absolute reticulocyte counts below $25\,000/\mu l$. A few patients with AA do show a significant reticulocytosis, but this is usually inappropriately low when the level of haemoglobin is taken into account. Persistent evidence of haemolysis should prompt tests for paroxysmal nocturnal haemoglobinuria. The level of the reticulocyte count is of some prognostic importance.

Attempts at marrow aspiration are often unsuccessful or yield only fatty particles. Trephine biopsy is essential in a case of suspected AA, both to prove hypocellularity and to exclude infiltrative or fibrotic disorders. Sometimes islands of active haemopoiesis are seen, and a second trephine from another site is required to show that the marrow is predominantly hypocellular. Occasionally bone marrow scanning with Indlium III or ^{52}Fe are required to assess total cellularity. It should not be forgotten that the marrow becomes less cellular in old age.

Clinical course of the disease

AA is not an inexorably progressive disease like leukaemia or lymphoma. The clinical and haematological features seem, often, to result from a single episode of damage to the marrow. Thee is often a latent period of weeks between exposure to a putative toxic agent and clinical onset of marrow failure (Gordon-Smith, 1979a). The subsequent course (provided the patient is not re-exposed to the myelotoxin) depends on the number of residual stem cells and their proliferative capacity. In the short term, bone marrow function can be further depressed by infection, an inflammatory disorder, uraemia, nutritional deficiency or alcoholism. Clinical remissions, and even apparent cures, occur as a result of treatment, or occasionally spontaneously.

Nevertheless, the prognosis in a newly diagnosed case is serious. The overall mortality is 70 per cent and even worse for patients presenting with profound pancytopenia (granulocyte count less than $500/\mu l$, platelet count less than $20\,000/\mu l$ and corrected reticulocyte count less than 1 per cent); these bad-risk patients are further defined as having fewer than 30 per cent 'non-myeloid' cells in the marrow (Camitta et al, 1979). Hepatitis-related AA is also associated with a very poor prognosis. Few of these patients survive more than a year. There is some evidence from analysis of survival curves of two classes of aplastic anaemia of different severity, but there are no published data on the effect of age on survival using therapies other than bone marrow transplantation. Death is usually due to infection or haemorrhage, or a combination of the two; evolution into paroxysmal nocturnal haemoglobinuria, and rarely myeloblastic leukaemia, are recognised sequelae. Both these diseases are believed to occur as a result of abnormal clones of haemopoietic cells erupting from the damaged marrow. They are discussed elsewhere in this book.

Differential diagnosis

AA is an uncommon disorder, and distinction from other, commoner, causes of pancytopenia is not always easy (Table 6.3). The anaemia in AA is normochromic and normocytic, with, occasionally, slight macrocytosis. The presence of significant aniso- and poikilocytosis, of nucleated red cells or primitive granulocytic cells (leuco-erythroblastic picture), or megaplatelets should alert the physician to an alternative diagnosis. An adequate bone marrow trephine biopsy will usually help to exclude marrow infiltrative disorders or fibrosis.

Clinically, aplastic anaemia is often associated with a paucity of clinical signs, and the presence of splenomegaly or lymphadenopathy should suggest some other diagnosis. The other diseases listed in Table 6.1 as causes of pancytopenia can usually be excluded on clinical grounds, but tuberculosis can sometimes cause marrow hypoplasia (as well as other unusual blood

Table 6.3   The differential diagnosis of aplastic anaemia (Heimpel, 1970)

Blood picture	Disease	Discriminating features
Pancytopenia	Acute leukaemia	Usually some atypical cells in blood
	Severe vitamin B_{12} or	$MCV > 110\ \mu l$
	folic acid deficiency	$MCH > 40$ pg
		Bone marrow diagnostic Low folic acid or
		vitamin B_{12} plasma levels
	Hypersplenism	Large spleen; reticulocytosis
		Bone marrow hypercellular
	Aplasia induced by	History
	cytostatics	Early haemopoietic regeneration
	Bone marrow	Erythroblasts and immature granulocytes in
	metastases	blood
		Bone marrow: fibrosis, neoplastic infiltration
Anaemia and	Evans' syndrome	Marked reticulocytosis, positive
thrombocytopenia	(haemolytic anaemia)	antiglobulin-test.
		Megaplatelets
	Bleeding from ITP	Reticulocytosis
		Megaplatelets
		Low plasma iron
Anaemia and	Acute	Platelets normal to high; very low neutrophil
leucopenia	agranulocytosis	count
		Bone marrow: absence or maturation arrest of
		granulocytes
	Preleukaemia	Bone marrow: hyperplastic, often Pelger-cells,
		micromegakaryocytes

pictures) without producing the more conventional clinical signs of miliary tuberculosis. Marrow fibrosis is often present even if not granulomata are visible on biopsy; the ESR is usually very high, and slight to moderate splenomegaly may be found, or appear later.

Another difficult problem is the distinction of AA from certain forms of myeloblastic leukaemia and potentially preleukaemic marrow dysplasias, which may present with marrow hypoplasia and pancytopenia, and are fairly common in the elderly. Again, careful examination of the blood and marrow will usually reveal small numbers of atypical myeloid cells, or abnormal megakaryocytes ('micromegakaryocytes') on biopsy. In cases of great difficulty, chromsome analysis or studies of the proliferative pattern of granulocytic colonies and 'clusters' may provide evidence of an underlying leukaemia. In practice, the distinction between the two conditions is not always helpful therapeutically; patients with an underlying oligoblastic leukaemia may occasionally benefit from chemotherapy (see Chapter), but ATG therapy is unlikely to help.

Management of AA

This has been reviewed by Lewis & Gordon-Smith (1982) and Gordon-Smith (1979b). Here points particularly relevant to treatment of the older patient are emphasised.

It is important to discover any known aetiological agent to which the patient had been exposed. Idiopathic disease seems to be more common in older subjects; however, this may reflect difficulty in identifying a specific substance as toxic when it is widely used and the risk of aplasia is very small. Identification requires careful history-taking; elderly patients are especially likely to have been exposed to more than one potentially myelotoxic drugs, but their memory may be poor, or they may not recall the name of the drug! It is wise to ask a relative to bring in for inspection all tablets and medications which the patient has taken within six months of the onset of marrow failure. The physician must enquire about hobbies, (e.g. gardening) which might be associated with exposure to chemical agents. Obviously, in the case of multiple drug exposure it may be impossible to decide which has caused marrow damage, but any drugs not essential to life should be stopped.

If a high-risk drug is identified (e.g. chloramphenicol, sulphonamides, carbimazole), it should not be used again. If gold is suspected, it should be removed from the body using a chelating agent. Occasionally, marrow hypoplasia may result from the disease under treatment and not the drug itself. Bone marrow transplantation, the treatment of choice in severe AA, is not at present feasible in elderly patients. Apart from the difficulties in recruiting suitable, HLA- compatible donors amongst their siblings, the risk of graft-verus-host disease is much increased in patients over the age of 40.

All patients with hypoplastic anaemia must be given advice about changes in lifestyle designed to reduce the risk of infection, and this is particularly true of older patients in whom, for example, infections following minor skin abrasions are often troublesome, and may rapidly evolve into life-threatening emergencies. All patients with chronic AA should be kept out of hospital as much as possible to minimise the risk of infection.

Supportive therapy

Blood transfusions are given only as frequently as required to relieve symptoms and signs related to cardiovascular insufficiency; it is a mistake to aim at maintaining the haemoglobin at an arbitrary level. Even in old age, the body can adapt to a surprisingly low packed-cell volume (PCV). In a given patient, the pattern of transfusion requirement is often remarkably stable. Sudden deviation form the pattern may indicate blood loss, infection or, conversely, an improvement in bone marrow function. Frozen packed cells are recommended, as there is then less risk of sensitisation or transmission of virus infection.

Profound thrombocytopenia requires support with platelet infusions, but again it is wise to formulate a strategy for their use in the light of availability and the patient's clinical state. Serious bleeding rarely occurs with platelet counts of over 30 000/μl. Skin purpura alone is not an indication for platelet support, unless associated with a sudden fall in the platelet count, but fresh retinal haemorrhages, or bleeding from mucous surfaces usually are. The onset of infection is often associated with a profound fall in a previously stable platelet count, and is usually an indication for platelet support. The difficulties which arise in connection with development of platelet-specific and/or HLA antibodies are discussed in Chapter 9.

Again, most haematologists do not recommend prophylactic antibiotics for patients with chronic neutropenic states in the absence of fever, though this policy might be modified for an elderly person with some persistent focus of infection such as bronchiectasis of pyelonephritis. Infections demand immediate identification of the organism involved and institution of appropriate antibiotic therapy which, in the case of a gram-negative organism, will usually require intravenous therapy with a combination of drugs, such as gentamycin and cephaloridine, depending on the bacteriologist's report on sensitivities. Granulocyte infusions from a random or HLA-compatible donor may be necessary in severe infection not responding to appropriate antibiotics, and may be combined with isolation in a sterile environment, but their efficacy in prolonging life in chronic hypoplastic marrow disorders is not yet fully documented.

Androgen therapy

Androgenic steroids were introduced for the treatment of AA in children in the early 1960s, and were later used for adult patients (Gardner, 1978). There is still controversy as to their efficacy. Androgens stimulate the production of erythropoietin (already high in aplasia), and probably increase the replication rate of the erythropoietin-sensitive stem cell. In normal individuals, androgens increase the PCV, and this is also observed in some patients with aplastic anaemia and dysplastic marrow disorders. However, effects on the platelet and granulocyte counts are often less impressive, and some studies have suggested that survival is not improved by the use of androgens. An important minority, nevertheless, show partial or complete dependency on androgen therapy, and oxymethalone should probably be tried for a period of up to three months in any patient requiring blood transfusions. The usual dose of 200–300 mg/day may be modified in the light of side-effects, such as cholestatic jaundice, fluid retention, virilism and psychic changes which may be particularly troublesome in the elderly. Good results were observed in at least one study (Besa et al, 1977) using the non-virilising metabolite of testosterore, aetiocholanolone. Corticosteroids at continuous low dosage seem to be of no value in aplastic anaemia, but have been advocated as a form of immunosuppressive therapy in severe disease given at high dosage (see next section).

Treatment with antithymocyte globulin (ATG)

The evidence, cited above, of abnormal immunological processes at work in AA have prompted attempts to treat the disease with immunosuppressive drugs. Cytotoxic drugs, such as cyclophosphamide, have occasionally been tried, but the additional myelosuppression produced can be dangerous. There have been several trials using equine antithymoyocyte globulin, which does not cause marrow suppression, though it often produces thrombocytopenia. Results have differed reather widely: some workers claim that this therapy is as good as, if not superior, to allogeneic transplantation in younger individuals (Speck et al, 1981). Others have recorded less impressive results. Difficulties include the lack of standardisation and specificity of the final product. Nevertheless, this therapy is probably worth a trial fairly early in the natural history of the disease; beneficial effects are rarely seen in long-established cases.

The usual procedure is to infuse the ATG at a dose of 10–40 mg/kg in a period of up to two hours, after first ascertaining that the patient is not sensitive to the carrier horse protein by intradermal testing, or instillation into the conjunctival sac. Infusions are repeated for up to five days. (Other species of ATG, such as rabbit, are also available). Some authorities recommend larger doses than this, but side-effects are common. Apart from anaphylactic reactions (not always predicted by skin testing!), fever, skin rashes, arthralgia, headache, abdominal pain, vomiting and haemorrhage due to excerbation of thrombocytopenia are troublesome and sometimes dangerous. It is prudent to give platelet support to patients who already have profound thrombocytopenia. There is some evidence that ATG is most likely to be effective in patients who are also receiving androgens. Improvement, when it occurs, is gradual and may not be observed for several weeks; often a reduction in transfusion requirements is the first obvious sign, but the platelet and granulocyte counts may also respond.

Although low-dose corticosteroids are of little value in AA, some workers have recorded improvement after short courses of very high-dose schedules of methylprednisolone, and have postulated a similar abrogation of an abnormal immune process (Bacigalupo et al, 1981). This therapy has obvious dangers in the elderly.

ISOLATED CYTOPENIAS

AA is a disease of the pluripotent haemopoietic stem cell but damage to a more mature cell compartment will characteristically produce a mono- or bicytopenia. Here the stem cell compartment is assumed to be intact, and the observed cell deficiency is due to hypoplasia or defective maturtion of the specific cell-line ('ineffective' myelopoiesis) or to peripheral consumption or destruction of the cells as fast as they are formed.

RED CELL APLASIA

This is less common than AA, but in its chronic form occurs particularly in the elderly. An aetiological classification of the chronic disease is shown in

Table 6.4   Clinical classification of chronic red cell aplasia

---

Idiopathic
    presumed auto-immune pathogenesis*
    pathogenesis obscure

Associated with:
    thymic tumour*
    auto-immune disease* e.g. SLE, AIHA
    thyroiditis etc.
    carcinoma*, lymphomata*, myeloma
    drugs?
    pre-leukaemic dysplasias
    severe nutritional deficiency

---

*Humoral auto-antibodies to erythroid cells or erythropoietin demonstrated in some cases. Lymphocytotoxic antibodies have also been identified in a few cases. Note that chronic renal failure, though associated with depression of haemopoiesis, rarely leads to morphological erythroid aplasia

Table 6.4. The patient presents with a refractory normochromic anaemia, without the other signs of AA, such as haemorrhage. Slight splenomegaly may be present. In secondary forms of the disease there may be signs of a connective tissue disorder, or of lymphoma, etc. Thymoma is a well-documented association, especially in women. The blood picture is characterised by profound reticulocytopenia without, in a typical case, any disturbance of granulopoiesis or thrombopoiesis. The marrow, often of normal cellularity, shows either a complete absence of erythroblasts or a few pro-erythroblasts. There may be a marrow lymphocytosis. Immunological investigation may show either hypo- or hypergammaglobulinaemia; occasionally the red cell antiglobulin test is positive, or a paraprotein may be present (Geary, 1979; Sieff, 1983).

Pathogenesis

Acute, self-limiting red cell aplasia is mainly a syndrome of children and young adults and is thought to be due to infection with a parvovirus. The syndrome seen in adults over the age of 50 is often of slow onset and tends to be chronic, although spontaneous remissions to occur. Some cases represent a clonal disorder following mutation of the haemopoietic stem cell, and, in this group, myeloblastic leukaemia may evolve after a period of months or years. Here, although the main deficiency is of red cells, examination of the blood and marrow often shows dysplastic features in granulocytes and mega-karyocytes, and other cytopenias may appear later.

Chromosome abnormalities provide further evidence that a preleukaemic disorder is present. This form of the disease does not undergo spontaneous remission. The other major group of chronic cases represent the results of auto-immune damage to the erythroid cell line. Experimental evidence provides support for antibody or immune complex mediated suppression of erythropoiesis in some cases (Krantz, 1974). Sometimes, erthroblasts are the target for an IgG inhibitor which binds to the cells; in a few erythropoietin itself is the antigen.

Immune suppression of haemopoiesis by lymphocyte-mediated mechanisms have been described. These patients may show other clinical or serological evidence of auto-immunity, such as a positive DCT, or antibodies to smooth muscle. The syndrome may also occur within the clinical context of a lymphoproliferative disease such as chronic lymphatic leukaemia, non-Hodgkin lymphoma or myeloma. The relationship with thymoma, described many years ago, remains obscure; about 50 per cent of the published reports of red cell aplasia have also had thymoma. The most likely explanation is that both tumour and anaemia represent epiphenonemena of a chronic immunological disturbance; the thymic tumour usually precedes the onset of red cell aplasia, and remission of the anaemia may follow its surgical removal.

Management

As with other cytopenias, any environmental agent to which the patient has recently been exposed is identified and removed if possible. A number of drugs have been incriminated as causes of red cell aplasia, including many of those causing AA. If there is circumstantial clinical or serological evidence of an auto-immune disease, immunosuppressive therapy is worth a trial. A thymoma should be removed surgically if possible, as remission occurs in about 30 per cent of cases, and there is some evidence that immunosuppressive therapy is more likely to be effective after thymectomy. Androgens have occasionally been reported to be of value, and, interestingly, once remission has occurred, maintenance therapy may not be required.

Various forms of immunosuppressive therapy have been used. A few patients respond to corticosteroids, but usually cytotoxic drugs such as cyclophosphamide (150 mg/24th) or antimetabolites such as azathioprine (100 mg/24th) are required. Inevitably some myelosuppression will occur; in a few cases antilymphocyte globulin has produced remission, either alone or following previous chemotherapy. There are anecdotal reports of remission following plasmaphoresis (Messner et al, 1981), and occasionally splenectomy is effective.

NEUTROPENIA

Neutropenia is defined as a total neutrophil count of less than $1500/\mu l$. The term 'agranulocytosis' is often used with a clinical connotation to denote a profound neutropenia of explosive onset. Like pancytopenia it has many causes, only some of which represent intrinsic marrow disease. Neutropenia can result from reduced marrow production (either due to hypoplasia of the granulocyte cell line, or to ineffective granulopoiesis) or to accelerated removal of cells from the blood. The latter can in turn be due to immunological or non-immune processes. As with red cell aplasia, some cases of chronic neutropenia seem to be due to abnormal T-lymphocyte function (Bagby et al, 1983). Virus infections are frequently associated with neutropenia and transient thrombocytopenia; less frequently, bacteria and rickettsial infections.

Reduced granulopoiesis is a feature of chronic bone marrow hypoplasia, but it can also occur as a solitary cytopenia in bone marrow infiltrative conditions, and after the use of cytotoxic drugs. Marrow failure thus results in reduced production of granulocytes, while the body's storage and marginal granulocyte pools (in blood vessels and spleen) are also depleted. In such cases neutrophil survival is normal, though occasional immature cells may appear in the blood. Production of granulocytes may be reduced in certain constitutional and acquired disorders which may only be diagnosed later in life. These syndromes include cyclical neutropenia and so-called benign familial neutropenia, chronic hypoplastic neutropenia and chronic idiopathic neutropenia.

A neutropenic syndrome seen especially frequently in West Indian negroes appears to be due to abnormal sequestration of granulocytes in the storage pools rather than reduced production. This 'pseudoneutropenia' is not associated with a decrease in the total body granulocyte mass, and patients seem able to amount a neutrophilic leucocytosis to infection. Many of these syndromes are associated with relatively little morbidity (Wintrobe, 1981).

Drug-induced neutropenia

As is the case with red cell aplasia, drugs which cause aplasia are also incriminated as causes of neutropenia. It is not clear why the same drug should produce pancytopenia in one individual and an isolated cytopenia in another. In addition to cytotoxic and antimetabolic drugs, and drugs which produce unheralded marrow damage, a separate group has been identified as a frequent cause of neutropenia. This is exemplified by phenothiazine, which was found to cause neutropenia quite frequently in psychiatric hospitals (Pisciotta, 1973). The drug impairs DNA synthesis in only a proportion of individuals, but the severity of the neutropenia is related to total dose.

Other drugs in this group may include certain thyreostatics, anticonvulsants and antibiotics, including penicillin and other beta-lactans. With penicillin, high doses are usually required to cause neutropenia, which is associated with maturation arrest in the marrow rather than hypoplasia, and is reversible (Neftel et al, 1983). Here the neutropenia is due to a genetically determined metabolic defect, and there is often warning of an impending neutropenia. The more explosive onset of agranulocytosis appears to be an immunological syndrome, and is discussed in Chapter 15.

Management

This will depend on the severity of the clinical picture. Vulnerability to infection increases as the count falls below 1000/μl, and is extreme below

$500/\mu l$ except in some of the benign neutropenic syndromes listed above. Acute agranulocytosis is a medical emergency requiring intensive care; its management is described in Chapter 15. Less severe neutropenia due to bone marrow insufficiency requires identification of any underlying cause, such as drug exposure, or an immunological disorder, before therapy is considered. Bone marrow examination will determine whether there is hypoplasia of granulocytopoiesis, or maturation arrest. The latter is more likely to result from chronic immune damage, and auto-immune neutropenia has been recognised as an entity. Corticosteroids are worth a trial for a limited period in this group. Plasmaphoresis is sometimes attempted, and there are anecdotal reports of success. Splenectomy is sometimes of value. Lithium salts have been advocated for chronic hypoplastic neutropenic states (Barrett & Faille, 1980) but results are rather disappointing except in the short term, and there is a risk of renal toxicity, requiring careful monitoring of plasma levels.

THROMBOCYTOPENIA DUE TO MARROW FAILURE

In the elderly, thrombocytopenia of this type is most likely to be due to marrow infiltration by neoplasms such as carcinoma, lymphoma and leukaemia. Chronic thrombocytopenia is a not infrequent precursor of myeloid leukaemia. Sometimes other morphological features of a pre-leukaemic myelodysplasia are present, but in any case the morphology of marrow megakaryocytes (which may be increased or decreased in numbers) is frequently bizarre. Occasionally amegakaryocytic thrombocytopenia remains after partial remission of aplastic anaemia, the haemoglobin and neutrophil counts achieving normal levels.

Amongst bone marrow 'toxins' reported to cause selective damage to megakaryocytes are thiazides, and high doses of oestrogen. Occasionally chronic alcoholism is accompanied by thrombocytopenia due in part to reduced numbers of megakaryocytes in the marrow (Aster, 1977).

HYPERSPLENISM

The spleen can be regarded as a lymphoid organ modified for certain haematological functions. Its functions in the normal individual, however, are incompletely understood, though they include lymphopoiesis and antibody production, haemopoiesis, filtration, surveillance and destruction of defective or aged red cells, phagocytosis and removal of particulate matter and immune complexes from the blood, storage of iron, factor VIII and certain lipids, and probably generation of certain stimulants of phagocytic activity, such as tuftsin (Bowdler, 1983; Lockwood, 1983). A hormonal function, modulating marrow production, has been postulated, but the evidence is inconclusive.

The main haematological features of hypersplenism relate to a perversion of the organ's capacity for filtration and storage of blood cells, and to the consequences of splenic enlargement on the splanchnic venous system. Sequestration of blood cells is certainly important in some cases (in giant splenomegaly more than 80 per cent of the body's platelet pool, and up to 40 per cent of the red cell mass may be located in the spleen) but the increased blood flow through splenic and portal veins is often the dominant mechanism in causing anaemia. The hyperkinetic portal venous hypertension which results is associated with an increased blood volume: in patients with partial marrow failure, this is translated into expansion of the plasma volume, with consequent dilutional anaemia.

Hypersplenism is sometimes divided into two categories: primary, where disease intrinsic to the spleen causes it to behave abnormally; and secondary, where the spleen is involved by a disease process arising elsewhere in the body (Table 6.1). 'Occult' hypersplenism might be defined as a functional variant in which cytopenia is fully compensated by marrow hyperplasia. In addition there are conditions such as hereditary spherocytosis in which the spleen is intrinsically normal but undergoes 'work hypertrophy'. An interesting example of work hypertrophy is the slight splenic enlargement which often occurs in patients with chronic renal failure, especially on long-term dialysis. Here, because bone marrow function is depressed, the additional element of haemolysis contributed by splenic destruction of slightly abnormal red cells cannot be compensated for. Splenectormy may result in a useful increase in haemoglobin levels. Isotopic studies have enabled the haematologist to distinguish different patterns of red cell accumulation in the spleen, according to whether the primary defect exists in the organ itself or in the red cells.

Clinical definition

No definition is entirely satisfactory. The conventional criteria are (a) deficiency of one or more cellular elements in the blood, (b) marrow hyperplasia of the corresponding cell line(s) with, often, morphological evidence of increased cell turnover such as persistent reticulocytosis, (c) splenomegaly, (d) correction of cytopenia following surgery (Dameshek, 1955). However, hypersplenism may be associated with a hypocellular marrow, as, for example, in cases of marrow infiltration or fibrosis, or even occasionally in chronic aplastic anaemia. Again, the beneficial effects of splenectomy may result as much from reduction in splanchnic blood flow and plasma volume expansion as from the abolition of physical 'sequestration' of blood cells.

Splenectomy in blood diseases

Many of the diseases causing secondary hypersplenism are described elsewhere in this book; the more important are listed in Table 6.1 'Primary' hypersplenism is seen particularly in the tropics (cryptogenic splenomegaly) and is related in many areas to hyper-immunisation to the malarial parasite. A form of non-tropical idiopathic splenomegaly has been described in Europe (Dacie et al, 1967) and appears often, though not invariably, to be pre-lymphomatous. There is a natural disinclination to subject elderly patients to splenectomy, in the knowledge that the operation is palliative and seldom curative, and is inevitably associated with an operative risk, such as sub-phrenic abscess or thromboembolism.

Crosby (1966) has emphasised, however, that the indications for splenectomy on haematological grounds are not necessarily vitiated by age alone. The operation and its risks must be considered in the context of the severity of the hypersplenism, of its rate of progression, the likely natural history of the underlying disorder and concomitant disease in other systems. Thus, splenectomy in chronic immune thrombocytopenia may be preferable to long-term crticosteroid therapy. In chronic lymphatic leukaemia and some types of non-Hodgkin lymphoma, massive splenomegaly may be best dealt with by surgical removal rather than intensive chemotherapy or radiother-apy, especially if this is limited by thrombocytopenia. However, there is no evidence that the operation prolongs life in these patients.

In malignant disorders, it is important to assess the relative contributions made by hypersplenism and bone marrow failure to chronic cytopenias. For example, in hairy-cell leukaemia, splenectomy is often indicated for profound pancytopenia. In this disease hypersplenism seems to be associated with distortion of the splenic architecture (Eichner, 1979) by the neoplastic cells, but bone marrow failure is usually also present. In congestive splenomegaly associated only with granulocyto-and/or thrombocytopenia, splenectomy is rarely indicated. The patient is usually able to mount a granulocytic response from the body's granulocyte pool, and thrombocytopenia is rarely severe enough to be the only cause of bleeding. In Felty's syndrome, results of splenectomy are often disappointing because the cytopenias are due to a number of different mechanisms (see p. 70).

Radio-isotopic studies are frequently performed in assessing the value of splenectomy in auto-immune haemolytic anaemia but are of limited value; probably splenectomy should be considered even in an elderly patient if this disease does not remit after a reasonable trial of immunosuppressive therapy. In myelofibrosis, plasma volume expansion often dominates the blood changes. Although it might be thought that removal of a mass of myeloid tissue would deprive the patient of functional haemopoietic capacity, in fact few patients actually become more anaemic after surgery (Milner et al, 1973). Although there are many anecdotal reports of clinical improvement following splenectomy in myeloid metaplasia, it has not yet been proved that the operation prolongs life, and it is undoubtedly hazardous in an elderly patient. Finally, splenectomy may result in clinical improvement in ways which are at present undefined, but may relate to abrogation of an abnormal immunolo-gical process. Examples include red cell aplasia, thrombotic thrombocy-topenic purpura and idiopathic pulmonary haemosiderosis.

Any patient who has undergone splenectomy is probably at risk of pneumococcal septicaemia, and some authorities now recommend active immunisation against this organism.

REFERENCES

Aoki A, Fujiki N, Schimizu H, Ohno Y 1980 Geographic and ethnic differences of aplastic anaemia in medullary aplasia. In: Medullary aplasia. Masson, New York, Najean Y (ed) p 79–88

Arneborn P, Palmblad J 1982 Drug-induced neutropenia — a survey for Stockholm 1973–78. Acta Medica Scandinavica 212: 289–292

Ascensao J, Kagan W, Moore M, Pahwa R, Hansen J, Good R 1976 Aplastic anaemia: evidence for an immunological mechanism. Lancet 1: 669

Aster R H 1977 Disorders of hemostasis — quantitative platelet disorders. In: Williams W J, Beutler E, Erslev A J, Rundles R W Haematalogy, 2nd edn. McGraw Hill, New York: p 1320–1321

Aymard J P, Guerci O, Herbeuval 1980 Infection induced aplastic anaemia. In: Najean Y (ed) Medullary aplasia Masson, New York, p 43–52

Bacigalupo A et al 1981 Severe aplastic anaemia: correlation of *in vitro* tests with clinical response to immunosuppressants in 20 patients. British Journal of Haematology 47: 423–33

Bagby G G, Lawrence H F, Neerhaut R C (1983) T-lymphocyte-mediated granulopoietic failure. New England Journal of Medicine 309: 1073–1075.

Barrett A J Faille A 1980 Clinical studies with lithium. In: Najean Y (ed), Medullary aplasia. Masson, New York, p 241–244

Benested H B 1974 Aplastic anaemia: considerations on the pathogenesis. Acta Medica Scandinavica 196: 255

Benestad H B 1979 Drug mechanisms in marrow aplasia. In: Geary C G (ed) Aplastic anaemia. Bailliere Tindall, London, p 26–42

Bernard J, Najean Y 1965 Evolution and prognosis of the idiopathic pancytopenias. Series Haematologica 5:1

Besa E C, Dale D C, Wolff S M, Gardner F H 1977 Aetiocholanolone and Prednisolone therapy in patients with severe bone marrow failure. Lancet 1: 728

Bottiger L E 1979 Epidemiology and aetiology of aplastic anaemia. In: Aplastic anaemia: pathophysiology and approaches to treatment. Heimpel H, Gordon-Smith E C, Heit W Kubanek B (eds) Springer, Berlin, p 27–37

Bowdler A J 1983 Splenomegaly and hypersplenism. Clinics in Haematology 12: 467–488

Camitta B M 1979 The role of viral infections in aplastic anaemia. In: (eds) Aplastic anaemia: pathophysiology and approaches to therapy. Heimpel H, Gordon-Smith E C, Heit W Kubanek B. Springer, Berlin, p 39–46

Camitta B M, Thomas E D, Nathan D G 1979 A prospective study of androgens and bone marrow transplantation for treatment of severe aplastic anaemia. Blood 53: 504–14

Camitta B M, Storb R and Thomas E D 1982 Aplastic anaemia. New England Journal of Medicine 306: 645–652 and 712–718

Cline M J, Golde D W 1978 Immune suppression of hematopoiesis. American Journal of Medicine 64: 301

Crosby W H, Whelan T J, Heaton L D 1966 Splenectomy in the elderly. Medical Clinics of North America 50: 1533

Curzon P G D, Muers M F, Rajah S M 1983 Aplastic anaemia associated with influenza A infection. Scandinavia Journal of Haematology 30: 232–234

Dacie J V et al 1967 Non-tropical idiopathic splenomegaly (primary hypersplenism): a review of ten cases and their relationship to malignant lymphomas. British Journal of Haematology 17: 317–333

Damashek W 1955 Hypersplenism. Bulletin of the New York Academy of Medicine 31: 113–126

Eichner E R 1979 Splenic function: normal, too much, too little. American Journal of Medicine 66: 311–320

Fraunfelden F T, Bagby G D, Kelly D J 1982 Fatal aplastic anemia following topical administration of opthalmic chloramphenicol. American Journal of Opthalmology 93: 356–60

Gardner F H 1978 Androgen therapy of aplastic anaemia. Clinics in Haematology 1: 571

Geary C G 1979 Red cell aplasia: In Aplastic Anaemia. Baillière Tindall, London, p 195–229

Gordon-Smith E C 1979a Clinical features of aplastic anaemia. In: Heimpel H, Gordon-Smith E C, Heit W, Kubanek B, (eds) Aplastic anaemia: pathophysiology and approaches to therapy. Springer, Berlin, p 9–14

Gordon-Smith E C 1979b Treatment of aplastic anaemia I: conservative management. In: Geary C G (ed) Aplastic anaemia. Baillière Tindall, London, p 108–130

Heimpel H 1979 Laboratory aspects of aplastic anaemia. In: (ed) Geary C G Aplastic Anaemia, Baillière Tindall, London, p 63–81

Hoffman R et al 1979 Antibody mediated aplastic anemia and diffuse fasciitis. New England Journal of Medicine 300: 718

Krantz S B 1974 Pure red cell aplasia. New England Journal of Medicine 291: 345

Lewis S M, Gordon-Smith E C 1982 Aplastic and dysplastic anaemias. In: Blood and its disorders, 2nd edn. Blackwell, London, p 1229–1268. Hardisty R M, Weatherall D J, (eds)

Lockwood C M 1983 Immunological functions of the spleen. Clinics in Haematology 12: 449–466

Messner H A, Fauser A A, Cutis J E, Dotten D 1981 Control of antibody mediated pure red cell aplasia by plasmapheresis. New Zealand Journal of Medicine 304: 1334–1338

Milner G R, Geary C G, Wadsworth L, Doss A 1973 Erythrokinetic studies as a guide to the value of splenectomy in primary myeloid metaplasia. British Journal of Haematology 25: 467–485

Mir A, Geary C G, Delamore I W 1977 Hypoimmunoglobulinaemia and aplastic anaemia. Scandanavian Journal of Haematology 19: 725–730

Morley A, Trainor K, Black J 1975 A primary stem cell lesion in experimental hypoplastic marrow failure. Blood 45: 681

Neftel K A, Muller M R, Hausser S P 1983 More on penicillin induced leukopenia. New England Journal of Medicine 308: 901

Pisciotta A V 1973 Immune and toxic mechanisms in drug-induced agranulocytosis. Seminars in Haematology 10: 279

Saita G 1973 Benzene induced hypoplastic anaemias and leukaemia. In: Girdwood R H (ed) Blood disorders due to drugs and other agents Excerpta Medica, Amsterdam, p 132

Schofield R 1979 Mechanism of damage to the stem cell population. In: Heimpel H, Gordon Smith E C, Heit W, Kubanek B (eds): Aplastic anaemia pathophysiology and approach to therapy. Springer, Berlin, p 63–72

Sieff C 1985 Pure red cell aplasia (annotation). British Journal of Haematology 54: 331–336

Speck B et al 1981 Treatment of severe aplastic anaemia with antilymphocyte globulin or bone marrow transplantation. British Medical Journal 282: 860–3

Williams D M, Lynch R E, Cartwright G E 1973 Drug-induced aplastic anaemia. Seminars in Haematology 10: 195

Wintrobe MM 1981 Clinical hematology, 8th edn. Lea & Febiger, New York, p 1287–1291 and 1326–1329

Yunis A A 1973 Chloramphenicol-induced bone marrow suppression Seminars in Haematology 10: 225

Screening for anaemia and its prevention

SCREENING

Anaemia, particularly its most common forms, iron-deficiency anaemia and pernicious anaemia, would seem to be common enough in the elderly for us to examine the question as to whether routine screening would be advantageous.

The general requirements for worthwhile screening programmes have been well examined, for example, by Holland (1974) and Whitby (1974). The salient points can be summarised as follows:

1. Is the condition important? — This rating would embody both its frequency and seriousness.
2. Is it treatable? — Is its response to treatment better if diagnosed early and are resources for treatment available?
3. Is the condition clearly defined?
4. Have we a sound strategy for dealing with borderline results?
5. Have we a satisfactory test which is acceptable, reliable and affordable?

IMPORTANCE OF ANAEMIA

On the face of it, the importance of anaemia in the elderly would seem to be easily established. Hyams (1978) summarises previous work on the prevalence of anaemia in the elderly in the community where usual figures are around 10–12 per cent (though the range is 1–55 per cent) and in elderly inpatients where rates are of the order of 20 per cent. Iron-deficiency anaemia is the commonest type and is quite readily treatable, and so the case for screening might be thought to be strong. However, the reported prevalences of anaemia vary partly because of different criteria being used. These were variably 11.9, 12.5, 13.0, 13.8 and 14.0 g/dl as the lower limit for men, 10.4 and 12.0 for women and 11.7, 11.8, 11.9 and 12.7 g/dl for the sexes combined! However, 12 g/100dl for women and for the sexes together and 13 g/dl for men were the modes and medians for the 21 quoted community surveys. Obviously, anaemia cannot be regarded as being clearly defined!

Even if a criterion were generally agreed, say 12 g/dl, does the possession of a haemoglobin value modestly lower than this represent disease and call for treatment or investigation? This is the key question, for community surveys find considerable prevalence of haemoglobin in the 10–12g/dl range, but few lower than this. Thus, for example, McLennan et al (1973) found that whilst 7.5 per cent of men and 20 per cent of women in a large partly stratified community sample had haemoglobin values below 12 g/dl, only 2.4 per cent overall had values below 10 g/dl. Elwood et al (1971), in a similar survey, found only 1 percent of subjects with haemoglobin below 10 g/dl, all of whom were female. They found these lower haemoglobins to be strongly associated with evidence of iron deficiency, and it could be argued that treatment is justifiable either because anaemia has deleterious effects or that iron deficiency is deterious quite apart from the associated anaemia. Both these possibilities have been quite extensively investigated, though not specifically in elderly subjects.

Furthermore, the effect of haemoglobin on prognosis has been examined in community samples, including studies of the elderly specifically. Elwood (1973) reviews the evidence relating various degrees of anaemia to symptoms or to objective changes such as cardiac output. Studies have only shown an association of symptoms with haemoglobin levels below 7–8 g/dl. Similarly, tachycardia, increased cardiac output and reduced vascular resistance have only been shown in association with anaemia below 7–8 g/dl. Furthermore, controlled trials found no evidence of symptomatic benefit for treatment of iron-deficiency anaemia of above 8 g/dl. The question of a general effect of iron deficiency has also been examined by Elwood & Hughes (1970) who found no benefits to motor or psychomotor function in a controlled trial in iron-deficient women.

Haemoglobin levels have been shown to predict mortality in adult community samples, but it is high, not low, haemoglobin levels which are associated with excess deaths (Waters et al, 1969). This may have been due to the association of high haemoglobin levels with respiratory disease or due to increased blood viscosity favouring thromboembolic disease. In a study of 852 elderly in the community, Hodkinson & Exton-Smith (1976) found no association between haemoglobin values and mortality over the ensuing five years. So there is no support for the idea that the many somewhat low haemoglobin values in the elderly which are classified as anaemia by many authors are deleterious either in terms of symptoms, cardiovascular effects or mortality. Positive evidence of harm comes only with haemoglobin values below, say 8 g/dl, and such values are rare in community samples.

IS ANAEMIA TREATABLE?

The majority of anaemias found in elderly people in the community can be firmly ascribed to iron deficiency (DHSS, 1972; McLennan et al, 1973; Elwood et al, 1971). The anaemia is easily treated by iron supplements, but, as discussed above, such treatment confers no benefit when the anaemia is of modest degree and, if it were left untreated and were to become more severe, would still remain equally well responsive to treatment later. Is it, however, of value to recognise minor degrees of iron-deficiency anaemia because of their ability to identify other diseases which are giving rise to the anaemia by virtue of increased blood loss and which might benefit from earlier recognition and treatment? Table 7.1 lists the commonly recognised underlying causes of iron-deficiency anaemia, pure dietary deficiency probably being a very rare explanation. Among these, drug-induced bleeding and peptic ulceration are probably the most common, and their prompt recognition could be helpful. Early recognition of carcinoma, particularly of the colon, could also be helpful, but the pick-up from anaemia screening would be very small and could not justify the procedure. (Elwood, 1974).

The second most common type of anaemia found in community surveys is pernicious anaemia. Here again, more marked degrees of anaemia remain fully responsive to treatment, so that the only advantage of treatment at a presymptomatic stage would be that the occurrence of subacute combined degeneration of the cord might be prevented, which, when fully developed, may not be completely reversed by B_{12} treatment. However, this is an extremely rare condition so that the potential for benefit is very small one.

IS ANAEMIA CLEARLY DEFINED?

It will already be obvious that anaemia has no clear definition. Haemoglobin values from community samples are not bimodal but are a continuous distribution which, indeed, fails to show any negative skewing as would be expected if there were a small abnormal anaemic population hidden in the lower tail of the overall distribution. On the other hand, McLennan et al (1973) showed a strong relationship between low serum iron and iron saturation and low haemoglobin values; the DHSS study (1972) also found a significant association. The data of McLennan et al (1973) show that, whilst low iron values are strongly associated with lower haemoglobin, they are spread well up the range of haemoglobin. Indeed, less than half of the

Table 7.1   The more important causes of iron-deficiency anaemia in the elderly

1. GIT bleeding associated with aspirin, phenylbutazone and other non-steroidal anti-inflammatory drugs
2. GIT bleeding associated with corticosteroid therapy
3. Peptic ulcer
4. Hiatus hernia
5. GIT carcinomata (stomach, colon)
6. Gut angiodysphasias
7. Previous gastric surgery
8. Diverticulitis of large gut

subjects judged iron-deficient had haemoglobin values below 12 g/dl. There is thus no clearly definable iron deficiency anaemia subgroup.

BORDERLINE RESULTS

We are left, therefore, with a very considerable problem of borderline results. Anaemia itself is an essentially arbitrary attempt to categorise into two groups (anaemic and non-anaemic) a continuous distribution of results which is not bimodal — a problem which may be compared to that of defining hypertension. Moreover, even is we try to improve matters by addressing ourselves to more circumscribed disease concepts, most importantly iron-deficiency anaemia and B_{12}-deficiency anaemia (pernicious anaemia), we remain in great difficulties as iron, ferritin, iron saturation and B_{12} results similarly show continuous distributions of results which are not bimodal. Arbitrary cut-off points are commonly used and result in totally artificial categories which cannot be equated with the clinical diagnostic categories. The finding that, for example, both haemoglobin and B_{12} are a little below our defined limits does not prove that the patient has pernicious anaemia. We could only substantiate that diagnosis if we also demonstrated other features such as achlorhydria, parietal cell antibodies, abnormal B_{12} absorbtion corrected by administration of intrinsic factor or a clinical response to B_{12} therapy.

The experimental evidence with respect to iron-deficiency anaemia, already mentioned, strongly suggests that no benefits are likely to arise from treatment of such borderline cases. We are thus likely to involve ourselves in extensive and expensive follow-up of large numbers of patients with borderline results and these will very greatly outnumber the undeniable cases for which treatment is clearly necessary. Alternatively, one must accept the need to treat very substantial numbers of individuals unnecessarily in order to be sure of treating those who are truly abnormal.

THE TESTS

Are the tests themselves satisfactory? Haemoglobin determinations are cheap and reasonably accurate. Their main problem is that of physiological variation due to posture. In the erect posture, ultra-filtration of the blood takes place to a greater extent, water and small molecular constituents of plasma leaving the venous vascular compartment under the influence of the increased hydrostatic pressure in the lower parts of the body. This has the effect of increasing the concentrations of all macromolecular and cellular constituents of the blood (Statland et al, 1973). The process is partially counteracted by the opposing influence of oncotic pressure of the plasma proteins and other macromolecules, of which albumin, with his high concentration and relatively low molecular weight (c 64 000) is by far the most important. The effects of posture are thus exaggerated when hypoalbuminaemia exists and albumin values fall with age, particularly when there is coexisting illness (Hodkinson, 1977). In these circumstances the changes from lying to standing may be as high as +20 per cent, whereas with normal albumin levels changes of around +10 per cent can be expected. These postural effects occur within 30 minutes of standing. Sitting up produces smaller increases than standing. Clearly, these changes are of a sufficient magnitude to move an individual's haemoglobin result from one which might be classified as anaemic too one considered normal, for example a lying haemoglobin of 11.5 g/dl judged anaemic might well rise to 12.6 g/dl after standing and be accepted as 'normal'. This problem can best be dealt with by standardisation of specimen-taking so that the criterion set for anaemia is applied to one posture.

Even with this proviso, however, we are left with considerable difficulties in using haemoglobin as our screening test which are not solely due to the uncertainties regarding criteria. We may suppose that the probable state of affairs is as shown diagrammatically in Figure 7.1, where a small subpopulation (illustrated as 5 per cent of the total population) of 'anaemic' results is buried in the lower tail of the overall distribution. There is no cut-off point which separates 'anaemic' from 'non-anaemic' values, but the probability of any given haemoglobin value being 'anaemic' is given by the proportion of the height under the total curve contributed by the 'anaemic' curve.

Our present problem is that we do not know the size, means and standard deviation of the two component curves, but even if we did, the method would still have inherent difficulties. We could even then never classify any result as due to 'anaemia', though we could calculate an exact probability of this being so, as long as the prevalence of anaemia for the population (and thus relative size of the two curves) was known. Unfortunately, we are currently in a logical circle, for we cannot determine prevalence without interpreting haemoglobin results, and we cannot interpret haemoglobin results without knowing the prevalence of anaemia!

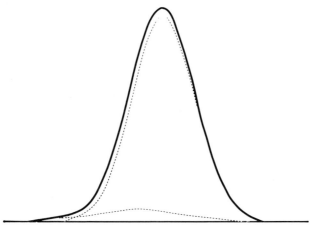

Fig. 7.1 Two normally distributed populations of results (dotted lines) which together (solid line) give a unimodal distribution.

TYPES OF ANAEMIA

Where haemoglobin estimates are included in such multiphasic profiles applied to groups of patients, clinicians will, nowadays, almost always use a Coulter counter which will also provide information to show haemological indices. Particularly useful are the mean corpuscular volume (MCV) and mean corpuscular haemoglobin (MCH) as these, together with the haemoglobin value, will allow patients to be roughly classified as follows so that the direction of their further investigation can be determined.

Thus, a normal MCV and MCH coupled with a low haemoglobin value will suggest either anaemia of chronic disease, e.g. of renal failure, or haemolytic anaemia. High MCV and MCH coupled with anaemia suggest megaloblastic anaemia, such as those of pernicious anaemia or folate deficiency, but may also be seen less commonly with aplastic anaemia or sideroblastic anaemia. High MCV without anaemia may indicate heavy recent alcohol intake or hypothyroidism. Low MCV and MCH with low haemoglobin levels usually indicate iron-deficiency anaemia, but may also be seen in anaemia of chronic disease or in thalassaemia. The screening value of the Coulter result is thus considerably greater in suggesting possible diagnoses than measurement of haemoglobin levels alone.

SCREENING PATIENT GROUPS FOR ANAEMIA

Whilst we may conclude that screening of the well elderly for anaemia is not justifiable, we need to examine the rather different situation of the inclusion of haemoglobin in multiphasic screening (or admission) profiles of tests applied to patient groups. Here pick-up of anaemia (however defined) will be much greater, and much more severe degrees are likely to be encountered. Much of the importance of the finding of anaemia now rests on its value as an indicator of serious diseases to which it may be secondary, and few people would therefore argue against the inclusion of haemoglobin determinations in profiles.

The powers of anaemia as an indicator of underlying disease in elderly patients are demonstrated by its powerful contribution to prediction of short-term mortality in geriatric inpatients of both sexes (Hodkinson, 1981), values at either extreme being associated with significantly higher mortalities. Elevated values presumably owe their predictive power to associations with dehydration and severe chronic respiratory disease, whilst low values are associated with many conditions giving rise to blood loss (Table 7.1) but also, as the 'anaemia of chronic disease', with malignancy, renal failure and many other serious underlying medical conditions which may carry an unfavourable prognosis.

Groups at special risk of anaemia

There remain a number of specific groups of patients where regular monitoring for anaemia (as opposed to single screening surveys) would seem to be indicated.

Post-gastric surgery patients are one such at-risk group. Total gastrectomy can be expected to lead to B_{12} deficiency megaloblastic anaemia, but partial gastrectomy also carries an increased risk. Gastric surgery is also often associated with impairment of iron absorption, so that there is an increased risk of iron deficiency anaemia even in those who do not have chronic blood loss secondary to stomach ulceration. Ideally, therefore, patients who have had gastric surgery should have regular life-long medical monitoring which should include measurement of haemoglobin levels.

Epileptic patients are also at risk, as anti-epileptic drugs are potent hepatic enzyme inducers. The increased enzyme activity leads to more rapid destruction of folate, and folate deficiency megaloblastic anaemia may be a consequence (as is osteomalacia because of increased destruction of vitamin D metabolites). Regular monitoring for the development of anaemia is thus advisable in this group of patients.

Patients on aspirin and other non-steroidal anti-inflammatory drugs have an increased likelihood of chronic gastric blood loss. Indeed, surveys of the elderly in the community indicate that regular use of such drugs is an important explanation of low haemoglobin levels. Thus McLennan et al (1973) found a significant excess of subjects taking regular salicylate preparations among the elderly whose haemogloblin values were below 12 g/dl. It could therefore be argued that elderly subjects who take such drugs should have their haemoglobin levels checked regularly.

Vegans are also at special risk of developing B_{12} deficiency megaloblastic anaemia, as B_{12} is largely confined to foods of animal origin. Many vegans are now aware of this and take B_{12} supplements but, if this is not so, regular surveillance for the development of megaloblastic anaemia would be advisable, particularly as there is also a risk of subacute combined degeneration of the cord as a far more serious development.

Other special diets may also give rise to some concern if they are deficient in iron, B_{12} or folate and may call for appropriate monitoring, though it seems likely that iron deficiency is very rarely due solely to inadequate intake, some abnormal loss almost always playing a part.

Patients with auto-immune diseases such as hypothyroidism, vitiligo and rheumatoid arthritis have an increased likelihood of developing pernicious anaemia. However, with the exception of hypothyroidism it is doubtful if this increased risk if of such a magnitude as to justify regular surveillance for this reason alone, although haemoglobin determination would be a sensible addition to any other medical monitoring considered necessary.

PREVENTION OF ANAEMIA

So far we have been considering the early detection of anaemia rather than true prevention. The only exception to this is the use of B_{12} supplements in vegans. Opportunities for the true prevention would otherwise seem rather few, apart from in isolated specific circumstances such as prophylactic B_{12} injections after total gastrectomy, for example. The broadly-based preventive approach would need to address the commonest type of anaemia, iron-deficiency anaemia. There has been the suggestion that food supplementation, for example fortification of bread, with iron so as to increase iron intake for the whole community might be advantageous. On current evidence, this must be regarded as an extremely dubious proposition. The extra amounts of iron which could in practice be added to individual intakes would be limited and would doubtless be insufficient to compensate for severe losses associated with bleeding diseases such as listed in Table 7.1. They might achieve elevation of haemoglobin in individuals with borderline values, but we have already noted that present evidence indicates that this will not be associated with any symptomatic improvement. Indeed, the increased mortality associated with high haemoglobin values indicates the need for considerable caution.

Higher haemoglobin values are associated with higher cholesterol values (reviewed by Elwood, 1973), a well-recognised risk factor for ischaemic heart disease, and raised packed-cell volume results in increased blood viscosity which may also have deleterious effects with respect to vascular disease. Nor is it clear whether correction of iron deficiency is advantageous per se, for, whilst immune function is impaired when iron is low, bacterial resistance may be improved, as iron is an essential nutrient for bacteria. The balance of advantages has not been adequately assessed.

CONCLUSION

Screening of the elderly community for anaemia cannot be justified on present evidence, despite the high reported prevalences from community surveys. By contrast, the inclusion of haemoglobin determinations as a part of screening profiles applied to elderly patients seems well worthwhile.

Opportunities for true prevention of anaemia would appear to be highly circumscribed, and any community-wide attempt at prevention of iron deficiency anaemia in the elderly by dietary supplementation cannot be supported by available research findings.

REFERENCES

Department of Health and Social 1972 A nutrition survey of the elderly: report by the panel on nutrition of the elderly. (Reports on Health and Social Security No.3) HMSO, London
Elwood P C 1973 Evaluation of the clinical importance of anemia. American Journal of Clinical Nutrition 26: 958–964
Elwood P C 1974 Anaemia. Lancet 2: 1364–1369
Elwood P C, Hughes 1970 Clinical trial of iron therapy on psychomotor function in anaemic women. British Medical Journal 3: 254–255
Elwood P C, Shinton C I D, Wilson P, Sweetnam P, Franzer A C 1971 Haemoglobin, vitamin B_{12} and folate levels in the elderly. British Journal of Haemotology 21: 557–563

Hodkinson H M 1977 Biochemical diagnosis of the elderly. Chapman & Hall, London
Hodkinson H M 1981 Value of admission profile tests for prognosis in elderly patients. Journal of the American Geriatrics Society 29: 206–210
Hodkinson H M, Exton-Smith A N 1976 Factors predicting mortality in the elderly in the community. Age and Ageing 5: 110–115
Holland W W 1974 Taking stock. Lancet 2: 1494–1497
Hyams D E 1978 The blood. In: Brocklehurst J C (ed) Textbook of geriatric medicine and gerontology, 2nd edn. Churchill Livingstone, Edinburgh p 560–625
McLennan W J, Andrews G R, Macleod Catriona, Caird F I 1973 Anaemia in the elderly. Quarterly Journal of Medicine 165: 1–13
Statland B E, Winkel P, Bokelund H 1973 Factors contributing to intra-individual variation of serum constituents: 1 within-day variation of serum constituents in healthy subjects. Clinical Chemistry 19: 1374–1379
Waters W E, Withey J E, Kilpatrick G S, Wood P H N, Abernethy 1969 Ten-year haematological follow-up: mortality and haematological changes. British Medical Journal 4: 761–764
Whitby L G 1974 Definitions and criteria. Lancet 2: 819–822

Haemolytic disease

DEFINITION

Haemolytic anaemia is anaemia due to an increased rate of red cell destruction when the ability of the bone marrow to respond to the stimulus of anaemia is inimpaired (Wintrobe et al, 1981). This is differentiated from those anaemias with a 'haemolytic component' where the primary defect is the underproduction of erythrocytes. In geriatric medicine the underproduction anaemias are very common and include the anaemia of chronic disease, sideroblastic anaemias and the deficiency states (folate, B_{12} and iron). These may co-exist with a true haemolytic anemia and can confuse the picture by obscuring red cell regeneration. The haemolytic anaemia that is normally accompanied by vigorous red cell regeneration is discussed here.

In young persons, the marrow is capable of undergoing hyperplasia to increase its production of erythrocytes 6–8-fold. Thus, it is possible for the survival of red cells in the circulation to decrease to 15–20 days from the normal of 120 days without the appearance of anaemia. This would then be a 'compensated haemolytic disease'. There is evidence that human bone marrow proliferation may wane significantly with age, but careful studies of the bone marrow response to haemolysis in the elderly has not yet been done (Freedman, 1982).

CLASSIFICATION

When considering evidence for a haemolytic process, one looks for signs of increased red cell destruction and signs of accelerated erythropoiesis. These are summarised in Table 8.1. Not all of these tests are necessary to confirm the diagnosis. Usually a reticulocyte count, serial observations of the anaemia and a serum unconjugated bilirubin determination will approximate the degree of red cell destruction. The finding of anaemia, elevated reticulocyte count and a raised serum unconjugated bilirubin (but less than 75μmol/l (5 mg/dl)) is suggestive of a haemolytic anaemia as long as occult haemorrhage into an organ or tissue to recovery from a nutritional anaemia are excluded. Other tests are confirmatory and are helpful in defining the type of haemoly-

Table 8.1   Laboratory signs of haemolysis (Wintrobe et al, 1981)

Signs of accelerated red cell destruction
a. Decreased red blood cell lifespan
b. Increased catabolism of haem
     increased serum unconjugated bilirubin
     increased endogenous carbon monoxide production
     increased rate of bilirubin production
     increased rate of urobilinogen excretion

c. Increased serum lactate dehydrogenase activity (LDH-2 predominantly)

d. Signs of intravascular haemolysis
     haemoglobinaemia
     decreased or absent free haptoglobin (occurs in extravascular haemolysis also)
     haemoglobinuria
     haemosiderinuria
     methaemalbuminaemia
     reduced serum haemopexin

Signs of accelerated erythropoiesis
a. Peripheral blood smear
     reticulocytosis (polychromatophilia, basophilic stipling)
     polychromatophilic macrocytes
     nucleated RBC
     leukocytosis and thrombocytosis

b. Bone marrow
     erythroid hyperplasia

c. Ferrokinetics
     increased plasma iron turnover
     increased erythrocyte iron turnover

d. Biochemical
     increased red blood cell creatinine
     increased red blood cell enzyme activities (uroporphyrin I synthetase, hexokinase and
     glutamate oxalate transaminase)

tic anaemia (e.g., is it extravascular or intravascular ?). The determination of red cell survival is useful in those patients presenting with a difficult diagnostic picture.

Evidence of intravascular haemolysis including haemoglobinaemia, haemoglobinuria (Ham, 1955), haemosiderinuria (Crosby & Dameshek, 1951), methaemalbuminaemia (Fairley, 1941), reduced serum haemopexin (Muller-Eberhard, 1970) and absence of haptoglobin (Brus & Lewis, 1959), indicates red cell destruction even if there are no other signs. Table 8.2 summarises the conditions that may be mistaken for a haemolytic anaemia.

Haemolytic anaemia may be acquired or inherited (Table 8.3). Most of the inherited types are diagnosed at a young age, but occasionally they may be mild enough and the diagnosis made in later life (hereditary spherocytosis, elliptocytosis and glucose-6-phosphate dehydrogenase (G6PD) deficiency). The acquired varieties are much more common in elderly people and for the most part are due to extrinsic agents acting on the red cell. The exceptions to this rule are paroxysmal nocturnal haemoglobinuria and thermal injury, which are characterised by an acquired intrinsic defect. In the inherited forms the defect is usually intrinsic, the exception being the common type of G6PD deficiency where there are no ill effects until the patient is exposed to an extrinsic agent, usually a drug.

Haemolytic anaemia can present either as an acute or chronic illness. If this condition presents acutely (Wallerstein & Aggeler, 1964), as in a patient with glucose-6-phosphate dehydrogenase deficiency given an oxidant drug or after the transfusion of incompatible blood, the symptoms will resemble that of an acute febrile illness. The patient will have aching pains in the back, limbs or abdomen along with headache, vomiting, shaking chills and fever. The

Table 8.2 Conditions which may be confused with haemolytic anaemias

With anaemia and reticulocytosis
  haemorrhage
  recovery from iron, B_{12} or folate deficiency

With anaemia and unconjugated hyperbilirubinaemia
  ineffective erythroporesis
  loss of blood into body cavity or tissue

Unconjugated hyperbilirubinaemia without anaemia
  Gilbert's syndrome
  defects in bilirubin conjugation (e.g. by steroids)
  severe fasting
  severe exercise

Marrow invasion
  myelofibrosis
  myelophthisis (metastatic disease)

Myoglobinuria

Table 8.3 Classification of the haemolytic anaemias seen in the elderly

Aquired Haemolytic anaemia
1. Immunohaemolytic anaemia
      transfusion of incompatible blood
      auto-immune haemolytic anaemia due to warm reacting antibodies
      auto-immune haemolytic anaemia due to cold reacting antibodies
      drug-induced auto-immune haemolytic anaemia
2. Red cell fragmentation syndromes
      traumatic haemolytic anaemia
      microangiopathic haemolytic anaemia
3. Infectious agents
4. Chemicals, drugs and venoms
5. Physical agents
6. Hypophosphatemia
7. 'Spur-cell' anaemia in liver disease
8. Paroxysmal nocturnal haemoglobinuria

Inherited haemolytic disorders (usually diagnosed earlier in life)
1. Glucose-6-phosphate dehydrogenase deficiency
2. Hereditary elliptocytosis
3. Hereditary spherocytosis
4. Haemoglobinopathies, thalassaemias

patient may go into shock followed by oliguria or anuria. Symptoms of severe anaemia will also be prominent.

In the chronic form, such as with auto-immune haemolytic anaemia, the symptoms develop slowly over a few weeks or months. Pallor, scleral icterus or a jaundiced complexion may be noted. Many times in the geriatric patient the first symptoms are cardiovascular, either with angina or congestive heart failure. Other common presentations in the elderly are weakness, fatigue, mental confusion or depression. In some instances the clinical presentation may be predominantly that of the underlying illness to which the haemolytic anaemia is secondary. It is also important to remember that in all haemolytic anaemias folic acid requirements are increased and should be replaced. In chronic intravascular haemolysis iron is lost in the urine and may have to be given as well (Sears et al, 1966).

ACQUIRED HAEMOLYTIC ANAEMIAS

Acquired haemolytic anaemias due to infectious, chemical or physical agents

Haemolysis may develop with exposure to many infectious, chemical or physical agents. In most such instances auto-antibodies against RBC will be found, and this subject will be discussed later. Exposure to oxidant drugs and chemicals may precipitate haemolysis in patients with G6PD deficiency (or unstable haemoglobins) and will also be discussed later. In this section only those agents most likely to cause a haemolytic anaemia without an intrinsic red cell defect or antibody-mediated damage will be considered. Table 8.4 lists these agents.

A number of drugs and chemicals can produce oxidant damage to the erythrocyte with resultant denaturation of haemoglobin, and formation of methaemoglobin, sulphaemoglobin and Heinz bodies. Apparently in some cases the chemical itself acts as an oxidising agent, but the usual mechanism is interaction with oxygen to form the free radicals or peroxides. These then, if produced in quantities too great to be detoxified by the glutathione-dependent reduction system, will damage the red cells, haemoglobin and other structures.

People deficient in G6PD or other components of the glutahione-dependent reduction system are much more susceptible to the effects of these drugs. However, if high doses of these drugs are given, of if there is decreased renal function as seen with ageing, and there are unusually high blood levels, haemolysis can result in normal people.

Chemicals can cause haemolysis directly by non-oxidative mechanisms. Many of these have been reported in industrial settings and produce an acute picture of intravascular haemolysis (Fowler & Weissberg, 1974).

Haemoglobinuria and even death from renal failure have been observed in association with transurethral resection of the prostate, apparently due to the

Table 8.4 Infectious, chemical and physical agents causing haemolytic anaemia (Wintrobe et al, 1981)

Oxidant drus and chemicals
  naphthalene (mothballs)
  Nitrofurantoin
  Salicylazosulphidine
  Sulphamethoxypiridine
  Aminosalicylic acid
  Sodium sulphone
  Sulphonamides
  Phenazopyridine
  Phenacetin
  Dapsone and other sulphones
  Phenylhydrazine and its derivatives
  Aniline
  Phenylsemicarbozide
  Resorcin
  Hydroxylamine
  Nitrobenzene
  Phenol derivatives
  Potassium and sodium chlorates
  Stibine
  Lead
  Trimettalic anhydride
  Isolated reports of propylthiouracil, apiol, mephenesin, intravenous glycol, zinc ethylene, bisidithiocarbamate
  Inorganic copper (Wilson's disease)
  Distilled water
  Haemodialysis

Venoms
  Snake bites
  Spider bites
  Bee stings (rare)

Physical agents
  Thermal injury

Hypophosphataemia

Infectious agents

  Malaria
  Other protozoans (kalaazar, trypanosomiasis)
  Bartonellosis
  Clostridial sepsis
  Rarely in other bacterial infections

irrigating distilled water entering the bloodstream through venous and lymphatic channels opened by the operation. If more than 0.6 litres of water enter the circulation, osmotic haemolysis will result (Landsteiner & Finch, 1947). This can also occur in survivors from near drowning (Rath, 1953).

Haemodialysis has also been associated with haemolytic anaemias as a result of the presence of chloramines (an oxidant chemical) used as bactericidal agents in water supplies (Eaton et al, 1973), formaldehyde in a water filtration system (Orringer & Mattern, 1976), overheated dialysate (Lynn et al, 1979) or other contaminants such as copper (Oski, 1970) or nitrates (Carlson & Shapiro, 1970).

Venoms such as those produced by certain snakes (Condrea et al, 1964) and spiders (Nance, 1961) can cause haemolytic anaemias at any age. Similarly, following extensive burn injuries, intravascular haemolysis may occur (Shen et al, 1943).

Severe hypophosphatemia (less than 0.2 mg/dl) can also result in a haemolytic anaemia. This can occur in patients undergoing prolonged therapy with antacids, those receiving hyperalimentation without phosphorus supplementation and in severely debilitated and starved people. The predominant picture in those people is confusion, weakness, anorexia, malaise, paresthesias and EEG and EMG changes (Jacob & Amsden, 1971; Klock et al, 1974).

Infectious agents may be a direct cause of haemolysis at any age. These include malaria (Woodruff et al, 1979), bartonella (Reynafarje & Ramos, 1961) and clostridia (Ikezawa & Murata, 1964). Other agents have also been implicated in rare patients and include many of the gram-positive and gram-negative bacteria and even tuberculosis. Viruses and mycoplasms cause haemolytic diseases, but these are thought to be due to immunological mechanisms.

Immunohaemolytic anaemia

Immune haemolytic anaemia due to warm-reactive antibodies

Warm-reactive auto-antibodies causing haemolytic anaemia may arise as a primary or idiopathic disorder or as a secondary phenomenon in people with a variety of illnesses (Table 8.5) This condition is more common in women, and the incidence of the secondary varieties rises with age (Dacie & Worlledge, 1969). Auto-immune haemolytic anaemia appears to arise in people with a genetic predisposition and a disorder of immunological regulation (Waldmann et al, 1978). Particularly in older people, a secondary disease or drug aetiology must be carefully considered.

Auto-immune haemolytic anaemia of the warm antibody type has a variable clinical onset and cause. In the varieties secondary to malignancies, the onset is usually gradual and insidious and the course correlates with that of the underlying disease. In the primary type the illness is quite variable in presentation and may be so mild as to be barely discernible or fulminant and fatal. The presenting symptoms are usually referable to the anaemia and include weakness and dizziness. Hepatomegaly, lymphadenopathy and particularly splenomegaly are common signs, but clinically detectable jaundice is not (Dacie, 1962; Pirofsky, 1976).

We are heavily dependent on the laboratory to diagnose auto-immune haemolytic anaemia. There is usually an anaemia, the red cell indices are

Table 8.5   Immunohaemolytic anaemia

Associated with warm-reactive antibodies
a. Idiopathic autoimmune haemolytic anaemia
b. Secondary to:
    1. Systemic lupus erythaematosus and other collagen vascular disorders
    2. Chronic lymphocytic leukaemia and other lymphoreticular malignancies including
        multiple myeloma
    3. Other tumours and malignancies
    4. Viral infections
    5. Immune deficiency syndromes

Associated with cold-reactive antibodies
a. Primary — idiopathic cold agglutinin disease
b. Secondary — associated with:
    1. Infections, particularly mycoplasm pneumoniae
    2. Chronic lymphocytic leukaemia, lymphomas
c. Paroxysmal cold haemoglobinuria
    1. Idiopathic
    2. secondary to syphilis and viral infections

Drug-induced immune haemolytic anaemia
a. Penicillin-type
b. Stibophen ('innocent bystander') type
c. α-methyldopa-type
d. Streptomycin-type

normocytic, normochromic, but may be macrocytic depending upon the degree of reticulocytosis. The reticulocyte count is usually high, but co-existing anaemia of chronic disease, a deficiency state or myelophthisis can markedly reduce the degree of reticulocytosis (Pirofsky, 1976). In some cases, perhaps as many as 25 per cent, there is reticulocytopenia thought to be due to reticulocyte-specific antibodies (Hedge et al, 1977). The peripheral smear classically shows microspherocytes, poikilocytosis, polychromatophilia, anisocytosis and polychromatophilic macrocytes. Nucleated red cells are common. The white count may be low, normal or elevated if the onset is acute, and the platelet count is usually normal (Pirofsky, 1976). The occurrence of auto-immune haemolytic anaemia and 'auto-immune' thrombocytopenia is referred to as Evans' syndrome and may be seen together with a lymphoma (Jones, 1973; Kaden et al, 1979). The serum bilirubin is usually modestly increased and the haemolysis is usually extravascular, except in the acute fulminant cases where intravascular haemolysis also occurs (Pirofsky, 1976).

The hallmark of the auto-immune nature of the illness is the antiglobulin or 'Coombs' test (Coombs et al, 1945). The presence of a direct reacting antiglobulin test indicates antibody on the red cell surface and is the expected finding in virtually all patients with an auto-immune haemolytic anaemia. This test may be modified to yield information about the immunoglobulin clas and subclass as well as the presence of complement components (Dacie & Worlledge, 1969; Chaplin, 1973; Lalezari, 1976). The indirect antiglobulin test may be used to demonstrate auto-antibodies in the patient's serum (Dacie & Worlledge, 1969). Theoretically, the only deficiency of the Coombs' test is its relative insensitivity. Commercially available reagents commonly in use in blood banks will yield a positive reaction when 100–500 antibodies are attached to each red cell (Lalezari, 1976). However, since only 10 anti-Rh antibodies can reduce the red cell T half survival time to three days, severe haemolytic disease can exist in patients with a negative antiglobulin test (Mallison & Hugh-Jones, 1967). However, this is not a common situation. Recently, new techniques have been developed to increase the sensitivity of this test, including the addition of proteins, polyvinyl pyrrolidone or polybrene to the suspending medium to narrow the intracellular distance between red cells (Lalezari, 1976). In particular, polybrene with automated techniques using continuous flow systems has proven much more sensitive (Lalezari, 1976). Methods using proteolytic enzyme-treated cells are also more sensitive and are in wide use (Dacie, 1962; Lalezari, 1976).

In auto-immune haemolytic anaemia due to warm-reacting antibodies, about 30–40 per cent of patients will have only IgG on their red cells; 40–50 per cent will have IgG and complement and 10 per cent will have complement alone (usually in patients with systemic lupus erythematosus) (Dacie & Worlledge, 1969; Chaplin, 1973; Morgan et al, 1967). Many of the antibodies are directed against Rh antigenic determinants which may make typing and cross-matching of blood difficult (Vos et al, 1971; Issit et al, 1976). The IgG antibodies are usually polyclonal (Lalezari, 1976).

The treatment of auto-immune haemolytic anaemia of the warm antibody type must always include that of any associated disease. In many instances if the illness if due to lymphoma, particularly chromic lymphocytic leukaemia, or tumour, treatment of the primary illness will result in a remission of the haemolytic anaemia (Jones, 1973). In emergency situations with fulminant haemolysis, blood tranfusion may be necessary but is difficult due to the typing and cross-matching problems. In these cases red cells which give the 'best match' are used (Rosenfield & Jagathombal, 1976). When imperfectly matched blood is given, it must be done under constant supervision and given slowly. Adrenocorticosteroids should be used concomitantly.

Adrenocorticosteroids are the initial treatment of choice. Usally one starts with a dose of prednisone of 40 mg/m^2 of body surface per day, but higher doses may be needed. Haematological improvement usually occurs within 3–7 days, and in subsequent weeks there should be an increase in haemoglobin of 2–3 g/dl blood per week. When the haemoglobin level reaches 10 g/dl, the dose may be reduced gradually. In general one should try to halve the dose over a 4–6 week period and then slowly try to withdraw prednisone during the next 3–4 months (Murphy & LoBuglio, 1976). About 15–20 per cent of patients will be unresponsive to corticosteroids and will require splenectomy or cytotoxic drugs. In about one-fourth of cases the corticosteroid can be completely withdrawn, and in the remainder of the patients steroids may be necessary for maintenance, with all of its attendant risks in the elderly,

Splenectomy is recommended for those patients whose anaemia cannot be controlled by steroids, for those who require continuous high dose steroids, or for those who have developed serious complications due to the steroids (Dacie and Worlledge, 1969). The success rate of splenectomy will be increased if patients are selected who have demonstrated excessive sequestration of ^{51}Cr-labelled red cells in the spleen (Goldberg et al, 1966; Christensen, 1973). However, this operation should never be taken lightly, as there is a not inconsiderable morbidity in the elderly (Dacie, 1962). Before the operation, patients should receive pneumococcal vaccine to attempt to reduce the post-splenectomy pneumococcal sepsis.

In most older people cytotoxic drugs are given only after failure to respond to steroids, or splenectomy, or in those who have relapsed following splenectomy, or if they are poor candidates for the operation. The drugs most commonly used have been cyclophosphamide and azothioprine, both combined with prednisone (Murphy & LoBuglio, 1976).

Immune haemolytic anaemias due to cold-reactive antibodies

Auto-antibodies that react with red cells below 32°C are termed cold-reactive antibodies. They give rise to two clinical syndromes: the cold agglutinin syndrome, and paroxysmal cold haemoglobinuria (Table 8.5). The latter condition is very rare and is usually seen in association with syphilis.

Cold agglutinins are usually of the IgM class (Pruzanski & Shuma, 1977). They may either be polyclonal or monoclonal (Table 8.6), and almost all of them bind complement (Dacie, 1950). The majority have specificity for one of the Ii antigens of the erythrocyte. Ii antigens also exist on other cells, and any of the formed elements of the blood may be decreased by anti-Ii cold agglutinins (Pruzanski & Shumak, 1977).

Cold agglutinin disease of the polyclonal variety is most ofen due to *Mycoplasma pneumoniae* infection and is most commonly seen in young adults (Pruzanski & Shumak, 1977) but can occur in the elderly. The other conditions associated with it are seen only rarely. On the other hand, the monoc-

Table 8.6 Diseases associated with cold agglutinins

Polyclonal cold agglutinins	Monoclonal cold agglutinins
Mycoplasma pneumonia	Chronic cold agglutinin disease
Rarely:	Waldenström's macroglobulinaemia
Angio-immunoblastic lymphadenopathy	Lymphomas
Collagen vascular and immune complex	Chronic lymphocytic leukaemia
disease	Kaposi's sarcoma
Subacute bacterial endocarditis	Multiple myeloma
Other infections	Mycoplasma pneumonia (rare)

lonal chronic, cold agglutinin disease is predominantly a disease of the elderly, with a peak incidence in the seventh and eighth decades of life (Dacie, 1962; Schubothe, 1966). The cold agglutinins associated with lymphoreticular malignancies are also seen almost exclusively in the elderly (Dacie, 1962).

The clinical manifestations are due to intravascular agglutination of cells or haemolysis (Schubothe, 1966). As blood flows through the capillaries of the skin and subcutaneous tissues, the temperature of the blood may fall to 28°C or even lower. If the cold-reactive antibody is active at this temperature, it agglutinates the cells and fixes complement. Agglutination will obstruct the vasculature, and complement activation may lead to intravascular haemolysis or hepatic sequestration (Pruzanski & Shumak, 1977).

Acrocyanosis, or a striking discoloration of the skin varying from white to a deep blue, results from the intracapillary agglutination of red cells in areas of the body cooled sufficiently to be in the range of the antibody's activity. These colour changes are often accompanied by numbness or pain and are seen most commonly in the distal extremities, the tip of the nose and the earlobes (Nelson & Marshall, 1953). Acrocyanosis may be induced by placing an ice cube in the palm of the hand (Schubothe, 1966).

The chronic haemolytic anaemia in idiopathic cold agglutinin disease is usually of moderate severity and is usually extravascular (Evans et al, 1965). The haemoglobin concentration is commonly maintained above 7 g/dl. In many instances the illness is worse in cold weather. The C_3b inactivator system may be overwhelmed with cold stress or when there is high antibody titre or high thermal reactivity. If the patient develops an acute cold-induced episode of intravascular haemolysis, haemoglobinuria, fever, chills and even renal shutdown can occur. The 'Ehrlich finger test' may be used to demonstrate haemolysis in the cold. A rubber band is placed around a finger to occlude venous return and the finger is dipped in cold water (20°C) for fifteen minutes. A control is done at the same time with another finger kept in water at 37°C. The centrifuged capillary blood from the finger in cold water will be haemolysed, while the blood from the control finger will not.

The patient usually shows no other physical findings other than acrocyanosis, pallor and perhaps mild jaundice. The spleen may be barely palpable and the liver may be slightly enlarged.

The blood shows anaemia, modest reticulocytosis, and perhaps a slight hyperbilirubinaemia. The specific findings for intravascular haemolysis may be present. The blood may agglutinate at room temperature, and the diagnosis is first suspected because of difficulty in performing red cell counts or peripheral smears. The diagnosis is confirmed by demonstrating elevated titres of the cold agglutinins. The antiglobulin test is positive but specific only for complement components, while anti-γ globulin sera give no reaction. Complement levels are low while haemolysis is brisk (Pruzanski & Shumak, 1977).

Treatment of this condition is mainly to advise the patient how to maintain temperatures above that at which the antibody reacts. Blood transfusions are usually not necessary and may even be dangerous, as they can accelerate the haemolysis (Evans et al, 1967). If blood is needed, cross-matching must be carried out at 37°C and the blood should be warmed by an 'in-line' blood warmer (Rosenfield & Jagathambal, 1976). Plasmapheresis to remove the intravascular IgM is useful (as opposed to the warm-reacting IgG auto-antibodies which are extravascular and not removed by this procedure) (Murphy & LoBuglio, 1976). Corticosteroids and splenectomy have not proven beneficial. The experience with cytotoxic drugs has been limited but low-dose chlorambucil (2–4 mg daily) may be useful. To date, maintenance of body warmth and avoidance of cold has proved the best therapy.

Drug-induced immune haemolytic anaemia

The number of reported cases of drug-induced immune haemolytic anaemia is small, but most people believe that it is a more common problem than is usually diagnosed. Particularly in the elderly with superimposed chronic disease, the usual signs and symptoms of haemolysis may be overlooked and the diagnosis missed. In addition, the types of haemolysis induced by drugs give an insight into mechanisms of auto-immune phenomena in general. The types of drug-induced haemolysis are listed in Table 8.7.

In the penicillin type the drug acts as a hapten and binds firmly to the red cell membrane (Petz & Fudenberg, 1966). The antibody produced reacts with the drug itself and not with any other component of the red cell membrane. This type of reaction is uncommon and occurs only when re-latively high doses of penicillin are used, of the order of 20 million units or more for a prolonged period (Petz, 1980). The antibodies are usually IgG, warm-reacting and non-complement-binding, but complement activation has been reported (Ries et al, 1975). This type of absorption reaction has also been seen with cephalosporin therapy but less commonly than with penicillin (Gralnick et al, 1971; Jeannet et al, 1976).

The patients with penicillin-induced haemolysis usually show extra-vascular haemolysis with most of the destruction of red cells occurring in the spleen. The direct antiglobulin test is strongly positive, and if the antibody is eluted it has specificity for penicillin derivatives and not the red cell mem-brane components. Treatment is to stop the penicillin, and haemolysis usual-ly stops in a few days or weeks (Petz, 1980). At times, blood transfusion or corticosteroids may be necessary.

The Stibophen or 'innocent bystander' type of haemolysis occurs with a wide variety of drugs (Table 8.8). In this reaction, antibodies form against the drug and combine with a complex of drug and a soluble macromolecule to form a large antigen–antibody aggregate. This complex then settles out on cell surfaces. Thus, the red cell is an 'innocent bystander', as no antibody is formed against the red cell components nor is there any interaction between the red cell and the drug (Petz & Garratty, 1975). Drug antibodies are IgG or

Table 8.7 Types of drug-induced immune haemolytic anaemias

Prototype Drug	Role of Drug	Antibody Attachment to RBC	Antiglobulin Reaction	Site of Cell Destruction
Penicillin	Hapten bound to RBC	Binds to drug on cell	IgG	Extravascular
Stibophen	Antigen in antigen-antibody complex	Immune complex	Complement	Intravascular
∝-methyldopa	Inhibits suppressor T-cells	Rh site on RBC	IgG	Extravascular
Streptomycin	Hapten bound to RBC	Binds to drug on cell	IgG and complement	Intravascular
Cephalosporins ('pseudohaemolysis')	Serum proteins absorb to RBC; non-immunological	None	IgG	No haemolysis

Table 8.8   Drugs reported to cause the stibophen or'innocent bystander' type of immunohaemolytic anaemia

Stibophen	Isoniazid (INH)
Quinidine	Insecticides
Quinine	Dipyrone
p-aminosalicylic acid	Anhistine
Phenacetin	Antazoline
Sulphonamides	Pyramidon
Sulphonylureas	Ibuprofen
Thiazides	Triamterene
Chlorpromazine	

IgM or both and usually have the ability to bind complement. The haemolytic anaemia that results is, therefore, usually intravascular (Worlledge, 1969).

The dose of drug causing this type of immunohaemolytic anaemia is usually small and the drug must be present to cause haemolysis. The haemolytic anaemia may be very severe and, since it is intravascular, haemoglobinaemia and haemoglobinuria occur. There is a high incidence of renal failure. Leukopenia and thrombocytopenia may be found, and diffuse intravascular haemolysis may also be seen. The direct antiglobulin test is positive, but reagent containing complement must be used. This reaction may remain positive for up to two months after the drug is stopped (Worlledge, 1973).

Treatment is to stop the drug. Steroids are of no use, as the haemolysis is intravascular. Blood transfusions may be needed, but the transfused cells will be destroyed as rapidly as the patient's own cells. The renal failure must be treated properly or death will ensue (Worlledge, 1969).

The haemolytic anaemia caused by α-methyldopa is the most common of the drug-induced immunohaemolytic anaemias. While 15 per cent of all patients who receive the drug will develop a positive direct antiglobulin test, haemolytic anaemia occurs probably in less than 1 per cent (Worlledge, 1969; Petz, 1980).

It is known that α-methyldopa inhibits T-suppressor cells both *in vitro* and *in vivo* (Kirtland et al, 1980). The drug apparently causes a rise in lymphocyte cyclic AMP which is thought then to cause the T-cell abnormalities. It is postulated that this decrease in T-suppressor cells leads to unregulated autoantibody production by a subset of B-cells in some people. Those with HLA-B$_7$ seem to be most at risk. There is also a decrease in total T-cells in patients who develop a positive antiglobulin test while on α-methyldopa (Kirtland et al, 1980).

The positive antiglobulin test apparently does not arise from any reaction between the drug and the red cell membrane. The antibody that forms is often in part directed against an Rh component of the erythrocyte (Worlledge, 1973). In addition, other auto-antibodies are found in patients on α-methyldopa including antinuclear antibodies, rheumatoid factor and anti-gastric mucosa (Worlledge, 1969). It appears that this drug should be used with caution in the elderly, who often show similar auto-immune phenomena (Shenkman et al, 1980).

The antibody produced is an IgG, warm reacting and appears identical to that described in auto-immune haemolytic anaemia of the warm-reactive type. Indeed, many investigators consider that this drug may be the prototype of many other agents that cause auto-immune phenomena by altering the immune system without participating in the immune response directly (Petz, 1980). Other drugs have now been shown also to cause this type of haemolytic anaemia, namely mefenamic acid (Scott et al, 1968) and levodopa (Bernstein, 1979).

Clinically the haemolytic anaemia usually begins 18 weeks to four years after the beginning of treatment with ∝-methyldopa. The course is usually mild to moderate and is similar to that of auto-immune haemolytic anaemia of the warm-reactive antibody type (Worlledge, 1969). Most patients do not require therapy other than discontinuation of the drug. However, death can occur, and blood transfusions may be necessary in those with compromised cardiopulmonary systems.

Immune haemolytic anaemia and renal failure have been reported in patients treated with streptomycin (Martinez et al, 1977). Here the drug seems to act as a hapten binding to the red cell membrane. Haemolysis is due to an IgG-complement fixing antibody that is specific for streptomycin. Intravascular haemolysis results because of the complement fixation. The clinical picture therefore is very similar to that seen with stibophen ('innocent bystander' type) and the treatment would be the same. Discontinuation of the drug is essential (Martinez et al, 1977).

A positive direct antiglobulin test may result from non-specific and non-immune absorption of serum proteins to the red cell. This is commonly seen with cephalothin therpay and does not lead to haemolysis ('pseudohaemolysis'). This type of reaction apparently occurs with other drugs also (Petz, 1980). It is seen in severe megaloblastic anaemia.

Traumatic haemolytic anaemias (red cell fragmentation syndromes)

When erythrocytes are subjected to excessive physical trauma within the cardiovascular system, they may undergo premature fragmentation and haemolysis (Nevaril et al, 1968). This will occur when the shear stress exceeds the elastic limits of the membrane (Grasse-Brockhoff & Gehrman 1967). In these conditions the haemolysis is intravascular and the hallmark is the schistocyte or the fragmented red cell. Schistocytes are fragmented erythrocytes that have sealed off their membrane and will circulate briefly before being removed by the reticuloendothelial system. They will resemble helmet cells, microspherocytes, triangles and crescents (Dameshek, 1964). A classification of these syndromes is given in Table 8.9.

Many cardiovascular abnormalities (Table 10.9) can give rise to intravascular haemolysis. Early red cell death is due mainly to turbulence and secondarily to the direct trauma to the erythrocyte caused by impact on an abnormal natural or artificial vascular structure (Grasse-Brockhoff & Gehrman 1967). Haemolysis rises as patient activity and cardiac output increase. A vicious cycle of greater haemolysis, more severe anaemia, cardiac hyperkinesis and progressive anaemia result.

The severity of the anaemia is variable. The peripheral smear shows fragmentation and reticulocytosis. The signs of intravascular haemolysis are present, and the patient may become iron-deficient and folate-deficient (Santinga et al, 1976). If the anaemia is tolerated by the patient and stable, treatment with iron and folate is all that is necessary. If, however, the patient shows progressive anaemia and cardiovascular compromise, operative intervention is necessary.

Microangiopathic haemolytic anaemia is usually associated either with deposition of fibrin within the microvasculature (Bull et al, 1968; Rubenberg et al, 1968), severe systemic hypertension or vasoconstriction (Venkatachalam et al, 1968). In these conditions red cells are fragmented as they course through a fibrin mesh network under applied pressure or when there is a direct vascular lesion. If the endothelium is inflamed, distorted and proliferating, red cell fragmentation will result as the forceful column of arterial blood moves past red cells attached to the abnormal endothelium (Brain, 1972). Here again diagnosis is made by demonstrating schistocytes and intravascular haemolyis. However, the anaemia is usually not the predominant problem in these conditions and treatment is mainly that of the underlying disease.

In the elderly, microangiopathic haemolytic anaemia is probably most commonly seen with disseminated intravascular coagulation. This may be secondary to sepsis (Rosner & Rubenberg, 1969), malignancies (Antman et

Table 8.9   Classification of the red cell fragmentation syndromes — traumatic haemolytic anaemia

Large vessel and heart disease
  Synthetic valve prostheses
  Valve homografts
  Autograft valvuloplasties
  Ruptured chordae tendinae
  Intracardiac patch repairs
  Valvular disease (unoperated)
  Arteriovenous fistulas
  Coarctation of the aorta

Microangiopathic haemolytic anaemia
  Disseminated intravascular coagulation
  Microangiopathy due to immune mechanisms
  Haemangiomas
  Disseminated carcinomas
  Malignant hypertension
  Pulmonary hypertension
  Others (not usually in the elderly)

  a. Thrombotic thrombocytopenic purpura
  b. Haemolytic–uremic syndrome
  c. Pregnancy

Table 8.10   Substances causing haemolytic anaemia in G6PD deficiency

Analgesics
    Acetanilid
	Sulphones
	    Dapsone
	    Thiazolesulphone

Antibacterials
    Nitrofurantoin
    Nalidixic acid
	Miscellaneous
	    Methylene blue
	    Napthalene

Antimalarials
    Primaquine
    Pamaquine
    Pentaquine
	Niridazole
	    Phenylhydrazine
	    Toluidine blue
	    Trinitotoluene

Sulphonamides
    Sulphanilamide
    Sulphacetamide
    Sulphapyridine
    Sulphamethoxazole	

al, 1979), heat stroke (Stefanini & Spicer, 1971, insertion of pre-clotted vascular grafts (Myers & Hill, 1977), purpura fulminans (Hollingsworth & Mohler, 1968), and immune damage of the microvasculature (Brain, 1970).

'Spur cell' anaemia in liver disease

Spur cells or acanthocytes may be seen in severe hepatocellular disease. The spur cell is a dense, contracted red cell having several irregularly placed 'thorny' projections on its surface. It has fewer projections than 'burr' cells seen in uraemia, and in addition the projections are variable in width and length (Kayden & Bessis, 1970). In liver disease the spur cell is due to an increase in the cholesterol content and the cholesterol/phospholipid ratio of red cell membranes (Cooper et al, 1969). The haemolysis appears to result from the distorted cells becoming trapped by macrophages.

Paroxysmal nocturnal haemoglobinuria

Paroxysmal nocturnal haemoglobinuria (PNH) is an uncommon acquired intrinsic disorder of the red cell membrane characterised by chronic haemolytic anaemia, intermittent or persistent haemoglobinuria and haemosiderinuria, thrombotic phenomena and bone marrow hypoplasia (Dacie, 1963, 1968). It is usually an illness first diagnosed in the third to fifth decade of life but can occur in the elderly (Dacie, 1967; Dacie & Lewis, 1972).

PNH is thought to evolve from a defective bone marrow stem cell clone producing at least three red cell populations that vary in their sensitivity to activated complement components (Rosse, 1972; 1973; 1980). Increased complement susceptibility is greatest among the young circulating erythrocytes (Hinz et al, 1956).

The clinical course is quite variable from a mild benign course to a severe aggressive one (Dacie, 1967; Dacie & Lewis, 1972). In the classic form the patients will haemolyse when they sleep (nocturnal haemoglobinuria). This may be due to mild reduction of blood pH at night. Only about 25 per cent of patients, however, have haemoglobinuria, and many of these do not have it at night. In the majority of cases the illness usually presents with signs and symptoms of anaemia. Haemolytic episodes may follow infection, strenuous exercise, surgery, menstruation, blood transfusion and therapeutic ingestion of iron. Often, the haemolysis is associated with bone and muscle aching, malaise and fever (Dacie & Lewis, 1972). The patient usually has pallor, jaundice, bronzing of the skin and moderate splenomegaly. Many patients complain of difficulty or painful swallowing (Rosse, 1980), and spontaneous intravascular haemolysis and infections are common (Peytermann et al, 1972).

PNH is also associated with aplastic anaemia (Gardner & Blum, 1967), preleukaemia, myeloproliferative disorders and acute myelogenous leukaemia. The finding of splenomegaly in a patient with aplastic anaemia should alert the clinician that the patient may have PNH (Rosse, 1980).

These is usually severe anaemia with haemoglobin levels of 6 g/dl or less. Leukopenia and thrombocytopenia are common (Rosse, 1980). Peripheral smear is usually normocytic but accordingly shows anisocytosis and the microcytic, hypochromic cells of iron deficiency secondary to the prolonged haemosiderinuria (Rosse & Gutterman, 1970). The reticulocyte count is high, except in those with accompanying marrow failure. The bone marrow is usually initially hyperplastic, but hypoplasia and even aplasia may develop during the course of the illness.

The neutrophil alkaline phosphatase level is low to absent (Lewis & Dacie, 1965). The parameters of intravascular haemolysis may all be present, but haemosiderinuria is usually severe and leads to iron deficiency. In addition, the chronic haemosiderinuria leads to renal tubular iron deposition and proximal tubular dysfunction (Clark et al, 1981). The antiglobulin test is usually negative (Dacie, 1967).

The diagnosis should be considered in any patient with a puzzling haemolytic anaemia, iron deficiency, combined iron and folate deficiency, pancytopenia, splenomegaly and thrombotic episodes. The diagnostic tests are the 'Ham' test (Ham, 1939) and the sucrose water test (Hartmann et al, 1970). In these tests, the red cell resistance to small amounts of complement is challenged.

Treatment is symptomatic, as there is no cure for the illness. If blood transfusions are necessary, saline-washed (Dacie, 1948) or preferably thawed frozen deglycerolised packed cells (Gockerman & Brouillard, 1977) should be used, as fresh donor plasma may accelerate haemolysis. Iron treatment is usually tolerated well, but it sometimes may precipitate haemolysis (Hartmann et al, 1966). Iron often given after transfusion has suppressed erythropoiesis (Hartmann & Kolhouse, 1972). High doses of corticosteroids have reportedly helped some patients (Firken et al, 1968). Androgen therapy may be useful (Rosse, 1980). Anticoagulation is useful following surgery, but has not proven useful on a long-term basis (Hartmann & Kolhouse, 1972). Some investigators have been reported haemolytic episodes being precipitated by heparin (Crosby, 1953). Splenectomy is of no proven use and carries a high morbidity.

INHERITED HEMOLYTIC DISORDERS

These disorders are usually, but not alway, diagnosed in younger subjects. Standard textbooks of haematology review these syndromes in detail.

One condition though that should be kept in mind in the elderly is glucose-6-phosphate dehydrogenase (G6PD) deficiency. This condition is asymptomatic until the patient is exposed to an infection, drug, fava beans or various illnesses such as acidosis, renal disease, uraemia and diabetic coma (Burka et al, 1966).

Glucose-6-phosphate dehydrogenase is the first enzyme in the hexose monophosphate shunt which generates NADPH for the maintenance of glutathione. It thus serves as the mechanism that prevents oxidative denaturation of intracellular and membrane components of the erthrocyte (Carson et al, 1956).

G6PD deficiency causes a hereditary, sex-linked haemolytic anaemia (Kirkman & Hendrickson, 1963) which occurs under oxidative stress. The defect is due to a coded gene on the X-chromosome and is completely expressed in male homozygotes, observed in rare female homozygotes, but, uncommonly may be expressed in female heterozygotes. About 10 per cent of American blacks and 8–20% of West African blacks harbour the deficiency (Burka et al, 1966).

There are over a hundred forms of G6PD isoenzymes described, but only a few have clinical significance (Beutler, 1978). The normal enzyme (GdB+) represents the 100 per cent standard activity. It is present in over 99 per cent of all whites and about 70 per cent of normal blacks. GdA+ is another normal variant and is present in 30 per cent of normal blacks. GdA− is the most frequent clinically significant abnormal form in blacks, and the enzyme activity is reduced to about 25 per cent of the normal. GdA− is relatively unstable, and the activity diminishes with cell ageing (Piomelli et al, 1968). The intracellular red cell enzyme concentration is therefore usually only 5–15 per cent of normal, with the reticulocytes having most activity and the oldest cell very little, if any.

The most common abnormal variant in whites is Gd Mediterranean. This enzyme concentration is less than 1 per cent of normal, which results in a mild subclinical haemolytic state in affected people. Overt haemolysis in all types usually occurs only when there is stress (Beutler, 1978). The most common stress probably is infection but the next in importance in exposure to drugs (Gordon-Smith, 1980) (Table 8.10). Although drugs are often implicated, the haemolysis might have been due to the stress of the illness for which they prescribed. Some drugs given in therapeutic amounts may cause a very mild and clinically insignificant haemolysis.

Clinically, in GdA− the patient is normal until exposed to stress. There will then be an acute intravascular haemolytic event which will last about one week, even if the precipitating event persists (Dern et al, 1954). This is because the recticulocytes and young red cells contain enough enzyme activity to resist haemolysis (Piomelli et al, 1968). The blood will then return to normal and the patient will have a compensated haemolytic state.

In the Gd-Mediterranean variety the haemolysis is more severe, as greater numbers of the red cells are susceptible to haemolysis (Pannacciulli et al, 1969). Because of the massive intravascular haemolysis, death can occur.

Diagnosis is made by demonstrating impaired enzyme activity. Assay should not be done when there are many young cells, as these contain enough activity to give a 'normal' result (Piomelli et al, 1969). One can circumvent this by only assaying old cells separated by differential sedimentation or by waiting until the haemolysis is over.

Treatment is, of course, to stop and avoid the offending stress or agent. If there is only a mild haemolytic state, the drug may be continued. In severe cases or if there is cardiovascular compromise, blood transfusions are necessary.

REFERENCES

Antman K H, Skarin A T, Mayer R J, Hargreaves H K, Canellos G P 1979 Microangiopathic hemolytic anaemia and cancer: a review. Medicine 58: 377–384

Atkinson J A, Frank M M 1974 Studies on the *in vivo* effects of antibody: interaction of IgM antibody and complement in the immune clearance and destruction of erythrocytes in man. Journal of Clinical Investigation 54: 339–348

Bernstein A M 1979 Reversible hemolytic anaemia after levodopa-carbidopa. British Medical Journal 1: 1461–1462

Beutler E 1978 Hemolytic anemia. In: Disorders of red cell metabolism. Plenum, New York

Brain M C 1970 Microangiopathic hemolytic anaemia. Annals of Internal Medicine 21: 133–144

Brain M C 1972 Microangiopathic haemolytic anaemia. British Journal of Haematology 23 (supplement): 45–52

Brus I, Lewis S M 1959 The haptoglobin content of serum in haemolytic anaemia. British Journal of Haematology 5: 348–355

Bull B S, Rubenberg M L, Dacie J V, Brain M C 1968 Microangiopathic haemolytic anaemia: mechanisms of red cell fragmentation: *in vitro* studies. British Journal of Haematology 14: 643–652

Burka E R, Weaver Z III, Marks P A 1966 Clinical spectrum of hemolytic anaemia associated with glucose-6-phosphate dehydrogenase deficiency. Annals of Internal Medicine 64: 817–825

Carlson D J, Shapiro F L 1970 Methemoglobinemia from well water nitrates — a complication of hemodialysis. Annals of Internal Medicine 73: 757–759

Carson P E, Flanagan C L, Ickes C E, Alving A S 1956 Enzymatic deficiency in primaquine sensitive erythrocytes. Science 124: 484–485

Chaplin H Jr 1973 Clinical usefulness of specific antiglobulin reagents in autoimmune hemolytic anemia. Progress in Hematology 8: 25–49

Christensen B E 1973 The pattern of erythrocyte sequestration in immunohaemolysis. Scandinavian Journal of Haematology 10: 120–129

Clark D A, Butler S A, Broren V, Hartmann R C, Jenkins D E Jr 1981 The kidneys in paroxysmal nocturnal hemoglobinuria. Blood 57: 83–89

Condrea E, Mammon Z, Aloof S, DeVries A 1964 Susceptibility of erythrocytes of various animal species to the hemolytic and phospholipid splitting action of snake venom. Biochimica et Biophysica Acta 84: 365–375

Coombs R R A, Mourant A E, Race R R 1945 A new test for detection of weak and incomplete Rh agglutinins. British Journal of Experimental Pathology 26: 255–266

Cooper R A 1969 Anaemia with spur cells: a red cell defect acquired in serum and modified in the circulation. Journal of Clinical Investigation 48: 1820–1831

Crosby W H 1953 PNH: relation of the clinical manifestations to underlying pathogenic mechanisms. Blood 8: 769–812

Crosby W H, Dameshek W 1951 The significance of hemoglobinemia and associated hemosiderinuria, with particular reference to various types of hemolytic anemia. Journal of Laboratory and Clinical Medicine 38: 829–841

Dacie J V 1948 Transfusion of saline-washed red cells in nocturnal hemoglobinuria. Clinical Science 7: 65–75

Dacie J V 1950 The presence of cold hemolysins in sera containing cold hemagglutinins. Journal of Pathology 62: 241–257

Dacie J V 1962 The haemolytic anaemias, congenital and acquired, part II, 2nd edn. Churchill, London

Dacie J V 1963 Paroxysmal nocturnal haemoglobinuria. Proceedings of the Royal Society of Medicine 56: 587–596

Dacie J V 1967 The hemolytic anemias, congenital and acquired, part IV, Grune & Stratton, New York

Dacie J V 1968 Paroxysmal nocturnal hemoglobinuria: an acquired disorder of the red cell membrane. Proceedings of the XII Congress of the International Society of Hematology, New York, 102–112

Dacie J V, Worlledge S M 1969 Autoimmune hemolytic anemias. Progress in Hematology 6: 82–120

Dacie J V, Lewis S M 1972 Paroxysmal nocturnal haemoglobinuria: clinical manifestations, hematology and nature of the disease. Series Haematologica 5: 3–23

Dameshek W 1964 Case records of the Massachusetts General Hospital, Case 52–1964. New England Journal of Medicine 271: 898–905

Dern R J, Beutler E, Alving A S 1954 The hemolytic effect of primaquine. Journal of Laboratory and Clinical Medicine 43: 303–309; 44: 171–176; 176–184; 439–442

Eaton J W, Kolpin C F, Swoffard H S, Kgellstrand C M, Jacob H S 1973 Chlorinated urban water: a cause of dialysis-induced hemolytic anemia. Science 181: 463–464

Evans R S, Bingham M, Turner E 1965 Autoimmune hemolytic disease: observations of serological reactions and disease activity. Annals of the New York Academy of Science 124: 422–440

Evans R S, Turner E, Bingham M 1967 Chronic hemolytic anemia due to cold agglutinins. Journal of Clinical Investigation 46: 95–138

Forshaw J, Hardwood L 1963 Folic acid deficiency in haemolytic anaemia. Postgraduate Medical Journal 39: 661–662

Firkin F, Goldberg H and Firkin B G 1968 Glucocorticoid management of paroxysmal nocturnal haemoglobinuria. Australian Annals of Medicine 17: 127–134

Fowler B A, Weissberg J B 1974 Arsine poisoning. New England Journal of Medicine 291: 1171–1174

Frank M M, Schreiber A D, Atkinson J P, Jaffe C J 1977 Pathophysiology of immune hemolytic anemia. Annals of Internal Medicine 87: 210–222

Freedman M L 1982 Anemias in the elderly: Is it physiologic or pathologic? Hospital Practice 17: 121–136

Gardner F H, Blum S F 1967 Aplastic anemia in PNH: mechanisms and therapy. Seminars in Hematology 4: 250–264

Gockerman J P, Brouillard R P 1977 RBC transfusions in paroxysmal nocturnal hemoglobinuria. Archives of Internal Medicine 137: 536–538

Goldberg A, Hutchison H E, MacDonald E 1966 Radiochromium in the selection of patients with haemolytic anaemia for splenectomy. Lancet 1: 109–113

Gordon-Smith EC 1980 Drug-induced oxidative haemolysis. Clinics in Haematology 9: 557–586

Gralnick H R, McGinnis M, Elton W, McCurdy P 1971 Hemolytic anemia associated with cephalothin. Journal of the American Medical Association 217: 1193–1197

Grasse-Brockhoff F, Gehrman G 1967 Mechanical hemolysis in patients with valvular heart disease and valve prosthesis. American Heart Journal 74: 137–139

Ham T H 1939 Studies on the destruction of red blood cells. I. Chronic hemolytic anemia with paroxysmal nocturnal hemoglobinuria: An investigation of the mechanism of hemolysis with observations in five cases. Archives of Internal Medicine 64: 1271–1305

Ham T H 1955 Hemoglobinuria. American Journal of Medicine 18: 990–1006

Hartmann R C, Jenkins D E Jr, McKee L C, Heyssel R M 1966 Paroxysmal nocturnal hemoglobinuria: clinical and laboratory studies relating to iron metabolism and therapy with androgens and iron. Medicine 45: 331–363

Hartmann R C, Jenkins D E Jr, Arnold A B 1970 Diagnostic specificity of sucrose hemolysis test for paroxysmal nocturnal hemoglobinuria. Blood 35: 462–475

Hartmann R C, Kolhouse J F 1972 Viewpoints on the management of PNH. Series Haematologica 5(3): 42–60

Hedge U M, Gordon-Smith E C, Worlledge S M 1977 Reticulocytopenia and 'absence' of red cell autoantibodies in immune haemolytic anaemia. British Medical Journal 2: 1444–1447

Hinz C F Jr, Jordan W S, Pillener L 1956 The properdin system and immunity: IV. The hemolysis of erythrocytes from patients with paroxysmal nocturnal hemoglobinuria. Journal of Clinical Investigation 35: 453–457

Hollingsworth J M, Mohler D N 1968 Microangiopathic hemolytic anemia caused by purpura fulminans. Annals of Internal Medicine 68: 1310–1314

Ikezawa H, Murata R 1964 Comparative kinetics of hemolysis of mammalian erythrocytes by clostridium perfringens $\propto$-toxin (phosphlipase C). Journal of Biochemistry 55: 217–224

Issit P D, Pavone B G, Goldfinger D, Zwicker H, Issit C H, Tessel J A, Kroovand S W, Bell C A 1976 Anti-Wr[b] and other autoantibodies responsible for positive direct antiglobulin tests in 150 individuals. British Journal of Haematology 34: 5–18

Jacobs H S, Amsden T 1971 Acute hemolytic anemia with rigid red cells in hypophosphatemia. New England Journal of Medicine 285: 1446–1450

Jeannet M, Bloch A, Doyer J M, Forquet J J, Gerard J P, Cruchaud A 1976 Cephalothin-induced immune hemolytic anemia. Acta Haematologica 55: 109–117

Jones S E 1973 Autoimmune disorders and malignant lymphomas. Cancer 31: 1092–1098

Kaden B R, Rosse W F, Hauch T W 1979 Immune thrombocytopenia in lymphoproliferative diseases. Blood 53: 545–551

Kayden H J, Bessis M 1970 Morphology of normal erythrocytes and acanthocytes using Nomasski optics and the scanning electron microscope. Blood 35: 427–436

Kirkman H N, Hendrickson E M 1963 Sex-linked electrophoretic difference in glucose-6-phosphate dehydrogenase. American Journal of Human Genetics 15: 241–258

Kirtland H H III, Mohler D N, Horowitz D A 1980 Methyldopa inhibition of suppressor-lymphocyte function: a proposed cause of autoimmune hemolytic anaemia. New England Journal of Medicine 302: 825–832

Klock J C, Williams, H E, Mentzer W C 1974 Hemolytic anemia and somatic cell dysfunction in severe hypophosphatemia. Archives of Internal Medicine 134: 360–364

Lalezari, P 1976 Serologic profile in autoimmune hemolytic disease: pathophysiologic and clinical interpretations. Seminars in Hematology 13: 291–310

Landsteiner E K, Finch C A 1947 Hemoglobinemia accompanying transurethral resection of the prostate. New England Journal of Medicine 237: 310–312

Lewis S M, Dacie J V 1965 Neutrophil (leukocyte) alkaline phosphatase in paroxysmal nocturnal haemoglobinuria. British Journal of Haematology 11: 549–556

Logue G L, Rosse W F, Gockerman J P 1973 Measurement of the third component of complement bound to red cells in patients with the cold agglutinin syndrome. Journal of Clinical Investigation 52: 493–501

Lynn K L, Boots M A, Mitchell T R 1979 Haemolytic anaemia caused by overheated dialysate. British Medical Journal 1: 306–307

Martinez J, Letona L, Barbolla E, Frieyro E, Bouza E, Gilsanz F, Fernandez M N 1977 Immune haemolytic anaemia and renal failure induced by streptomycin. British Journal of Haematology 35: 561–571

Mollison, P L, Hugh-Jones N C 1967 Clearance of Rh-positive red cells by low concentrations of Rh antibody. Immunology 12: 63–73

Mollison P L 1970 The role of complement in antibody-mediated red cell destruction. British Journal of Haematology 18: 249–255

Morgan E S, Leddy J P, Atwater E C, Barnett E V 1967 Direct antiglobulin (Coombs) reaction in patients with connective tissue disorders. Arthritis and Rheumatism 10: 502–508

Müller-Eberhard U 1970 Hemopexin. New England Journal of Medicine 283: 1090–1094

Murphy S, LoBuglio A F 1976 Drug therapy in autoimmune hemolytic anemia. Seminars in Hematology 13: 323–334

Myers T J, Hild D H 1977 Consumption coagulopathy and microangiopathic hemolytic anemia with an axillo-femoral graft. Circulation 56: 891–893

Nance W E 1961 Hemolytic anemia of necrotic arachnidism. American Journal of Medicine 31: 801–807

Nelson M G, Marshall R J 1953 The syndrome of high titre cold haemagglutination. British Medical Journal 2: 314–317

Nevaril C G, Lynch E C, Alfrey D P Jr, Hellums J D 1968 Erythrocyte damage and destruction induced by shearing stress. Journal of Laboratory and Clinical Medicine 71: 784–790

Orringer E P, Mattern W D 1976 Formaldehyde-induced hemolysis during chronic hemodialysis. New England Journal of Medicine 294: 1416–1420

Oski F 1970 Chickee the copper. Annals of Internal Medicine 73: 485–486

Pannacciulli I, Salvidio E, Tizianello A, Parravidino G 1969 Hemolytic effects of standard single dosages of primaquine and chloroquine in G6PD deficient Caucasians. Journal of Laboratory and Clinical Medicine 74: 653–661

Petz L D, Fudenberg H H 1966 Coombs-positive hemolytic anemia caused by penicillin administration. New England Journal of Medicine 274: 171–178

Petz L D, Garratty G 1975 Drug-induced haemolytic anaemia. Clinics in Haematology 4: 181–197

Petz L D 1980 Drug-induced immune haemolytic anaemia. Clinics in Haematology 9: 455–482

Peytermann R, Rhodes R S, Hartmann R C 1972 Thrombosis in paroxysmal nocturnal haemoglobinuria with particular reference to progressive, diffuse hepatic venous thrombosis. Series Haematologica 5: 115–136

Piomelli S, Corash L M, Davenport D D, Miraglia J, Amorosi E L 1968. *In vivo* lability of glucose-6-phosphate dehydrogenase in GdA− and Gd Mediterranean deficiency. Journal of Clinical Investigation 47: 940–948

Pirofsky B 1976 Clinical aspects of autoimmune hemolytic anemia. Seminars in Hematology 13: 251–265

Pruzanski W, Shumak, K H 1977 Biologic activity of cold reactive autoantibodies. New England Journal of Medicine 297: 538–542: 583–589

Rath C E 1953 Drowning hemoglobinuria. Blood 8: 1099–1104

Reynafarje C, Rasmos J 1961 The hemolytic anemia of human bartonellosis. Blood 17: 562–578

Ries C A, Rosenbaum T J, Garratty G, Petz L D, Fudenberg H H 1975 Pencillin-induced immune haemolytic anaemia. Journal of the American Medical Association 233: 432–435

Rosenfield R E, Jagathamal 1976 Transfusion therapy for autoimmune hemolytic disease. Seminars in Hematology 13: 311–321

Rosner F, Rubenberg M L 1969 Erythrocyte fragmentation in consumption coagulopathy. New England Journal of Medicine 280: 219–220

Rosse W F 1972 The complement sensitivity of PNH cells. Series Haematologica 5: 101–114

Rosse W F 1973 Variations in the red cells in paroxysmal nocturnal haemoglobinuria. British Journal of Haematology 24: 327–342

Rosse W F 1980 Paroxysmal nocturnal hemoglobinuria — present status and future projects. Western Journal of Medicine 132: 219–228

Rosse W F, Gutterman L A 1970 The effect of iron therapy in paroxysmal nocturnal hemoglobinuria. Blood 36: 559–565

Rosse, W F, Adams J, Logue G 1977 Hemolysis by complement and cold reactive antibodies: time and temperature results. American Journal of Hematology 2: 259–270

Rubenberg M L, Regoeczi E, Bull B S, Dacie J V, Brain M C 1968 Microangiopathic haemolytic anaemia: the experimental production of haemolysis and red cell fragmentation by defibrination *in vivo*. British Journal of Haematology 14: 627–642

Santinga J T, Batsakis J T, Flora J D, Kirsh M M 1976 Hemolysis in the aortic prosthetic valve. Chest 69: 56–61

Schubothe H 1965 Current problems of chronic cold hemagglutinin disease. Annals of the New York Academy of Science 124: 484–490

Schubothe H 1966 The cold hemagglutinin disease. Seminars in Hematology 3: 27–47

Scott C L, Myles A B, Bacon P A 1968 Autoimmune haemolytic anaemia and mefenamic acid therapy. British Medical Journal 3: 534–535

Sears D A, Anderson P R, Fay A L, Williams H L, Crosby W H 1966 Urinary iron excretion and renal metabolism of hemoglobin in hemolytic disease. Blood 28: 708–725

Shen S C, Ham T H, Fleming E M 1943 Studies on the destruction of red blood cells. III. Mechanism and complication of hemoglobinuria in patients with thermal burns: spherocytosis and increased osmotic fragility of red blood cells. New England Journal of Medicine 229: 701–713

Shenkman L, Freedman M L, Finkelstein M S, Nadel H, Marcus D L 1980 Immune function in an ambulatory geriatric population. Clinical Research 28: 360

Stefanini M, Spicer D D 1971 Hemostatic breakdown, fibrinolysis and acquired hemolytic anemia in a patient with fatal heat stroke. American Journal of Clinical Pathology 55: 180–186

Venkatachalam M A, Jones D B, Nelson D A 1968 Microangiopathic hemolytic anaemia in rats with malignant hypertension. Blood 32: 278–291

Vos G H, Petz L D, Fudenberg H H 1971 Specificity and immunoglobulin characteristics of autoantibodies in acquired hemolytic anemia. Journal of Immunology 106: 1172–1176

Waldmann T A, Blaese R M, Broder S, Krakauer R S 1978 Disorders of suppressor immunoregulatory cells in the pathogenesis of immunodeficiency and autoimmunity. Annals of Internal Medicine 88: 226–238

Wallerstein, R O Aggeler P M 1964 Acute hemolytic anemia. American Journal of Medicine 37: 92–104

Wintrobe M M, Lee G R, Boggs D R, Bithell T C, Foerster J, Athens J W, Lukens J N 1981 The hemolytic disorders. In: Clinical Hematology, 8th edn. Lea & Febiger, Philadelphia, ch 29, p 734–754

Woodruff A W, Ansdell V E, Pettitt L E 1979 Cause of anaemia in malaria. Lancet i: 1055–1957

Worlledge S 1969 Immune drug-induced hemolytic anemias. Seminars in Hematology 6: 181–200

Worlledge S M 1973 Immune drug-induced hemolytic anemia. Seminars in Hematology 10: 327–344

Bleeding and coagulation disorders

PHYSIOLOGY OF HAEMOSTASIS

The process of haemostasis involves protecting blood floow through a virtually closed circuit of blood vessels at various pressures and re-establishing vascular patency if any segments become occluded. Haemostatic reactions can be classified into several overlapping and sequential events: localised vasoconstriction at the site of injury, platelet adhesion to exposed subendothelial basement membrane and collagen fibres, formation of a platelet aggregate or plug, activation of the coagulation cascade leading to formation of fibrin which reinforces the platelet plug, and finally activation of the fibrinolytic system which digests the haemostatic plug and allows growth of new vascular endothelial cells to complete the repair process (Sixma & Wester, 1977). Also a complex system of physiological inhibitors and feedback control mechanisms exists to control and limit any excessive or inappropriate activation of the haemostatic system (Bennett, 1977).

Following injury vasoconstriction is transient, lasting less than one minute and seems to have little influence on the rate of bleeding. The lumen is not even reduced below two-thirds of its original diameter. The mechanism of vasoconstriction is unclear but is probably related to neurogenic contraction of the vessel wall and the release of various humoral substances, such as serotonin and thromboxane A_2 from activated platelets.

The various blood components are not activated to any significant extent by the healthy vascular endothelial surface. Following vessel wall damage the subsequent interactions with circulating platelets are summarised in Figure 9.1. When the vessel wall is damaged, subendothelial structures are exposed, including basement membrane collagen and microfibrils. Circulating platelets react with exposed collagen fibres and adhere to the damaged surface aided by fibronectin and high molecular weight multimers of the factor VIII complex coating the platelet surface. The factor VIII complex consists of the factor VIII von Willebrand factor (VIIIvWf) which participates in the initial adhesion of circulating platelets to damaged subendothelial structures (Zimmerman & Ruggeri, 1983). The protein is synthesised in vascular endothelial cells and megakaryocytes and is present in normal

Damaged vessel wall

↓

Platelet adhesion and plasma VIIIvWf multimers inferaction

↓

Activation of platelet membrane receptors

↓

Platelet shape change and aggregation

↓

Platelet activation proceeds by:
1. Arachidonic acid metabolism
2. Increase of free cytoplasmic calcium ions
3. Release of PAF

↓

Release of granule contents

↓

Irreversible aggregate formed

↓

Flip-flop of outer membrane
promotes coagulation cascade

Fig. 9.1   Platelet involvement in the haemostatic process (Vermylen et al, 1983)

platelets. The VIIIvWf protein consists of subunits with a M.W. of approximately 200 000–240 000 which readily form dimers and subsequently large multimers with molecular weights ranging up to 20 million. It is the large multimeric forms of VIIIvWf with a M.W. in excess of 8 million in plasma which are essential for platelet adhesion to the damaged vessel wall.

In areas of non-linear blood flow, such as at the site of an injured vessel wall or atherosclerotic plaque, locally damaged red cells release adenosine-5-diphosphate (ADP), which further activates platelets and induces adhesion (Born et al, 1976).

Platelets circulate as non-nucleated discs and consist of a trilaminar phospholipoprotein membrane with submembrane circumferential contractile filaments, three types of granules and an irregular internal network of canaliculi whereby the granule contents can be released onto the platelet surface.

Following adhesion of a single layer of platelets to the damaged vascular endothelium, platelets stick to one another and form aggregates. Certain substances react with specific platelet membrane surface receptors and initiate platelet aggregation and further activation. These include exposed collagen fibres, ADP released from damaged red cells and other aggregated platelets, adrenaline, serotonin, thrombin and certain arachidonic acid metabolites including thromboxane A_2 (TXA_2). Upon the initiation of aggregation, platelets immediately change shape losing their discoid appearance and form tiny spheres with numerous projecting pseudopods.

Human platelet aggregation may be activated by at least two and possibly three independent but related pathways. The first pathway of activation concerns arachidonic acid metabolism (Smith, 1981). Activation of phospholipase enzymes releases free arachidonic acid from the membrane phospholipids. Approximately 50 per cent of free arachidonic acid is converted initially by a lipoxygenase enzyme to a series of products including various leukotrienes which probably play very little role in the control of haemostasis. The remaining arachidonic acid is converted by the enzyme cyclo-oxygenase into the cyclic endoperoxides, PGG_2 and PGH_2, which are very labile products. Most of the endoperoxides are then rapidly converted by the thromboxane synthetase enzyme complex into thromboxane A_2 (TXA_2). TXA_2 has profound biological activity causing platelet granule release, local vasoconstriction and stimulating other platelets to aggregate locally.

Platelet granules are composed of three distinct groups — dense granules which release ADP, ATP and serotonin; alpha granules which release several constituents including a smooth-muscle stimulating factor, platelet factor 4 with heparin neutralising ability, beta thromboglobulin, factor VIIIRAg, factor V and fibrinogen; and lysosomal granules. The release of these various granule contents further support platelet aggregate formation. TXA_2 is a very labile product, with a half-life *in vivo* of approximately 45 seconds before being degraded to the inactive compounds thromboxane B_2 (TXB_3) and malondialdehyde. A small proportion of the cyclic endoperoxides are converted to the primary prostaglandins, PGE_2, PGD_2, and $PGF_2\propto$. Platelet arachidonic acid metabolism is summarised in Figure 9.2.

The second pathway of platelet activation is completely independent of arachidonic acid metabolism and thromboxane A_2 generation. Various platelet activators, including thrombin and collagen, bring about a sudden increase in the amount of free cytoplasmic calcium (White, 1980). Calcium is released from the dense tubular system and forms a complex with calmodulin, and the calcium–calmodulin complex acts as a co-enzyme in a series of platelet reactions. It initiates granule release, liberates arachidonic acid from the membrane phospholipids so it is available for conversion into thromboxane A_2 and activates the actomyosin contractile system of filaments beneath the platelet membrane.

The third pathway involves the release of a lysolecithin compound called PAF (platelet activating factor) from the platelet membrane phospholipids which seems to activate platelets independently of thromboxane A_2 generation and calcium release (Chignard et al, 1980). The actual importance of PAF activation of human platelets has not been fully determined.

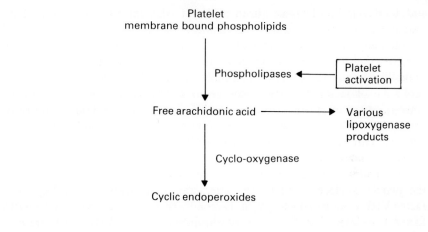

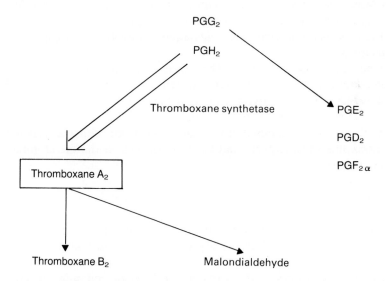

Fig. 9.2   Platelet arachidonic acid metabolism

The aggregating platelets align together into initially a rather loose reversible aggregate, but following the release reaction of the platelet granule constituents a larger interdigitating irreversible plug is formed. Changes in the platelet membrane configuration now occur which involves a flip-flop arrangement of the membrane surface so that certain coagulation reactions may proceed considerably faster on the platelet surface (Zwaal & Hemker, 1982).

The coagulation mechanism, which consists of a multicomponent enzyme system of pro-enzymes, co-factors and inhibitors, is activated by contact with the negatively charged damaged endothelial surface (the intrinsic pathway) and local release of tissue thromboplastin (the extrinsic pathway). The coagulation reaction is shown schematically in Figure 9.3. The complex interaction of factor XII and high molecular-weight kininogen, which are adsorbed onto the negatively charged endothelial surface, and the binding of prekallikrein and factor XI to high molecular-weight kininogen leads to the activation of factor XI (Thompson et al, 1977). Then follows a series of conversions of inert precursors into active serine proteases leading to fibrin formation. Diffusion of tissue juices into the circulation will activate the extrinsic pathways by converting factor VII into factor VIIa, which subsequently activates factor X.

Two main clotting reactions are accelerated by phospholipid micelles on the platelet surface — firstly the interaction of activated factor IXa with factor VIII to activate factor X, and secondly that of activated factor Xa with factor V to form thrombin from prothrombin. Factors VIII and V are not serine proteases but play a role in orienting clotting factors on the platelet surface so as to accelerate proteolysis of factor X and prothrombin respectively. Platelets may also actually trigger coagulation by directly activating factor XI and factor X.

Following thrombin formation, fibrinogen is cleaved to form fibrin monomers. These monomers polymerise to form a weak fibrin clot which is stabilised by factor XIII activity. Thrombin further reinforces the haemostatic mechanism by increasing factor VIII and V activity and causing platelet activation. Finally the stabilised fibrin clot intertwines with the platelet clump, entrapping some red cells and forms a firm plug at the site of initial vessel wall damage.

Once the haemostatic mechanism outlined above has been activated, it is important that the reaction should be limited to the initial damaged area and that subsequent repair should be initiated with eventual regrowth of healthy endothelial cells. The digestion of the fibrin clot depends on activation of the fibrinolytic enzyme system which is shown schematically in Figure 9.4.

Plasminogen circulates as an inactive pro-enzyme and is converted by various different activators to the active serine protease, plasmin. Several different pathways of plasminogen activation exist.

Vascular activator, which is released by vascular endothelial cells into the bloodstream, is the main physiological activator, and higher levels are released by various stimuli such as venous occlusion, vaso-active agents, exercise and hyperpyrexia. Tissue activator, particularly rich in the uterus and prostate, is not normally released into the bloodstream but becomes available locally after extensive trauma and extravascular fibrin deposition. The renal parenchymal cells synthesise and release a urinary activator, urokinase, which is excreted continuously in the urine and is probably important in maintaining patency of the urinary tract. Other activating systems include a factor XII-mediated pathway which follows activation of the intrinsic coagulation system and is interrelated with co-activation of kallikrein–kinin and complement systems (Stormorken, 1977).

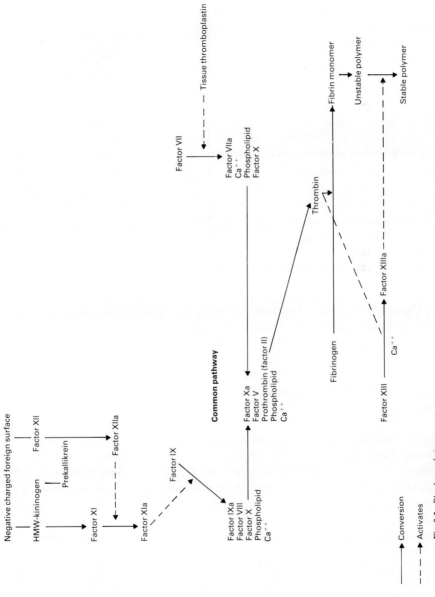

Fig. 9.3 Blood coagulation process

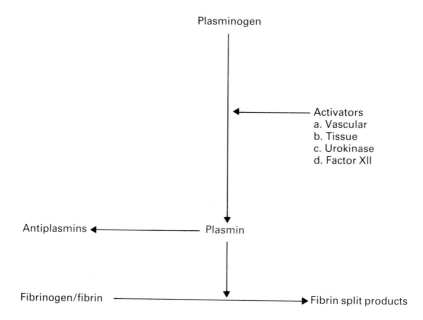

Fig. 9.4   The fibrinolytic sysem (Gaffney, 1981)

Physiological levels of plasma activators are rapidly inactivated by anti-activators and are also degraded in the liver. Only at the site of thrombus formation is plasminogen converted to plasmin in appreciable amounts. Any plasmin that is released into the general circulation is rapidly inactivated by complex formation with antiplasmins (Collen, 1980). Plasmin hydrolyses fibrin into soluble split products and brings about gradual thrombus dissolution.

To prevent uncontrolled activity in blood of the large number of interrelated reactions leading to fibrin formation, a powerful natural system of coagulation inhibitors exists. Antithrombin III is the major inhibitor of thrombin but also inhibits activated factor IXa, Xa, XIa, kallikrein and plasmin (Seegers, 1978). Heparin binds to antithrombin III and alters its molecular configuration so that inhibition of thrombin and factor Xa in particular are markedly accelerated (Rosenberg, 1978). The other main plasma thrombin inhibitors are alpha$_2$-macroglobulin and alpha$_2$-antitrypsin. A recently described vitamin-K dependent protein, protein C, inactivates factors V and VIII and thus probably also prevents excess thrombin generation (Esmon, 1983). As well as these inhibitory agents it seems likely that both coagulation pathways can control their own activity to some extent by a series of feedback mechanisms.

Platelets do not adhere to undamaged endothelial cells, and in the last decade it has been shown that vascular endothelial cells play an important role in the control of the haemostatic process (Thorgeirsson & Robertson, 1978). Endothelial cells synthesise prostacyclin from arachidonic acid which when released into the circulation causes local vasodilation and is the most potent known natural inhibitor of platelet adhesion and aggregation (Whittle & Moncada, 1983). Prostacyclin probably does not circulate in biological quantities but is released locally when the vessel wall is stressed or injured so as to control any excessive platelet activation. Upon binding to specific platelet membrane receptors it activates membrane-bound adenylate cyclase which produces increased levels of cAMP. This inhibits platelet aggregation by inhibiting arachidonic acid metabolism and internal calcium flux. The endothelial cells also synthesise plasminogen activator, a heparin-like anti-coagulant, and possess a thrombin-induced binding site for protein C. All these processes control interactions between the blood and vessel wall and thus help to maintain vascular integrity and patency.

CLINICAL AND LABORATORY APPROACH TO HAEMOSTATIC DISORDERS

The haemostatic process is carefully balanced so that haemorrhage is promptly arrested and inappropriate thrombosis does not occur. The causes of haemostatic failure are numerous, and it is useful to have a standardised approach to the clinical and laboratory diagnosis of any bleeding tendency.

The initial problem is to determine whether bleeding is due to a local factor, such as a peptic ulcer, or to an underlying haemostatic abnormality. Often a mild abnormality only becomes apparent after trauma or a local precipitating lesion. Any bleeding disorder may be inherited or acquired. This may result from one of the following mechanisms, as shown in Table 9.1.

A careful clinical history and physical examination should be undertaken, and special care must be taken in patients with multisystem disease to recognise any bleeding tendency. In particular, continual oozing from vene-puncture and drip sites, extensive petechiae and purpura at pressure areas and steady blood loss from drainage tubes are often signs of impending haemostatic failure. Often the cause of the bleeding will then be strongly suspected, but laboratory tests are always required to make a precise diagnosis and to define the severity of any abnormality.

Table 9.1 Pathogenesis of haemostatic failure

1. Thrombocytopenia
2. Functional platelet abnormality
3. Blood vessel defect
4. Coagulation factor (s) defect
5. Excess fibrinolysis
6. Combined defect

Initially a series of simple screening tests which are easy to perform and give reliable results should be undertaken. A suggested screening procedure is given in Table 9.2. The normal range for each test performed in the particular laboratory involved should be known before any results can be interpreted. If the screening tests suggest an abnormality, further specialised investigations, such as coagulant and immunological factor assays or platelet aggregation studies, should be carried out to define precisely the defect and its severity. The technical details of these tests are described in detail elsewhere (Austen & Rhymes, 1975; Thompson, 1980).

Most patients with an inherited disorder present in childhood, often with a family history of a bleeding tendency and excessive bleeding in response to minor operations, dental extractions, or trauma. However, mild defects may sometimes not present until adult life, and occasionally in old age, often as a result of minor trauma or operative procedure. If an inherited disorder is suspected, no effort should be spared to investigate other family members who might also be affected.

PLATELET DISORDERS

Excessive bleeding due to a deficiency in the circulating platelet mass or abnormal platelet function can usually be controlled by prolonged local pressure. Generally platelet bleeding starts immediately after the initiating event, but once controlled it does not recur. In comparison, bleeding primarily due to coagulation factor deficiency is not controlled by prolonged pressure but continues with a slow but steady loss of unclottable blood and large friable non-functioning fibrin clots. This type of bleeding classically occurs up to several hours after the initial trauma and if untreated will, in severe cases, continue unabated for prolonged periods. Surgical bleeding, in the presence of a normal haemostatic system, is usually more dramatic, with a much faster initial rate of blood loss, and is never generalised.

The peripheral platelet count and the bleeding time are the first-line basic

Table 9.2   Screening tests for a bleeding tendency

For platelet disorders
1. Bleeding time
2. Platelet count
3. Fresh blood film inspection

For vascular disorders
1. Bleeding time
2. Tourniquet test (Hess)

For coagulation disorders
1. Prothrombin time
2. Activated partial thromboplastin time
3. Thrombin time
4. Fibrinogen assay

laboratory tests of platelet involvement in the haemostatic process. If the results of these two tests are within normal limits, it is almost certain that a platelet defect is not responsible for excessive clinical bleeding. The normal range for the peripheral platelet count in adults of all ages is 150–400 × 10^9/l. Formerly platelets were routinely counted by phase contrast microscopy after suitable dilution of anticoagulated whole blood. However, the accuracy of this procedure is only about ± 15 per cent and the technique is rather laborious. Recently, several automated machines have become available which count platelets more reliably and considerably faster and also provide an assessment of mean platelet volume and total plateletcrit (Corash, 1983). However, all very low values, below approximately 20 × 10^9/l, should be checked manually and verified by inspection of a freshly stained peripheral blood film.

Although a platelet count of 150 × 10^9/l is the lower limit of the normal range, spontaneous bleeding due to thrombocytopenia alone is unlikely to occur until the count is below 50 × 10^9/l, and usually does not occur until it has fallen below 20 × 10^9/l. However, in the presence of a localised or generalised infection, serious platelet bleeding can occur when the count is at a higher level. Spontaneous platelet bleeding usually starts initially from the mucous membranes, especially the mouth and gums, often being exacerbated by poor oral hygiene, or as skin purpura around areas of local pressure such as tight socks around the ankles or under the application site of a sphygmomanometer cuff.

There are several methods for performing a bleeding time test (Ivy, Duke and template methods), all of which rely on the time taken for a standard skin incision of small subcutaneous vessels to stop bleeding. The normal range for the particular test performed by each laboratory should be clearly stated, along with the result. A prolonged bleeding time occurs when the platelet count falls below approximately 100 × 10^9/l, or, if found in the presence of a normal or raised platelet count, is suggestive of a platelet function defect. There is a progressive increase in the bleeding time as the platelet count falls below 100 × 10^9/l, and serial values correlate very well with the severity of clinical bleeding (Harker & Slichter, 1972).

Thrombocytopenia may occur as a result of diminished bone marrow production, excessive peripheral utilisation or destruction, or excessive peripheral pooling in an enlarged spleen. A bone marrow aspirate and trephine section will provide an assessment of megakaryocyte number and their form. Decreased platelet production due to a reduction in the megakaryocyte mass is a feature of aplastic anaemia and malignant infiltration of the marrow by leukaemia or secondary carcinoma. In severe megaloblastic anaemia, impaired megakaryocyte production and release of platelets rather than a reduction in megakaryocyte number are responsible for diminished marrow platelet production. Increased peripheral utilisation or destruction is associated with increased marrow megakaryocyte production of platelets.

Excess utilisation occurs in on-going disseminated intravascular coagulation (DIC) when continuing thrombus formation with platelet involvement causes thrombocytopenia due to the marrow being unable to compensate fully for the high platelet turnover. Following episodes of prolonged hypothermia, the elderly person may develop thrombocytopenia due to platelet sequestration in the liver and release of $\propto$-granule contents.

Increased peripheral destruction is caused by immune mechanisms. The platelet membrane is coated by IgG auto-antibodies, and premature platelet destruction occurs by phagocytosis in macrophages mainly in the spleen and liver. It is now possible to detect these antibodies directly on the platelet surface membrane or free in the plasma (McMillan, 1983). Plasma levels of antibodies are an unreliable indicator of clinical severity and disease progression. However, levels bound to the platelet surface have been found to be more helpful. *In vivo* platelet lifespan measurements with the patient's own platelets labelled with Cr^{51} or indium^{III} oxide will show reduced survival curves. Normal platelet lifespan is approximately ten days in the peripheral ciirculation, but in severe immune thrombocytopenia it may be reduced to only a few hours.

Three main forms of immune platelet destruction are recognised clinically. Acute thrombocytopenia occurs in children and is usually self-limiting. Chronic immune thrombocytopenia is often primary and idiopathic and may occur at any age. However, the idiopathic variety is a diagnosis of exclusion from associated diseases such as systemic lupus erythematosus and chronic lymphatic leukaemia, which may also develop platelet auto-antibodies that react with some, as yet undetermined, basic part of the platelet membrane.

The third type is drug-induced thrombocytopenia, where the drug or one of its metabolites combines with a plasma protein to form an antigen. Three criteria should be considered in this diagnosis: exclusion of other causes, recurrent thrombocytopenia after rechallenge with the drug and the demonstration of a specific drug-dependent effect on test platelets *in vitro* (Hackett et al, 1982). The antibody to this antigen forms an immune complex which is adsorbed secondarily onto the platelet surface, leading to premature platelet destruction. As soon as an offending drug is withdrawn, the platelet survival and count recover gradually over the next ten days.

Thrombocytopenia is commonly seen in patients with bacterial and viral infections. Selective platelet destruction may occur without the development of overt DIC. There is evidence that isolated thrombocytopenia may be due to immune complexes formed from antibody and bacterial or viral antigens which then bind to and result in increased platelet destruction (Kelton et al, 1980). A similar destructive thrombocytopenia occurs in malarial infections.

The normal-sized adult spleen, weighing 150–200 g, which may atrophy to a weight of approximately 50 g in the elderly, pools about 30 per cent of the total peripheral platelet mass, which exchanges freely with the platelets in the circulation. When a spleen becomes pathologically enlarged, the percentage of pooled platelets increases considerably and, especially if the bone marrow reserve capacity to increase platelet production is impaired, severe thrombopenia will result.

A platelet function disorder should be suspected in patients with abnormal skin or mucous membrane bleeding in whom the bleeding time is prolonged despite a normal platelet count. If a platelet function disorder is suspected, more detailed investigation, including platelet aggregation studies with several platelet agonists such as ADP, collagen, ristocetin and thrombin, platelet electronmicroscopy and quantitation of the products of arachidonic acid metabolism and and dense body release proteins, should be performed to characterise any defect (Thompson, 1980).

These disorders may be primarily due to an inherited abnormality of platelet function (Hardisty, 1983), but are much more likely in the elderly population to be secondary to some other disease process or related to side-effects of drug therapy (Rao & Walsh, 1983). The primary disease states associated with platelet dysfunction in the elderly are listed in Table 9.3.

The myeloproliferative disorders, comprising polycythaemia rubra vera, myelofibrosis and essential thrombocythaemia, are frequently associated with both bleeding and thrombotic events. The qualitative platelet defects which have been reported in these disorders are quite heterogeneous (Waddell et al, 1981). These include defective aggregation to ADP, collagen, adrenaline, ristocetin and thrombin, defects in arachidonic acid metabolism. resistance to the aggregation inhibitors PGD_2 and PGI_2 and abnormalities of the platelet membrane including glycoprotein deficiencies. Many studies have attempted to correlate these variations in platelet function with disease state and observed haemorrhagic and thrombotic complications. However, there is no clear correlation between any platelet dysfunction and disease state. Usually treatment with myelosuppressive agents, sometimes combined with venesection, improves the clinical bleeding and thrombotic problems and may be associated with correction of platelet function defects.

Although excess bleeding in patients with acute leukaemia and the pre-leukaemic states including myelodysplastic syndromes is usually associated with profound thrombocytopenia, isolated defects in platelet aggregation and granule release associated with serious bleeding have been reported (Russell et al, 1979).

Table 9.3 Disease states associated with platelet dysfunction in the elderly

Myeloproliferative disorders
Acute leukaemia
Myelodysplastic syndromes
Dysproteinaemias
Chronic renal failure
Chronic liver disease
Acute alcohol intoxication
Scurvy
Fibrin(ogen) degradation products (FDPs) in DIC

Several haemostatic abnormalities have been described in patients with dysproteinaemias and IgA myeloma. These include prolonged bleeding times, impaired platelet adhesion and aggregation. There seems to be a good correlation between the concentration of paraprotein and the platelet abnormality, and it is probable that coating of the platelet membrane by the protein results in the platelet abnormalities. Plasmapheresis to lower the paraprotein level usually corrects any platelet defects (Furie, 1982).

Uraemia is frequently associated with bleeding manifestations related to abnormal platelet function. These disorders are probably multifactorial and are partially corrected by dialysis. It has been suggested that the accumulation of some metabolites, possibly phenolic acids and guanidinosuccinic acid, coat the platelet surface and inhibit function. However, dialysis does not always shorten a prolonged bleeding time, and there is evidence that a plasma factor may stimulate excess vessel wall prostacyclin synthesis and release (Remuzzi et al, 1978). Recently cryoprecipitate infusions have been reported to correct on some occasions the bleeding defect, although the mechanism of action has not been determined (Janson et al, 1980).

Defects in platelet aggregation and prolonged bleeding times occur in patients with chronic liver disease. This is very common in alcoholics, in whom acute ethanol ingestion can cause thrombocytopenia associated with toxic damage of megakaryocytes and can also effect arachidonate metabolism and platelet membrane stability (Cowan, 1980). Patients with acute disseminated intravascular coagulation (DIC) and thrombocytopenia also have impaired platelet function, possibly due to the proteolytic products of fibrinogen/fibrin digestion (fragments X, Y, D and E) blocking the fibrin binding sites on the platelet membrane (Orloff & Michaeli, 1976).

The list of pharmacological agents which may affect platelet function is long (Packham & Mustard, 1977), and drugs are probably the commonest cause of platelet dysfunction in the elderly. Many of these drugs, if taken in high dosage or as an overdose, can lead to important clinical bleeding and in normal dosage will exacerbate any other defect in the haemostatic system. Clinically the most important of these drugs are listed in Table 9.4.

Aspirin (acetyl salicylic acid) irreversibly acetylates platelet cyclo-oxygenase and thus inhibits thromboxane A_2 synthesis. Even a relatively small dose such as 300 mg will prolong the bleeding time significantly and the effect will last for the next three to four days until sufficient circulating platelets with non-inhibited enzyme are produced from the bone marrow megakaryocytes. Aspirin also blocks vascular tissue cyclo-oxygenase activity and thus reduces prostacyclin synthesis and release, but requires a higher dose of aspirin, has a shorter duration of effect of between 12 and 24 hours, and in the elderly the capacity of vascular tissue to synthesise prostacyclin declines. Thus patients receiving even a small dose of aspirin experience gastrointestinal blood loss and are markedly susceptible to other bleeding complications. Other non-steroidal anti-inflammatory agents, such as indomethacin and phenylbutazone, reversibly inhibit cyclo-oxygenase activity,

Table 9.4 Drugs which affect platelet function

---

1. Membrane stabilising agents
   ∝-antagonists
   ß-blockers
   Local anaesthetics (procaine)
   Antihistamines
   Tricyclic antidepressants

2. Agents which affect prostanoid synthesis
   Aspirin
   Non-steroid anti-inflammatory
   Corticosteroids

3. Antibiotics
   Penicillin
   Cephalosporins

4. Agents which increase cyclic AMP levels
   Dipyridamole
   Aminophylline
   Prostanoids

5. Others
   Heparin
   Dextrans
   Ethanol
   Phenothiazine
   Clofibrate

---

but generally the effect is less pronounced and has disappeared approximately four hours after the drug has been eliminated from the circulation.

Penicillin and cephalosporin antibiotics when given in high dosage or in the presence of renal failure have been observed to cause purpura and a bleeding tendency. These antibiotics and related compounds such as carbenicillin, ampicillin, ticarcillin, piperacillin, mezlocillin and latamoxef coat the platelet membrane and inhibit platelet activators such as ADP and adrenaline from binding to their specific membrane receptors and inducing platelet stimulation (Smith & Lipsky, 1983).

The therapy of all patients with thrombocytopenia or an acquired platelet function defect depends on the severity of the clinical bleeding tendency. There should be two basic aims. First is the removal or correction of the primary cause of the defect. Obviously in some conditions correcting the primary condition will result in cessation of the bleeding tendency. Dialysis in chronic renal failure and plasmapheresis in dysproteinaemias are examples of such procedures. Second is the administration of blood products and in particular platelet concentrates to control the immediate bleeding tendency so as to allow the treatment of the predisposing condition time to be effective.

To control clinical bleeding in patients with thrombocytopenia, it is enough to raise the platelet count to between 40 and 60 × 10^9/l. This is usually achieved by giving one platelet concentrate per 10 kg of body weight (Menitove & Aster, 1983). Patients with massive splenomegaly, septicaemia or DIC may require larger doses. The effectiveness of each infusion can be assessed by platelet counts, one and 24 hours post infusion and by clinical control of any bleeding episodes. One area of controversy is whether platelet support should be given prophylactically to non-bleeding thrombocytopenic patients with platelet counts below $20 \times 10^9/l$. If the period of thrombocytopenia is expected to be for a short time of a few days only or to cover an invasive or surgical procedure, I would advocate platelet infusions, but otherwise in the elderly patient I would only use them to control severe haemorrhage. Similarly for patients with platelet function disorders, infusion of platelet concentrates should be given to control serious haemorrhage, and their effectiveness can be monitored by shortening of the bleeding time.

Patients with an immune mediated thrombocytopenia are generally unresponsive to platelet infusions. However, in life-threatening situations they may be helpful in conjunction with immunosuppressive agents, intravenous human gammaglobulin, plasma exchange and splenectomy (Rosse, 1983). Steroid therapy reduces the rate of removal of antibody-coated platelets by the reticuloendothelial system. In some non-immune conditions, steroids may also lessen platelet-induced bleeding, possibly by improving vascular integrity.

COAGULATION DEFECTS

Results of the three basic laboratory screening tests for the coagulation system usually suggest the nature of any deficiency. The significance of each test is shown in Table 9.5. The activated partial thromboplastin time is more sensitive to factor XII, XI, IX, and VIII abnormalities than the later factors of the common pathway and, like the prothrombin time, is especially insensitive to fibrinogen (factor I) deficiency. If a prolonged partial thromboplastin time is found by repeating the test with a 50:50 mixture of patient plasma and normal plasma, it can be shown whether the abnormality is caused by factor deficiency or an inhibitor, usually IgG in nature, which is inactivating one of the coagulation proteins. A factor deficiency will be significantly corrected by the normal plasma, whereas if an inhibitor is present very little correction of the prolonged time will occur. The nature and degree of any suggested deficiency should be ascertained by specific assays of the biological and immunological activity of the factors involved.

Coagulant factor defects can be produced in several ways. There may be reduced or absent synthesis of the coagulation protein, or a qualitatively

Table 9.5   Sensitivity of coagulation screening tests to factor deficiency

Test	Detect abnormalities
Prothrombin time	VII, X, V, II, I
Partial thromboplastin time	XII, XI, IX, VIII, X, V, II, I
Thrombin time	I, raised FDPs, circulating heparin

abnormal molecule may be produced which is deficient in the biological, active part of the molecule only. Defects can also arise from excess peripheral utilisation or loss, and inactivation can occur by way of circulating antibodies or inhibitors. All the coagulation factors apart from factor VIII are synthesised in the liver. Factor VIII related antigen (VIII:Rag) is synthesised in vascular endothelial cells and megakaryocytes and is present in the α-granules of circulating platelets. In the circulation large multimers of VIII-Rag protein express von Willebrand factor (VIII:vWF) activity. The procoagulant part of the factor VIII molecule (VIII:C) is a distinct protein with its own immunological characteristics (VIII:Cag) which complexes with VIII:vWF in the circulation. The site of VIII:C synthesis is unknown.

CONGENITAL COAGULATION DISORDERS

Most patients with congenital coagulation factor deficiency are diagnosed in childhood or early adult life. The diagnosis and treatment of these conditions are described in detail elsewhere (Bloom, 1981). However, with increasing experience in the management of these conditions and availability of blood products, these patients now have a near-normal median expectation of life, and patients with severe deficiencies, especially of factor VIII:C (haemophilia A) and factor IX (Christmas disease) are beginning to live into their seventies (Rizza & Spooner, 1983).

VITAMIN K DEFICIENCY

Vitamin K, a fat-soluble vitamin, is required by the liver for synthesis of factors II (prothrombin), VII, IX and X. The natural K vitamins are synthesised by intestinal bacteria and are present in green plants. As they are fat-soluble, they require bile for absorption and are not stored in the body to any extent.

Vitamin K acts at a post-ribosomal site and causes the carboxylation of glutamyl residues at the amino end of the molecule (Brozovic, 1976). This enables the factors to bind to a phospholipid surface in the presence of calcium ions and activate the next part of the coagulation cascade. In vitamin K deficiency the liver synthesises an abnormal protein which is unable to bind to phospholipid surfaces despite having the same immunological and amino acid composition as the normal protein. These immunologically detectable proteins are known as PIVKAs — protein induced by vitamin K absence or antagonism — and may themselves even inhibit coagulation.

However, in liver disease when the synthesis of all proteins is diminished, PIVKAs are not produced. When vitamin K becomes deficient, the activity of the dependent factors decreases according to their circulating half-life (factor VII 2-4 h, factor IX 25 h, factor X 40 h and factor II 60 h).

Vitamin K malabsorption will occur in obstructive jaundice due to the absence of bile. Various malabsorption syndromes such as sprue, prolonged diarrhoea, cystic fibrosis and medication with large doses of mineral oil may also result in vitamin K deficiency. Intestinal sterilisation will decrease the bacterial production of vitamin K. This is seen in patients receiving antibiotics to sterilise the colon prior to gastrointestinal surgery or during long-term parenteral feeding in combination with gut-sterilising antibiotics. Especially if the patient has previously had a poor diet, severe vitamin K deficiency may develop. In these circumstances the deficiency can be easily corrected by 10mg vitamin K_1IV at weekly intervals.

Oral anticoagulants of the coumarin and inandione derivatives probably inhibit the action of vitamin K in the carboxylation of glutamyl residues of factors II, VII, IX and X at a post-ribosomal site (Suttie, 1977). Many patients receiving long-term oral anti-coagulants are taking various other drugs, some of which may potentiate or antagonise oral anticoagulants. This may cause fluctuating control, and serious bleeding may occur spontaneously if the prothrombin time becomes grossly prolonged. An IV dose of vitamin K_I takes 6 hours before any synthesis of biologically active factors occurs. So to control acute bleeding immediately, an infusion of fresh frozen plasma or prothrombin complex concentrate is required.

Occasionally, psychiatrically disturbed patients may be encountered who are secretly taking oral anticoagulants themselves. They usually have a previous history of thrombosis, and are often associated with one of the paramedical professions. Despite an unexplained prolonged prothrombin time and fluctuating bleeding problems, they deny vigorously taking any drugs and go to great lengths to conceal and ingest their supply of tablets. If necessary, to prove drug ingestion the drug concentration in the blood may be measured (Gover et al, 1976).

LIVER DISEASE

Bleeding is a frequent complication of liver disease. As the circulating survival times of the clotting factors are much shorter than those of the other plasma proteins synthesised by the liver, laboratory clotting tests and specific factor assays give a most reliable index of the current state of liver cell synthesis. The vitamin K-dependent factors decrease first, and with more severe liver disease factor V activity falls. As factor V is not vitamin K-dependent, depression of factor V indicates liver synthetic failure rather than malabsorption of vitamin K. With more severe disease, fibrinogen levels decrease and in some cases an abnormal fibrinogen molecule with defective fibrin polymerisation is synthesised. It has been shown that in acute liver failure factor VII coagulant levels are an accurate prognostic indicator. In a small series, patients whose level fell below 8 per cent all died, whilst those with activity exceeding 8 per cent survived.

The liver also degrades activated clotting factors and the fibrinolytic enzymes. The failure to degrade activated clotting factors in liver disease may trigger off disseminated intravascular coagulation (DIC). Impaired breakdown of the fibrinolytic enzymes may result in abnormally excessive fibrinolysis. Surprisingly, factor VIII levels are often raised in liver failure due to the fact that it is synthesised outside the liver, and impaired clearance of activated factor VIII molecules by damaged liver cells may occur.

Thrombocytopenia commonly occurs due to hypersplenism secondary to cirrhosis and portal hypertension. Excessive alcohol intake may depress platelet production, and functional platelet abnormalities may occur.

Major bleeding complications are usually due to gastrointestinal haemorrhages related to portal hypertension. The management of any underlying coagulation defect involving the temporary correction of any abnormality may improve the chances of recovery of liver cell function.

Infusions of fresh frozen plasma and platelet concentrates will control for a short time haemorrhage due primarily to coagulation disorders. The use of prothrombin complexes instead of fresh frozen plasma has been associated with thromboembolic complications due to the presence of activated coagulation factors and should not routinely be used (Kasper, 1973). However, the Oxford product appears much safer, and no adverse thrombotic effects have been reported.

DISSEMINATED INTRAVASCULAR COAGULATION

Episodes of DIC result from intravascular activation of the coagulation system, with resultant widespread deposition of altered fibrinogen and platelets mainly in the microcirculation. In the majority of patients the process of diffuse DIC produces no clinical symptoms, but evidence of excess consumption of coagulation factors and platelets can be demonstrated by laboratory tests. However, in some patients the episode is severe enough to give rise to a generalised haemorrhagic state and/or end-organ failure following blockade of the microvasculature by thrombus formation. The organ most liable to ischaemic damage is the kidney, but the brain, heart and adrenals can also sustain severe ischaemic changes. Underlying triggering mechanisms are numerous, but DIC may be initiated in three basic ways (Cash, 1977):

1. Stimulation of the coagulation process by release of tissue factors into the bloodstream. This occurs, for example, following surgical trauma, during an acute intravascular haemolytic episode, or during dissemination of malignant tissue.
2. Induction of platelet aggregation, which occurs in septicaemia, viraemia and immune complex diseases and also by thrombin, which forms whenever the coagulation process is activated.
3. Severe endothelial injury of the vessel wall, which occurs in patients with extensive burns, widespread vasculitis, infections, prolonged hypotension, acidosis and hypoxia, and activates both intrinsic and extrinsic coagulation pathways.

It is likely that more than 60 per cent of clinical cases of DIC have a strong association with septicaemic infections, gram-negative bacteria being the most frequent micro-organism; but other agents including viruses, fungi, tubercle bacilli, and Rickettsia have also been clearly responsible. Partial blockage by fibrin of the microcirculation, particularly in the kidney, may cause damage to red cells as they pass through the obstructed vessels. Strands of fibrin act rather like a fine-mesh sieve and passing red cells are traumatised, leading to distorted microcytic red cells and an intravascular haemolytic process which has been called micro-angiopathic haemolytic anaemia.

In the acute state of DIC it is essential to demonstrate the abnormal laboratory parameters accurately and quickly. Ideally the screening tests should be available 30 minutes after the laboratory receives the sample. To demonstrate depletion or consumption of clotting factors and platelets and the degree of the process, a thrombin time, prothrombin time, fibrinogen assay, platelet count and haemoglobin estimation will give all the necessary information. The abnormalities are reflected by a prolonged thrombin time, hypofibrinogenaemia and thrombocytopenia. On these values therapy can be initiated and the progress of the consumptive coagulopathy monitored by frequent repeat estimations of these simple screening tests. Although patients will also often have a decreased level of prothrombin, factor V and factor VIII, specific coagulation factor assays, apart from a fibrinogen level, are of limited value in acute DIC. A fibrinogen level below 1.0 g/l and a platelet count below 100×10^9/l are regarded as almost diagnostic.

Following activation of the coagulation system and intravascular thrombosis, there is usually a localised secondary increase in fibrinolytic activity, leading to the formation of plasmin which degrades fibrin and fibrinogen progressively. Secondary fibrinolysis causes increased levels of circulating fibrin complexes and fibrin split products. A serum fibrinogen/fibrin degradation product (FDP) assay, which the provision of commercial kits has made readily available as a rapid screening technique, is usually raised above 100 μg/ml in acute DIC. However, some patients with severe DIC have no elevation of FDPs, due to inhibition of their fibrinolytic response, and they usually have a poor outcome due to irreversible organ failure. The thrombin time is prolonged by a deficiency of clottable fibrinogen, elevated serum FDPs which act as anticoagulants, or the presence of circulating heparin. The thrombin time acts as a practical guide to the clinical significance of raised FDPs and a low fibrinogen level. A prolonged thrombin time more than double the control time is usually indicative of impending overt clinical bleeding.

The management of acute DIC is extremely controversial, and several widely different approaches are currently advocated. The first essential, if at all possible, is to eliminate the precipitating factors. In particular, all antibiotics must be given i.v. and shock should be vigorously treated to avoid excess vascular stasis. If the bleeding diathesis is severe enough to warrant replacement therapy platelet concentrates, fresh frozen plasma and cryoprecipitate (which also contains fibrinogen) should be given. Volume expanders, such as dextrans, should not be used as they may exacerbate bleeding, but human plasma protein fractions which contain 5 per cent albumin can be safely given. The various factor IX concentrates and fibrinogen preparations should also not be used because of potential thrombogenicity. Excessive fibrinogen and platelet therapy may lead to their rapid consumption and further exacerbate microvasculature thrombosis. Frequent repetition of the basic laboratory screening tests should be undertaken and the response of the thrombin time, fibrinogen assay, and serum FDP level used to determine when future replacement therapy is required. The use of heparin in DIC remains particularly controversial, and there are many report in the literature of benefit and marked deterioration. As a general guideline I only advocate its use after a satisfactory trial of replacement therapy has failed to alleviate clinically severe bleeding and/or thrombosis. I begin with a low-dose continuous i.v. infusion of 500 units per hour, increasing the dose hourly by 500 units if no improvement of the clinical condition or serial laboratory results ensues.

Associated low levels of antithrombin III occur in acute DIC, which will make heparin therapy relatively ineffective. Infusions of antithrombin III or complexed antithrombin III-heparin may well be the therapy for severe DIC in the future.

PROBLEMS ASSOCIATED WITH BLOOD TRANSFUSION

When the patient's blood volume is replaced by the administration of large quantities of stored bank blood in a short period of time, haemorrhagic manifestations may well follow (Collins, 1976).

Bank blood that has been stored for more than 24 hours contains no functioning platelets, concentrations of factors V and VIII of approximately 10 per cent, and of factor XI of about 20 per cent. If a transfusion equal to the blood volume of the patient is given, a significant dilutional thrombocytopenia and clotting factor deficiency develop. These must be corrected by an infusion of platelet concentrates and fresh frozen plasma or clotting concentrates.

Bank blood may precipitate DIC due to a combination of partial activation of clotting factors during storage and breakdown of platelets, leucocytes and red cells releasing thromboplastic substances into the blood. There is also evidence that platelet function may be impaired in patients receiving massive transfusions.

Occasionally severe post-transfusion thrombocytopenia develops about one week after a transfusion. This is a self-limiting process due to the formation of platelet antibodies against infused platelet antigens with secondary destruction of the patient's own platelets as a result of attachment to the antigen–antibody complexes.

The use of dextrans or hydroxyethyl starch as volume expanders after severe blood loss is associated with haemostatic disorders. Haemodilution is common to all colloidal plasma expanders, but even small doses of low molecular-weight dextrans inhibit platelet function with a maximum effect about 4 hours after infusion. Higher doses precipitate factor VIII and give an acquired von Willebrand's type of syndrome and also inhibits the fibrinolytic system, so that fibrinolysis is retarded. If higher molecular-weight dextrans are used, coagulation factors are also affected, resulting in prolonged coagulation times. However, the various gelatin solutions do not interfere with any aspect of coagulation even when when very high clinical doses are used.

ACQUIRED INHIBITORS TO COAGULATION FACTORS

There are two basic groups of coagulation factor inhibitors which are encountered in the elderly. The first type is an inhibitor directed specifically against one coagulation factor. The most frequent is directed against VIII:C but inhibitors to factors VIII:vWf, IX, V, XI, XII and XIII have also been reported. The second type is the lupus-type anticoagulant which is of poorly defined specificity and inhibits coagulation reactions which occur on phospholipid surfaces.

Specific inhibitors to factor VIII:C present in old age and may be idiopathic or related to other auto-immune disorders and rheumatoid arthritis in particular. These inhibitors are IgG in nature and show the same characteristics as those identified in approximately 5–10 per cent of haemophiliacs. The non-haemophiliac patient presents with a severe spontaneous bleeding diathesis with extensive bruising and usually gastrointestinal bleeding. The diagnosis is confirmed by a prolonged activated partial thromboplastin time which is not corrected by added normal plasma or factor VIII. A specific factor VIII inhibitor assay allows quantitation of the defect and acts as an indicator of efficacy of therapy. Although some inhibitors disappear spontaneously, most patients present with troublesome bleeding which requires therapy. Control of acute bleeding episodes is attempted by infusions of high doses of factor VIII concentrate at 8-hourly intervals, and if this is not successful by plasma exchange and infusions of an activated factor IX concentrate. Immunosuppressive therapy with steroids, azathioprine and cyclophosphamide may be more beneficial in older patients, resulting in a gradual reduction in inhibitor concentration and cessation of bleeding episodes.

An acquired bleeding diathesis similar to inherited von Willebrand's disease is occasionally seen in association with auto-immune disorders, paraproteinaemias and lymphoproliferative disorders. These patients have an antibody to factor VIII von Willebrand factor activity, and bleeding episodes should be controlled by cryoprecipitate infusions. Acquired inhibitors to the other coagulation factors are encountered very rarely (Brozovic, 1981).

The non-specific lupus-type anticoagulant occurs in approximately 10 per cent of patients with systemic lupus erythematosus and related immune disorders. These inhibitors are diagnosed by a prolonged activated partial thromboplastin time, not corrected by normal plasma and a slightly prolonged prothrombin time which becomes disproportionally longer upon dilution of the thromboplastin (Shapiro & Thiagarajan, 1982). Paradoxically, these patients virtually never experience significant bleeding episodes but have an increased tendency to develop thrombotic events (Carreras et al, 1981).

VASCULAR DISORDERS

A diagnosis of a vascular defect is usually suspected when bleeding is confined to the skin and mucous membranes and the standard laboratory screening tests show no abnormality. The tourniquet (Hess) test is usually positive and occasionally the bleeding time may be prolonged. Bleeding is usually minor with an easy bruising tendency and spontaneous bleeding from small vessels, and is commonly seen in elderly people. The underlying defect is in the vessel wall which may be structurally weak or suffer damage due to inflammatory or immune processes, or in the supporting connective tissue.

Hereditary haemorrhagic telangiectasia is transmitted as an autosomal dominant trait and is clearly an inherited vascular abnormality. This is the only inherited disorder to present with increasing and more troublesome bleeding episodes in old age. These patients have multiple telangiectasia, which are abnormal dilatations of capillaries and arterioles, usually found on the skin and mucous membranes around the nose and mouth. The lesions blanch on pressure and become more numerous with advancing age, and they bleed easily because of vascular wall thinness and contract poorly, so that bleeding tends to be prolonged. Treatment consists of local pressure, but if bleeding becomes persistent, oestrogens or cautery may control bleeding from the nasal mucosa. Chronic mucosal blood loss will precipitate chronic iron deficiency, and persistent gastro-intestinal lesions may be very difficult to control.

Senile purpura is the commonest cause of an easy bruising and bleeding tendency in elderly people, being present to some extent in approximately 30–40 per cent of patients over 70 years of age when admitted to hospital. This is a benign condition in which purpuric spots appear spontaneously on the extensor surfaces of the forearms and hands and also on the face and neck (Forbes & Prentice, 1981). These spots tend to coalesce, giving the skin a reddish purple colour which may remain for several weeks, often leaving a brown stain when they eventually disappear. The lesions develop because the small skin capillary vessels lack the support of subendothelial collagen fibres which atrophy as part of the ageing process. This is associated with loss of supporting subcutaneous fat and elastic fibres which renders the vessels very fragile and liable to leakage of blood following the slightest touch or shearing stress. A similar form of purpura is seen in Cushing's syndrome and following excessive steroid administration. Steroids also cause atrophy of dermal connective tissue. If the purpuric bruising is widespread, it is important to exclude any other defect in the haemostatic system and avoid any form of steroid administration which will only exacerbate the bruising tendency. There is no specific therapy apart from avoiding excessive trauma and ensuring the patient is well nourished.

The severely malnourished or alcoholic patient may present with gingival bleeding, perifollicular skin haemorrhages and widespread purpura caused by vitamin C deficiency. This will cause defective collagen formation, making the skin capillary vessels more fragile, and abnormal platelet function predisposing to a bleeding tendency. This is easily corrected by regular vitamin C replacement therapy.

Damage of the vascular endothelium can be associated with infections, drug reactions and anaphylactoid purpura (Henoch–Schonlein syndrome). A variety of infective agents during the septicaemic or viraemic stage cause purpura by direct endothelial injury by an auto-immune process or by toxin-mediated damage. Organisms most frequently responsible in old age are meningococci, streptococci and salmonella. A wide variety of drugs have been reported to cause a vasculitis, and purpura develops due to changes in vessel permeability. A specific drug can be proved responsible by a positive patch test result. Anaphylactoid purpura may be occasionally encountered in old age due to a hypersensitivity reaction involving inflammatory changes in the small vessels. The dysproteinaemias including macroglobulinaemia, cryoglobulinaemia, multiple myeloma and amyloid may all present with vascular purpura. This results from infiltration of the abnormal protein into the endothelium and perivascular tissues causing vascular weakness.

Occasionally elderly patients present with excessive bruising for which no apparent cause can be found. In these circumstances one should always be aware of the possibility of the psychiatrically disturbed or senile person inflicting self-injury or that relatives or other people in close attendance are repeatedly mistreating them.

EXCESSIVE PATHOLOGICAL FIBRINOLYSIS

In certain conditions inappropriately large quantities of plasminogen activator are occasionally released into the circulation and may induce a bleeding tendency. This initially presents as progressive bleeding at sites of trauma, postoperative wound areas and venepunctures and, if severe and uncontrolled, generalised haemostatic failure may develop. Excess activator converts plasminogen to plasmin, which digests clotting factors before it can be inactivated by antiplasmins. For example, as a result of extensive tissue trauma following burns, postoperatively (especially after prostatic operations), or in patients with disseminated neoplams, large amounts of tissue activator may be released. Plasminogen activators are inactivated by the liver but in chronic liver disease impaired inactivation may also produce excessive bleeding. Thrombolytic therapy with streptokinase or urokinase infusions for acute thrombotic lesions may cause bleeding in up to 25 per cent of patients, usually at sites of skin incisions and venepunctures, and severe bleeding occasionally necessitates cessation of treatment. Both agents act by generating plasmin from plasminogen. Excess fibrinolysis is recognised by a prolonged thrombin time, due to decreased fibrinogen levels and raised FDPs. The euglobin clot lysis time, which is a measure of fibrinolytic potential of a patient's plasma to lyse a clot, is shortened considerably below the normal range.

Local release of excess activator may occur in the renal and urogenital tracts and be responsible for chronic blood loss. Antifibrinolytic agents, such as epsilon aminocaproic acid (EACA) and tranexamic acid, are inhibitors of plasminogen activation. They have proved effective in controlling clinical bleeding due to excessive fibrinolysis, especially in patients who have undergone prostatic surgery or have urinary tract bleeding.

REFERENCES

Austen D E G, Rhymes I L 1975 Laboratory manual of blood coagulation. Blackwell, Oxford
Bennett B 1977 Coagulation pathways: inter-relationship and control mechanisms. Seminars in hematology XIV 3: 301–318
Bloom A L 1981 Inherited disorders of blood coagulation. Haemostasis and thrombosis. Churchill Livingstone, Edinburgh, p 321–370
Born G V, Bergguist D, Arfors K E 1976 Evidence for inhibition of platelet activation in blood by a drug effect on erythrocytes. Nature 259: 233–235
Brozovic M 1976 Oral anticoagulants, vitamin K and prothrombin complex factors. British Journal of Haematology 32: 9–12
Brozovic M 1981 Acquired disorders of blood coagulation. In: Bloom A L, Thomas D P (eds) Haemostasis and thrombosis. Churchill Livingstone, Edinburgh, p 411–438
Carreras L O et al 1981 Arterial thrombosis, intrauterine death and lupus anticoagulant. Lancet I: 244–246
Cash J D 1977 Disseminated intravascular coagulation. In: Poller L (ed) Recent advances in blood coagulation, vol 2. Churchill Livingstone, Edinburgh, p 293–312
Chignard M, Le Couedic J P, Vergaftig B B, Benveniste J 1980 Platelet-activating factor (PAF-acether) secretion from platelets: effect of aggregating agents. British Journal of Haematology 46: 455–464
Collen D 1980 On the regulation and control of fibrinolysis. Thrombosis and Haemostasis 43: 77–89
Collins J A 1976 Massive transfusion. Clinics in Haematology 5: 201–227
Corash L 1983 Platelets sizing: techniques, biological significance and clinical applications. In: Liss A R (ed) Current topics in hematology, New York 4: 99–123
Cowan D H 1980 Effect of alcoholism on hemostasis. Seminars in Hematology 17: 137–147
Esmon C T 1983 Protein C: biochemistry, physiology and clinical implications. Blood 62: 1155–1158
Forbes C D, Prentice C R M 1981 Vascular and non-thrombocytopenic purpuras. In: Bloom A L, Thomas D P (eds) Haemostasis and thrombosis. Churchill Livingstone, Edinburgh, p 268–278
Furie B 1982 Acquired coagulation disorders and dysproteinaemias. In: Colman R W, Hirsh J, Marder V, Salzman E (eds) Thrombosis and hemostasis: basic principles and clinical practice. Lippincott, Philadelphia, p 577–603
Gaffney P J 1981 The fibrinolytic system. In: Bloom A L, Thomas D P T (eds) Haemostasis and thrombosis. Churchill Livingstone, Edinburgh, p 198–224
Gover P A, Ingram G I C, Cork M S, Holland L, Hopkins R P, Callaghan P, Barkhan P, Shearer M J 1976 Bleeding from self-administration of phenindione: a detailed case study. British Journal of Haematology, 33: 551–564
Hackett T, Kelton J G, Powers P 1982 Drug-induced platelet destruction. Seminars in Thrombosis and Haemostasis 8: 116–137

Hardisty R M 1983 Hereditary disorders of platelet function. Clinics in Haematology 12 (i): 153–174

Harker L A, Slichter S J 1972 The bleeding time as a screening test for evaluation of platelet function. New England Journal of Medicine 287: 999–1005

Janson P A, Jubelirer S J, Weinstein M, Deykin D 1980 Treatment of the bleeding tendency in uremia with cryoprecipitate. New England Journal of Medicine 303: 1318–1322

Kasper C K 1973 Post-operative thromboses in hemophilia B. New England Journal of Medicine 289: 160–161

Kelton J G, Neame P B, Gauldie J, Hirsh J 1980 Elevated platelet associated IgG in the thrombocytopenia of septicemia. New England Journal of Medicine 300: 760–764

McMillan R 1983 Immune thrombocytopenia. Clinics in Haematology 12: 69–88

Menitove J E, Aster R M 1983 Transfusion of platelets and plasma products. Clinics in Haematology 12 (i): 239–266

Orloff K G, Michaeli D 1976 Fibrin induced release of platelet serotonin. American Journal of Physiology 232: 344–351

Packham M A, Mustard J F 1977 Clinical pharmacology of platelets. Blood 50: 555–567

Rao A K, Walsh P N 1983 Acquired qualitative platelet disorders. Clinics in Haematology 12 (i): 201–238

Remuzzi G, Livio M, Cavenaghi A E, Marchesi D, Mecca G, Donati M B, de Gaetano G 1978 Unbalanced prostaglandin synthesis and plasma factors in uraemic bleeding. Thrombosis Research 13: 531–541

Rizza C R, Spooner R J D 1983 Treatment of haemophilia and related disorders in Britain during 1976–1980. British Medical Journal 286: 929–933

Rosenberg R D 1978 Heparin, antithrombin and abnormal clotting. Annual Review of Medicine 29: 367–378

Rosse W F 1983 Management of chronic immune thrombocytopenia. Clinics in Haematology 12 (i): 267–284

Russell N H, Keenan J P, Bellingham A J 1979 Thrombocytopathy in preleukaemia: association with a defect of thromboxane A_2 activity. British Journal of Haematology 41: 417–425

Seegers W H 1978 Antithrombin III: theory and clinical implications. American Journal of Clinical Pathology 69: 299–359

Shapiro S S, Thiagarajan P 1982 Lupus anticoagulants. In: Spaet T H (ed) Progress in hemostasis, vol 6. Grune & Stratton, New York, p 263–286

Sixma J J, Wester J 1977 The hemostatic plug. Seminars in Hematology XIV 3: 265–299

Smith C R, Lipsky J J 1983 Hypoprothrombinemia and platelet dysfunction caused by cephalosporin and oxalactam antibiotics. Journal of the American Medical Association 249: 69–71

Smith J B 1981 Involvement of prostaglandins in platelet aggregation and haemostasis. In: Bloom A L, Thomas D P (eds) Haemostasis and thrombosis. Churchill Livingstone, Edinburgh, p 61–72

Stormorken H 1977 Activation and interaction of some defence systems. Recent advances in blood coagulation, vol 2. Churchill Livingstone, Edinburgh, p 35–58

Suttie J W 1977 Oral anticoagulant therapy: the biosynthetic basis. Seminars in Hematology 14 (3): 365–374

Thompson J M 1980 Blood coagulation and haemostasis — a practical guide, 2nd edn. Churchill Livingstone, Edinburgh

Thompson R E, Mandle R T, Kaplan A P 1977 Association of factor XI and high molecular weight kininogen in human plasma. Journal of Clinical Investigations 60: 1376–1380

Thorgeirsson G, Robertson A L 1978 The vascular endothelium — pathobiologic significance. American Journal of Pathology 93: 803–848

Vermylen J, Badenhorst P N, Deckmyn H, Arnout J 1983 Normal mechanisms of platelet function. Clinics in Haematology 12: 107–152

Waddell C C, Brown J A, Repinecy Y A 1981 Abnormal platelet function in myeloproliferative disorders. Archives of Pathology and Laboratory Medicine 105: 432–443

White G C 1980 Calcium-dependent proteins in platelets. Biochimica Biophysica Acta 631: 130–139

Whittle B J R Moncada S 1983 Pharmacological interactions between prostacyclin and thromboxanes. British Medical Bulletin 39: 232–238

Zimmerman T S, Ruggeri Z N 1983 Von Willebrand's disease. Clinics in Haematology 12: 175–200

Zwaal R F A, Hemker H C 1982 Blood cell membranes and haemostasis. Haemostasis II: 12–39

Clinical Management of Venous Thromboembolism

INTRODUCTION

Venous thromboembolism is a very important clinical problem in the elderly population because of its high prevalence and because there are inherent problems related to the morbidity, diagnosis, prevention and treatment of this disease that are peculiar to older patients.

The high prevalence of venous thromboembolism in the elderly is explained by the fact that age itself (Hirsh et al, 1981b; Coon & Coller, 1959) is an important risk factor and also because elderly patients are prone to have illnesses such as congestive cardiac failure, malignant disease and hip fracture which are independent risk factors for the development of venous thromboembolism.

The direct consequences (mobidity) of venous thromboembolism may be more serious in elderly patients because they frequently have reduced cardiorespiratory reserve which renders them more vulnerable to the effect of even small or moderate-size pulmonary embolism.

The clinical diagnosis of venous thromboembolism may be particularly difficult in elderly patients if they are confused or if they have an associated disorder such as chronic obstructive lung disease, congestive cardiac failure, paralytic stroke with leg swelling or hip fracture which may mask some of the manifestations of this disease. In addition, non-invasive objective tests may be difficult to perform in uncooperative patients, and more invasive diagnostic procedures (e.g. pulmonary angiography) may be impossible to peform in the very sick patient.

Prophylaxis of venous thromboembolism constitutes a particular problem in elderly patients with hip fracture since there is no proven efficacious and safe method of prevention in this patient group (Hirsh & Salzman, 1982).

Finally, there is evidence that the risk of hemorrhage is increased in elderly patients on long-term oral anticoagulant therapy and in elderly females treated with intravenous heparin (Vieweg et al, 1970).

Despite these difficulties, there have been marked improvements during the last decade in the clinical management of venous thromboembolism in both the young and old patient. Important advances in diagnostic techniques and in clinical trial methodology (Hull, 1981) have provided the clinician with reliable information which forms the basis for a rational approach to the diagnosis, prevention and treatment of venous thromboembolism.

In this chapter, we will discuss the diagnosis, prevention and treatment of thrombosis and its consequences, which include acute deep-vein thrombosis, acute recurrent deep-vein thrombosis, the post-phlebitic syndrome, thromboneurosis and pulmonary embolism.

DIAGNOSIS OF DEEP-VEIN THROMBOSIS

Clinical diagnosis

It is now generally accepted that the clinical diagnosis of deep-vein thrombosis is inaccurate (Hirsh et al, 1981c; Hirsh, 1982). Many studies have demonstrated that less than 50 per cent of patients who present with clinically suspected deep-vein thrombosis do not have this condition confirmed when they are investigated with accurate objective tests (Hirsh et al, 1981c). Clinical diagnosis is non-specific because none of the symptoms and signs of venous thrombosis (Table 10.1) is unique to this condition and all can be caused by non-thrombotic disorders (e.g. cellulitis, ruptured Baker's cyst). Clinical diagnosis has a low sensitivity because many potentially dangerous venous thrombi are non-obstructive and not associated with inflammation of the vessel wall or surrounding perivascular tissues and therefore have few or no detectable clinical manifestations. Consequently, patients with relatively minor symptoms and signs may have large and extensive venous thrombi.

For these reasons, management of deep-vein thrombosis based on clinical diagnosis alone is no longer acceptable.

Diagnosis of venous thrombosis using objective tests

In recent years, objective tests have superseded clinical evaluation as the diagnostic standard for deep-vein thrombosis (Hirsh, 1982). The available objective diagnostic tests which have been adequately evaluated are: ascending venography (Hull et al, 1977, 1981a), impedance plethysmography (IPG)

Table 10.1   Clinical manifestations of venous thrombosis

Clinical feature	Mechanism
Pain and tenderness	Vascular and perivascular inflammation and venous distension
Swelling	Venous obstruction and inflammation
Venous distension	Raised venous pressure

Discoloration
  Pallor
  Cyanosis
	Arterial spasm
	Stagnant anoxia due to impaired venous return

Redness	Vascular and perivascular inflammation
Palpable cord	Thrombosed vein or thickened vein wall

(Hull et al, 1976, 1977; Taylor et al, 1980), Doppler ultrasound (Evans, 1971; Holmes, 1973; Sigel et al, 1972; Strandness & Summer, 1972; Barnes et al, 1972) and ^{125}I-fibrinogen leg scanning (Hull et al, 1977, 1981a). The choice of the objective test to be used depends on whether it is required for the detection of subclinical thrombosis in high-risk patients or whether it is required to confirm the diagnosis of clinically suspected deep-vein thrombosis.

Venography

Ascending venography is the recognised reference method for the diagnosis of deep-vein thrombosis. (Hull et al, 1977, 1981a) The aim of venography is to inject radio-opaquq contrast medium into a dorsal foot vein to outline the deep venous system of the leg. (Hirsh & Hull, 1978) The most reliable criterion for the diagnosis of acute deep-vein thrombosis is a constant intraluminal filling defect seen in two or more projections (Hull et al, 1977, 1981a). Other criteria, such as failure to fill a deep-vein segment, are less reliable and may be due to technical artefacts. In expert hands, this method yields very accurate results. Special care must be take to obtain adequate visualisation of the entire deep venous system of the leg (Fig. 10.1), including the external and common iliac veins, and also to minimise the frequency of artefacts such as incomplete filling of venous segments which may mimic deep-vein thrombosis. It is now accepted that the demonstration of a normal deep venous system by venography definitely excludes deep-vein thrombosis as a cause of the patient's symptoms (Hull et al, 1981a).

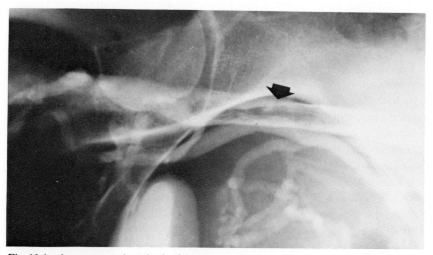

Fig. 10.1   Acute venous thrombosis of the external iliac vein, showing a large intraluminal filling defect in the distal external iliac vein. This venogram demonstrates the importance of adequate visualisation of the entire deep venous system

Venography has the disadvantage of being invasive and has a number of side-effects. The contrast material is irritating to venous endothelium and may produce pain in the foot at the time of injection or transient pain in the calf one to two days after (Hirsh & Hull, 1978). It may also induce a clinically significant deep-vein thrombosis in a small percentage (less than 5 per cent). (Hull & Hirsh, 1981).

The large bolus of dye necessary to obtain adequate visualisation of the proximal vein may cause fluid overload in elderly patients who have impaired cardiac function. Extravasation of contrast material at the site of injection may cause local skin and tissue necrosis (Hirsh & Hull, 1978) which may lead to serious consequences in elderly patients with peripheral arterial insuffi-ciency.

Finally, venography cannot be used for the screening of high-risk patients and cannot be conveniently used for follow-up. For these reasons, non-invasive diagnostic techniques have been developed to replace ascending venography for the diagnosis of deep-vein thrombosis (Hirsh, 1982).

Impedance plethysmography

Occlusive cuff impedance plethysmography (IPG) is a non-invasive techni-que based on the principle that blood volume changes in the calf produced by inflation and deflation of a pneumatic thigh cuff result in changes in electrical resistance (impedance) detected by skin eletrodes placed around the calf (Hirsh, 1982; Hull et al, 1976, 1977; Taylor et al, 1980). The change in impedance is recorded on an electrocardiographic paper strip and both the total rise during cuff inflation and the fall occurring during the first three seconds of deflation are plotted on a two-way IPG graph (Fig. 10.2). The graph includes a discriminant line separating normal and abnormal results. With this method, impedance plethysmography is 95 per cent sensitive and specific to thrombosis of the popliteal, femoral or iliac venins (Hull et al, 1975, 1977) but it is relatively insensitive to calf-vein thrombosis.

Impedance plethysmography does not distinguish between thrombotic and non-thrombotic obstruction to venous outflow. It may be falsely positive (Hirsh, 1982): (a) if the patient is positioned incorrectly or is inadequately relaxed (the vein is constricted by contracting muscles), (b) if the vein is compressed by an extrinsive mass (e.g. pelvic tumour) or (c) if the venous outflow is impaired by raised central venous pressure (Congestive heart failure, constrictive pericarditis, cardiac tamponade). Reduced arterial inflow to the limb due to severe obstructive peripheral arterial disease may also lead to reduced venous outflow and consequently produce a false-positive result. Finally, this test cannot be performed in patients who are uncooperative, with a leg in traction or wearing a plaster cast.

^{125}I-fibrinogen leg scanning

The diagnosis of venous thrombosis by radio-iodine labelled fibrinogen scan-

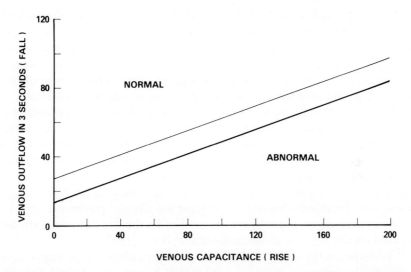

Fig. 10.2   For impedance plethysmography, the rise in blood volume during inflation of the thigh cuff and the fall in the three seconds after its release are plotted on a two-way IPG graph. The IPG graph contains a discriminant line (lower line) separating normal and abnormal results and a stop line (upper line) (Taylor et al, 1980)

ning depends upon incorporation of circulating labelled fibrinogen into a forming thrombus which is detected by measuring the increase in overlying surface radioactivity with an isotope detector (Fig. 10.3) (Hirsh, 1982; Kakkar, 1972; Kakkar et al, 1972). For this test 100 microcuries of labelled fibrinogen are administered intravenously and thyroid gland uptake is prevented by daily administration of 100mg of potassium iodine. For patients who cannot eat, 100mg of sodium iodine are given intravenously every 72 hours.

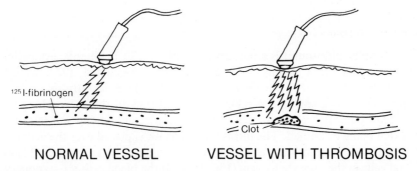

Fig. 10.3   Principle of ^{125}I-fribrinogen leg scanning: one hundred microcuries of radioactive fibrinogen are injected intravenously, and leg scanning is performed over specific points over the calf and thigh. Increased radioactivity can be detected in the region overlying a thrombus as fibrinogen is incorporated into the thrombus

The surface radioactivity is expressed as a percentage of the surface radioactivity measured over the heart. Readings are taken over both legs. Venous thrombosis is diagonsed if there is an increase in the radioactive reading of more than 20 per cent: (a) at any point compared with readings over adjacent points of the same leg or over the corresponding point on the opposite leg, and (b) if the scan remains abnormal at repeated examination 24 hours later. This test is very sensitive (95 per cent) for detection of calf-vein thrombosis in patients who have had symptoms for less than eight days (Hull et al, 1977). It is less sensitive for proximal deep-vein thrombosis and is unreliable in the upper thigh because of the close proximally of the bladder (containing radioactive urine) and the presence of large veins and arteries which produce and increase in the background count. It is insensitive to pelvic vein thrombosis because these veins are situated posterially and the relatively weak gamma rays which are emitted by the ^{125}I-fibrinogen are not detected on the anterior abdominal surface (Hirsh, 1982).

[125]I-fibrinogen leg scanning should never be used alone for the diagnosis of symptomatic deep-vein thrombosis because it is insensitive to high femoral and iliac vein thrombi and because there may be a 24–48 hour time delay before sufficient radioactivity is incorporated into the symptomatic thrombus (Hirsh, 1982). Falsely positive results are obtained when scanning is performed over haematoma or cellulitis. Patients with superficial varicosities may have a positive leg scan result, and when this occurs the test should be repeated after the leg has been wrapped in a compression bandage and elevated in order to decrease venous pooling. In elderly patients who are incontinent, radioactive urine may give a false-positive test result, and when this is suspected the test should be repeated after the leg has been thoroughly washed. Because of the lack of specificity of ^{125}I-fibrinogen leg scanning, a positive result with this test always requires confirmation by venography.

The major uses of ^{125}I-fibrinogen scanning are for screening high-risk patients and for the diagnosis of acute recurrent deep-vein thrombosis. These will be discussed later in the chapter.

Doppler ultrasound

The Doppler ultrasound is a non-invasive method for qualitative evaluation of venous blood flow (Evans, 1971; Holmes, 1973; Sigel et al, 1972; Strandness & Summer, 1972; Barnes et al, 1972). The Doppler ultrasound flow meter detects changes in the velocity of blood flow in the veins which are induced by normal respiratory excursions and by compressing and releasing the vein being examined. The ultrasound detector is placed over the vein and the 5mHz ultrasound beam is transmitted percutaneously and reflected from blood cells in the underlying vein (Fig. 10.4). If the blood cells are stationary, the frequency of the reflected beam is identical to the frequency of the incident beam and no sound is recorded. If the blood cells are moving, the beam is reflected at an altered frequency (the Doppler shift) that is prop-

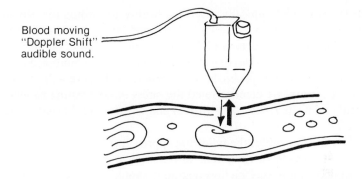

Blood moving
"Doppler Shift"
audible sound.

Fig. 10.4   Principle of Doppler ultrasound flow meter: the Doppler consists of a probe containing two pizolelectric crystals, one for emitting and the other for receiving the ultrasound beam. The reflected beam is transmitted at a different frequency than the incident beam if the red blood cells in the path are moving. This difference in frequency (known as the Doppler shift) is proportional to the velocity of flow. The difference in frequency between the incident and the reflected beam is translated into an audible signal

ortional to the velocity of blood flow. The difference in frequency between the incident and the reflected beam is translated into an audible signal. Venous blood flow produces a characteristic low-pitched sound that is phasic and changes in intensity with respiration, producing a 'windstorm effect'. The sound is abolished by venous occlusion and, when the compression is released, an augmented sound is heard as blood flow in the vein suddenly increases. An augmented sound is also obtained by compression of the vein being examined distal to the ultrasound probe.

For a Doppler ultrasound study, the following veins are examined indivdully: common femoral, superficial femoral, popliteal and posterior tibial. When deep-vein thrombosis is present, there will be a loss of phasicity of the venous signal during respiration if the probe is place proximal to the thrombus and there will be no augmented sound when the vein is compressed distal to the thrombus.

Venous Doppler is sensitive to proximal vein thrombosis but less sensitive to calf-vein thrombi (Hirsh et al, 1981c). The major pitfall of this technique is that it requires an experienced examiner and the interpretation is subjective. This technique is useful for the diagnosis of deep-vein thrombosis in patients in whom IPG cannot be performed. It is also a useful method for demonstrating deep venous incompetence in patients with the post-phlebitic syndrome.

A practical approach for the diagnosis of deep-vein thrombosis

Over the last decade, we have performed a number of studies evaluating non-invasive tests for the diagnosis of venous thrombosis. In the first of these studies, we evaluated the combined use of impedance plethysmography and ^{125}I-fibrinogen leg scanning, (Hull et al, 1977). In this study, consecutive patients referred with clinically suspected deep-vein thrombosis had an IPG on the day of referral and then daily for three days, concurrently with leg scanning. All patients underwent bilateral venography either on the third day or earlier (if either non-invasive tests was positive). This combined approach was highly sensitive and specific for the diagnosis of deep-vein thrombosis. In a subsequent study, we demonstrated the safety of not treating patients with anticoagulants if the results of both IPG and leg scan were negative (Hull et al, 1981c)

Based on the foregoing, the following approach (Fig. 10.5) for the diagnosis of a first episode of deep-vein thrombosis in symptomatic patients is recommended. Impedance plethysmography should be performed on the day of referral and, if positive in the absence of conditions known to produce a false-positive result, a diagnosis of deep-vein thrombosis can be made. In patients with a condition known to produce a falsely positive IPG result, ascending venography is required to confirm a diagnosis of deep-vein thrombosis.

If the IPG is negative on the day of referral, the clincian can either repeat the test at intervals to detect extending calf-vein thrombosis or inject the patient with ^{125}I-fibrionger and perform leg scanning. The first alternative, namely repeated examination with impedance plethysmography, is being used with apparent safety in many centres. Serial IPG testing should be performed the day following the initial test and then on day 3 and 5. If the patient has persistent symptoms which cannot be explained by an alternative cause, the IPG should be repeated on day 7 and 10. The second alternative, namely the addition of ^{125}I-fibrinogen leg scanning when impedance plethysmography is negative, is currently the most thoroughly evaluated approach.

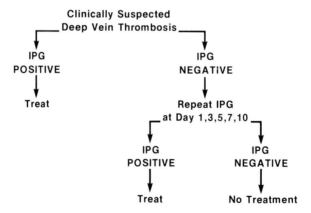

Fig 10.5 Practical non-invasive approach for patients with clinically suspected first episode of deep-vein thrombosis using serial impedance plethysmography. Patients with positive impedance plethysmography are treated in the absence of conditions known to produce a false-positive test result

Patients with deep-vein thrombosis should have their IPGs repeated at the time of discharge from the hospital and then three-monthly until the result of the IPG returns to normal. This provides a valuable baseline which can be used for diagnosis of acute recurrent deep-vein thrombosis. In our experience, 30 per cent of patients with deep vein thrombosis have a normal IPG after three weeks, 50 per cent after three months and 70 per cent after six months.

If impedance plethysmography is not available, then all patients with clinically suspected venous thrombosis should be tested by venography or by Doppler ultrasound. In the hands of an expert, Dopper ultrasound can probably be used interchangeably with impedance plethysmography, and a diagnostic algorithm similar to that described for impedance plethysmography should be followed.

This diagnostic approach is very cost-effective, since patients do not need to be hospitalised or treated with anticoagulants while undergoing serial IPG testing or leg scanning. For practical purposes a negative IPG and leg scanning result exclude the diagnosis of deep-vein thrombosis in symptomatic patients and there is no need for further investigation or treatment.

RECURRENT LEG SYMPTOMS FOLLOWING DEEP-VEIN THROMBOSIS

The short-term prognosis of patients with proximal deep-vein thrombosis is very good, provided that they are treated with adequate doses of heparin and oral anticoagulants for a period of three months. (Hull et al, 1979a). Less is known about the long-term prognosis of these patients, although follow-up studies indicate that a proportion will develop recurrent symptoms over the ensuing months or years (Hirsh et al, 1981a; Hull et al, 1983a). These recurrent symptoms may be persistent or intermittent in nature and they may be caused by acute recurrent deep vein thrombosis or they may be manifestations of either the post-phlebitic syndrome (leClerc et al, 198) or a variety of non-thrombotic disorders. It is important to differentiate between these three groups of disorders because their management differs, and in many patients differentiation on clinical grounds alone is difficult or impossible.

Clinically, patients present in one of three ways. These are:
1. The pain and swelling never completely subside after the initial episode of acute deep-vein thrombosis but persist with exacerbations and remissions for months or years. This presentation is compatible with the post-phlebitic syndrome, but when exacerbations are acute and severe it is difficult to differentiate clinically beween acute deep-vein thrombosis and a manifestation of the post-phlebitic syndrome.
2. The symptoms of acute venous thrombosis subside completely and new symptoms of pain and swelling develop gradually during the following months or years. This is characteristic of the post-phlebitic syndrome (see below). In this situation, the diagnosis of post-phlebitic syndrome is

usually evident on clinical grounds but needs confirmation by a variety of non-invasive tests.

3 .The symptoms and signs of acute deep-vein thrombosis subside complete-ly but recur either acutely or subacutely in the following weeks, months or years. In these patients, it is difficult to differentiate between acute recurrent venous thrombosis, the post-phlebitic syndrome or a non-thrombotic cause of leg pain and swelling without peforming as variety of diagnostic tests.

Diagnostic approach

If the patient has clinical manifestations which are compatible with acute recurrent venous thrombosis (i.e. either a new episode of leg pain and/or swelling or an acute or subacute exacerbation of leg pain and swelling) it is important first to exclude acute recurent venous thrombosis because this condition is potentially life-threatening (Hull et al, 1983a) and requires urgent treatment. If acute recurrence is excluded, a diagnosis of the post-phlebitic syndrome (LeClerc et al, 198) or a non-thrombotic cause of the patient's symptoms should be considered.

Diagnosis of acute recurrent venous thrombosis

Much like the situation with a first episode of deep-vein thrombosis, it is now clear (from the results of the study described below) that the clinical diagno-sis of acute recurrent venous thrombosis is also highly non-specific and that such a diagnosis should no longer be made on clinical grounds alone. Ascend-ing venography, the recognised diagnostic standard for patients with a first episode of suspected acute deep-vein thrombosis, is less useful for the diagno-sis of recurrent venous thrombosis. This is because a constant intraluminal filling defect, the diagnostic hallmark of acute thrombosis, may be difficult to visualise in vessels that have been obliterated by previous disease, and venography cannot be easily repeated in view of its invasive nature (many patients with clinically suspected recurrence have multiple episodes).

We have recently evaluated the use of combination of impedance plethys-morgaphy and ^{125}I-fibrinogen leg scanning in patients with clinically sus-pected recurrent deep-vein thrombosis (Hull et al, 1983a). In this prospective study, 270 patients considered by their physician to be experiencing symp-toms and signs of acute recurrent deep-vein thrombosis were evaluated by the combination of impedance plethysmography and fibrinogen leg scanning (Fig. 10.6).

Impedance plethysmography was performed at the initial visit and, if negative, the patient was injected with ^{125}I-fibrinogen. Leg scanning was performed 24 and 72 hours later, at which time impedance plethysmography was also repeated.

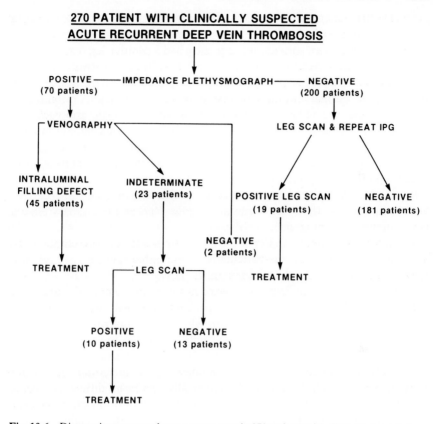

Fig. 10.6   Diagnostic process and outcome on entry in 270 patients with clinically suspected acute recurrent deep-vein thrombosis

If the impedance plethysmograph was positive at presentation, a venogram was peformed. If a new constant intraluminal filling defect was not seen (indetermine venogram), the patient was injected with ^{125}I-fibrinogen and leg scanning was performed 24 and 72 hours later.

Both tests negative. Both non-invasive tests were negative in 181 patients (67 per cent). These patients were considered not to have recurrent deep-vein thrombosis as the cause of their clinical manifestations and were not treated with anticoagulants.

Initial IPG negative — leg scan positive. In a small number (19) of patients with a negative impedance plethysmograph at presentation, the leg scan became positive at 24 or 72 hours and these patients were considered to have recurrent venous thrombosis and therefore were treated with anticoagulants.

IPG positive at presentation. In the group of patients with positive impedance plethysmograph at presentation, venography revealed three findings. An intraluminal filling defect was demonstrated in 45 patients (64.6 per cent) and this as considered diagnostic of acute recurrence. In 23 patients (32.8

percent), the venographic findings were consistent with previous disease (obliterated and recanalised vessels) and no intraluminal filling defect could be demonstrated. Ten patients subsequently had a positive leg scan and were considered to have recurrent venous thrombosis. In two patients (3 percent) with positive impedance plethysmograph at presentation, the venographic findings were normal and therefore excluded recurrent venous thrombosis.

Patients' outcome. The clinical validity of this diagnostic approach was verified by the long-term follow-up (one year) of all patients entered into the study. During the follow-up period, patients were seen at fixed intervals at a special clinic or on an emergency basis whenever necessary. During these follow-up visits, symptoms and signs of recurrent venous thromboembolism were sought. Objective tests were used to confirm the diagnosis of recurrent venous thrombosis (IPG, leg scanning, venography) and pulmonary embolism (pulmonary angiogram).

Patients in whom both non-invasive tests were negative at presentation had a different outcome than the patients in whom either non-invasive test was positive and who received anticoagulant therapy.

Only three of 181 patients who were negative by combined impedance plethysmography and leg scanning (1.7 per cent) returned with new signs and symptoms of venous thromboembolism which were confirmed by objective testing to be new episodes of venous thromboembolism. In contrast, 18 of 89 patients (20.8 per cent) with positive test results developed new episodes of objectively demonstrated venous thromboembolism, including four deaths from pulmonary embolism (a highly statistically significant difference). All of these 18 patients presented on an emergency basis with florid symptoms and signs and, at the time of entry into the study, each of these 18 patients had an intraluminal filling defect detected by initial venography. In the majority of these patients, recurrent venous thromboembolism occurred after anticoagulant therapy had been terminated inadvertently or following three months' therapy.

A practical approach to the diagnosis of acute recurrent venous thrombosis

A diagnosis of acute recurrent venous thrombosis can be made by impedance plethysmography if it can be demonstrated that the test result was negative prior to presentation and is positive at the time of presentation. The presence of a previously normal impedance plethysmograph result greatly simplified the practical diagnostic approach in patients subsequently presenting with clinically suspected acute recurrence.

Recurrent venous thromboembolism on adequate anticoagulant therapy is rare (less than 2 per cent), and the majority of patients who recur do so after discontinuation of three months of anticoagulant therapy. In our experience, 60 per cent of patients with their first episode of extensive proximal deep-vein thrombosis have a normal impedance plethysmograph result at the time of discontinuation of three months of anticoagulant therapy. For this reason, we perform a baseline impedance plethysmograph evaluation at the time of discontinuation of long-term anticoagulant therapy in all patients with deep-vein thrombosis.

Diagnostic approach in patients with a previously normal impedance plethysmograph result

The diagnostic algorithm for the diagnosis of clinically suspected recurrent deep-vein thrombosis in patients with a previously normal impedance plethysmograph is shown in Figure 10.7. We perform impedance plethysmography immediately on referral and, if negative, anticoagulant therapy is withheld. ^{125}I-fibrinogen leg scanning is performed daily for 72 hours together with repeat impedance plethysmography. If the results of both IPG and leg scanning remain negative, the diagnosis of acute recurrence is excluded and the need for anticoagulant therapy avoided.

   If the result of either IPG or leg scanning becomes positive, in the absence of conditions known to produce false-positive findings, a diagnosis of acute recurrent venous thrombosis is established and the patient is treated accordingly. A positive leg scan result in the presence of conditions known to produce a false-positive scan (e.g. haematoma) should be confirmed by venography. Venography should also be peformed in patients with a concur-

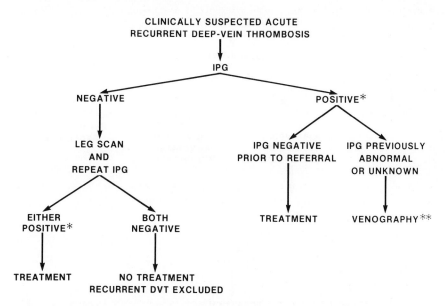

Fig 10.7 Practical diagnostic approach in patients with clinically suspected acute recurrent deep-vein thrombosis.
*In the absence of conditions known to produce a false-positive test result
**The management of the results by venography is shown in Figure 10.8

rent condition that is known to produce a false-positive result (e.g. congestive cardiac failure).

Diagnostic approach in patients with a previously abnormal or unknown impedance plethvsmograph result

The diagnostic algorithm for the diagnosis of suspected recurrent venous thrombosis in patients with a previously abnormal or unknown IPG result is shown in Figure 10.8. If, on referral, the result of IPG is positive in a patient in whom the IPG was previously abnormal, or if the result of the previous IPG is unknown, then venography should be performed because the abnormal IPG does not distinguish between acute recurrent deep-vein thrombosis and chronic venous outflow obstruction. If the venogram demonstrates a new, constant, intraluminal filling defect at a site not involved on the previous venogram, the diagnosis of acute recurrent deep-vein thrombosis is established. If the findings of venography are unchanged or indeterminate, but the common femoral and iliac veins are well visualised and normal, the patient should be injected with ^{125}I-fibrinogen and leg scanning peformed for 72 hours. If the results of leg scanning remain negative, acute recurrent venous thrombosis can be excluded and anticoagulant therapy withheld.

Patients with a positive IPG result, indeterminate findings by venography which include the common femoral or iliac veins (but in whom no new

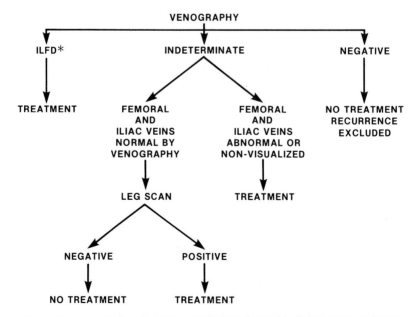

Fig. 10.8 Management of results by venography in patients with clinically suspected acute recurrent deep-vein thrombosis.
*ILFD = intraluminal filling defect

intraluminal filing defects can be seen) and a negative leg scan result present a diagnostic dilemma. In these patients, acute recurrence cannot be confidently excluded and, given the infrequency of this combination of test results, we prefer to err on the side of treatment rather than risk death from massive pulmonary embolism.

The management of patients with negative test results on referral in whom the previous IPG result was abnormal or unknown is the same as outlined above for patients with a previously negative IPG.

Diagnosis of the post-phlebitic syndrome

The post-phlebitic syndrome refers to a disorder caused by deep venous incompetence and/or persistent venous outflow obstruction following deep-vein thrombosis (LeClerc et al, 1985; Bauer, 1950; Negus, 1970; Johnson, 1980). The post-phlebitic syndrome occurs as a consequence of the generation of abnormally high pressure in the deep veins of the legs (DeCamp et al, 1951; Hojemsgard & Sturp, 1950). Chronic venous hypertension is secondary to deep-valve incompetence, with or without venous outflow obstruction. Incompetence of the deep-vein valves may be caused by their direct involvement by the thrombotic process or by dilatation of the distal veins as a consequence of proximal obstruction. It has been suggested that the competence of the popliteal valves is an important factor in determining the ambulatory venous pressure in post-thrombotic limbs (Shull et al, 1979). In more advanced cases, perforator valves become incompetent and cause direct transmission of the ambulatory venous hypertension to the superficial veins and dermal vessels (Burnand et al, 1977, 1979). The development of perforator incompetence is thought to be an important mechanism for the development of venous ulcers (Shull et al, 1979).

Classically, the post-phlebitic syndrome occurs several years after the initial thrombotic episode and its onset is gradual. The clinical mainfestations of the post-phlebitic syndrome are caused by chronic venous hypertension, perforator incompetence and incompetence of the superficial veins. The initial symptoms of the post-phlebitic syndrome are caused by *venous hypertension* and include swelling and edema of the ankle and calf which are most marked after the patient has been standing or walking (Negus, 1968). The swelling is usually relieved by rest and leg elevation. Marked swelling of the thigh may also occur after proximal vein thrombosis. Heavy, aching pain in the calf and thigh is typically present; it is exacerbated by standing up and relieved by rest and leg elevation. Venous caludication may occur after ilio-femoral thrombosis (tripolitis et al, 1980). Patients with this disorder complain of a bursting pain in the thigh or calf which is produced by walking and particularly by climbing. It can mimic arterial caludication. With time and the development of *incompetent perforators*, pigmentation, induration and prominent venules develop around the ankle and the lower third of the leg. The skin pigmentation is caused by repeated bleeding from dermal capillaries which results in the deposition of haemosiderin. There is also a thickening of the skin and subcutaneous tissue called lipodermatosclerosis. Venous ulceration is the most serious manifestation of the post-phlebitic syndrome and it is responsible for marked disability (Browse, 1982) It occurs as a late manifestation of the post-phlebitic syndrome. The uclers usually develop in the region of the medial malleolus. Venous ulcers respond to conservative management but have a tendency to recur. *Sperficial varicosities* may occur as a result of secondary destruction of the valves of the superficial veins.

Some patients with the post-phlebitic syndrome have intermittent symptoms of acute severeleg pain and swelling. These may occur on a background of chronic pain and swelling or less commonly in patients with few or no other manifestations of the post-phlebitic syndrome. This presentation is impossible to distinguish from acute recurrent deep-vein thrombosis without objective tests. It is thought to be caused by a sudden increase in venous pressure due to progressive valvular incompetence.

In the typical case, the clinical diagnosis of post-phlebitic syndrome is readily apparent and can be confirmed by demonstrating venous reflux and/or outflow obstruction. Detection of venous reflux with the Doppler ultrasound is presently the most simple and rapid method available for diagnosing valvular incompetence (Barues, 1982), which is the most common underlying abnormality in the post-phlebitic syndrome. With this technique, reflux is elicited by compressing the area proximal to the valve being examined and listening distally with the Doppler probe. Outflow obstruction is usually demonstrated by plethysmographic techniques of which strain-gauge plethysmography has been the most widely used.

In the group of patients with post-phlebitic syndrome who present with acute or subacute leg pain which mimics acute recurrent venous thrombosis, the diagnosis of post-phlebitic syndrome can only be established as the caused of the patient's symptoms after acute recurrence has been excluded (LeClerc et al, 198).

Other causes of leg pain

Other cause of leg pain are usually considered when acute recurrent venous thrombosis and the post-phlebitic syndrome have been ruled out by performing the appropriate objective tests. These non-thrombotic disorders in elderly patients include recurrent muscle strain, internal derangement of the knee, recurrent cellulitis, ruptured Baker's cyst and extrinsic compression of the vein by pelvic tumour. However, in many patients with recurrent leg pain not due to recurrent deep-vein thrombosis or the post-phlebitic syndrome, an alternate cause is not found and the symptoms can be attributed to thromboneurosis.

Thromboneurosis is a common but poorly recognised clinical syndrome which may simulate either acute venous thrombosis or acute recurrent venous thrombosis. It tends to occur in patients who have a morbid fear of the complications of venous thromboembolism and can be encountered in both the young and old patient. Patients usually present with pain and tenderness, and in its more severe form they may be incapacitated by the fear of recurrence, leg loss or death. This condition may occur both in patients with well-documented previous thrombosis or in patients who were misdiagnosed at their original presentation. Patients frequently have a history of multiple hospital admissions for treatment of 'recurrent venous thrombosis'. Most are on long-term anticoagulant therapy, with or without additional treatment with antiplatelet drugs, and some have had caval interruption procedures performed. It should be emphasised that thromboneurosis is a genuine syndrome which is often iatrogenic in origin, the fear of recurrence being reinforced by admission to hospital and treatment on clinical suspicion alone. Thromboneurosis is a different condition to treat, but it can be prevented by ensuring that a clinical suspicion of acute venous thrombosis (either the first episode or recurrent episodes) is always confirmed by appropriate objective tests.

SUB-CLINICAL THROMBOSIS IN HIGH RISK PATIENTS

The majority of venous thrombi which lead to fatal pulmonary embolism are asymptomatic (Bell & Simon, 1982). Therefore, prevention of fatal pulmonary embolism can only be achieved by detecting subclinical thrombi and treating them before they become dangerous or by using primary prophylaxis (Claggett & Salzman, 1975; kakkar et al, 1979; Gallus et al, 1976; Lancet, 1975; Circulation 1977). Of the two methods, primary prophylaxis is by far the most cost-effective (Hull et al, 1979b) and it is the method of choice in most clinical circumstances. Fatal pulmonary embolism is an important complication in the elderly because these patients frequently have comorbid conditions which predispose to venous thrombosis such as congestive cardiac failure, immobility, fractured hip, malignant disease, stroke.

PROPHYLAXIS OF VENOUS THROMBOEMBOLISM

A number of prophylactic methods are effective in preventing venous thrombosis and pulmonary embolism (Table 10.2). The most extensively tested methods are low-dose heparin (Kakkar et al, 1979; Gallus et al, 1976; Lancet 1975; Circulation, 1977), intermittent pneumatic compression of the leg (Hull et al, 1979b; Salzman et al, 1980; Skillman et al, 1978; Turpie et al, 1977), dextran (Gruber et al, 1980) and oral anticoagulants (Coventry et al, 1973). Low dose heparin is usually given in a dose of 5000 units two hours pre-operatively and then either twelve-hourly or eight-hourly post surgery (Circulation, 1977). This form of prophylaxis is effective in preventing calf-vein thrombi, proximal vein thrombi (Gallus et al, 1946; Circulation, 1977) and fatal pulmonary emboli (Lancet, 1975). It is the most convenient prophylactic method in high-risk medical and surgical patients. External

Table 10.2   Recommended prophylactic methods in the various high-risk groups

	Risk of thromboembolism	(%)	Recommended preventive measure
Elective abdominal or thoracic surgery Over 40, under general anesthesia for at least 30 minutes	Calf-vein thrombosis Proximal vein thrombosis Fatal pulmonary embolism	10–40 2–8 0.1–0.7	Low-dose heparin or external pneumatic compression
Over 40, previous venous thrombosis, or extensive surgery for malignant disease	Calf-vein thrombosis Proximal vein thrombosis Fatal pulmonary embolism	30–60 6–12 1–2	Low-dose heparin and postoperative ^{125}I-fibrinogen leg scanning
Genito-urinary surgery Transurethral Abdominal	Calf-vein thrombosis Calf-vein thrombosis	7–10 25–50	External pneumatic compression External pneumatic compression
Neurosurgery	Calf-vein thrombosis	20–25	External pneumatic compression
Orthopaedic Hip surgery	Calf-vein thrombosis Proximal vein thrombosis Fatal pulmonary embolism	50 20 1–5	External pneumatic compression prevents calf thrombosis but not proximal thrombosis. Screening with ^{125}I-fribrinogen leg scanning and IPG post-operatively.
Hip surgery			Oral anticoagulants commenced post operatively in patients with previous DVT.
Major knee surgery	Calf-vein thrombosis Proximal vein thrombosis	60–70 20	External pneumatic compression
High-risk medical patients Myocardial infarction Stroke	Calf-vein thrombosis Calf-vein thrombosis	20–40 60	Low-dose heparin Low-dose heparin or external pneumatic compression

pneumatic compression is a highly effective form of prophylaxiis which can be used as an alternative to low-dose heparin in patients in whom low-dose heparin is either contra-indicated or ineffective. Dextran is a useful method with demonstrated efficacy in orthopaedic patients with hip fracture (Gruber et al, 1980), but its use may be complicated by volume overload in elderly patients who have impaired cardiac function.

CHOICE OF PROPHYLAXIS IN THE VARIOUS HIGH RISK GROUPS

Elective abdominal and thoracic surgery

The risk of venous thromboembolism in patients undergoing abdominal or thoracic surgery is influenced by the patient's age, nature and extent of the operative procedure and on whether or not there is a history of previous thromboembolism. Without prophylaxis, elderly patients over the age of 60 who have abdominal or thoracic surgical procedures performed under general anaesthesia which last at least 30 minutes have a risk of developing calf-vein thrombosis which varies between 20 and 40 per cent of proximal vein thrombosis between 4 and 8 per cent and of fatal pulmonary embolism between 0.2 and 0.7 per cent. (Gallus et al, 1976; Lancet, 1975; Rosenberg, 1975). These patients should be given prophylaxis either with low-dose heparin or external pneumatic compression. Patients with a history of recent venous thromboembolism or who have extensive pelvic or abdominal surgery or advanced malignancy are even at higher risk (Roberts & Cotton, 1974). Without prophylaxis, these patients have a 30–60 per cent risk of developing ^{125}I-fibrinogen leg scan detected calf-vein thrombosis, a 6–12 per cent risk of developing proximal vein thrombi and a 1–2 per cent risk of fatal pulmonary embolism.

The best form of prophylaxis for this very high-risk category has not been established, but it is reasonable to suggest that an effective method of primary prophylaxis such as low-dose heparin or external pneumatic compression can be combined with ^{125}I-fibrinogen leg scanning to detect patients who break through primary prophylaxis.

Hip surgery

Without prophylaxis, over 50 per cent of patients who have elective hip surgery or who have a fractured hip develop venous thrombosis (Hirsh & Salzman, 1982; Hull et al, 1979c); 20 per cent develop proximal vein thrombosis (Hampson et al, 1974) and 1–5 per cent have a fatal pulmonary embolism embolism. (Eskeland et al, 1966). Two forms of prophylaxis, oral anticoagulants and dextran (Gruber et al, 1980) are effective in preventing venous thromboembolism in these patients. Oral anticoagulants are most effective when treatment is initiated before surgery or at the time of surgery, but this is associated with an increased risk of bleeding which is considered unacceptable by most orthopaedic surgeons. Bleeding is reduced if oral anticoagulants are started 48 hours after completing surgery in a dose which is aimed to prolong the prothrombin time to approximately 1.2–1.5 times control (rabbit-brain thromboplastin) on the fourth or fifth postoperative day. Although this approach needs to be evaluated further in properly designed studies, we use this method in fractured hip patients with a previous history of deep venous thrombosis. Dextran commenced pre-operatively is effective but, because of the risk of volume overload, it is not recommended in elderly patients. At the present time, the combination of screening tests (IPG and ^{125}I-fibrinogen leg scanning) although very cost-ineffective, is the most appropriate preventive measure in these patients until a safe and effective prophylactic method is available (Hull et al, 1979c).

Major knee surgery

Without protection, 60–70 per cent of patients undergoing major knee surgery develop calf-vein thrombosis and 20 per cent develop proximal vein thrombosis (Hull et al 1979b). External pneumatic compression is highly effective in these patients and is the prophylactic method of choice. In these patients, external pneumatic compression is continued postoperatively until patients are ambulatory. In patients with a plastercast, prophylaxis with oral anticoagulants or subcutaneous heparin started postoperatively is the method of choice and should be continued until the plastercast is removed.

Genito-urinary surgery

Transurethral resection of the prostate carries a 7–10 per cent risk of developing ^{125}I leg scan detected calf-vein thrombosis (Salzman et al, 1980; Coe et al, 1978). The risk is even higher in patients having retropubic prostatectomy or an equivalent operation, since 25–50 per cent develop leg scan detected calf-vein thrombosis. The results of low dose heparin have been inconsistent in this group. On the other hand, external pneumatic compression is effective and is the method of choice to prevent calf-vein thrombosis.

HIGH-RISK MEDICAL PATIENTS

Myocardial infarction

Between 20 and 40 per cent of patients who sustain an acute myocardial infarction develop calf-vein thrombosis, and the risk is higher in patients who also develop congestive heart failure (Habersberger et al, 1973). Low-dose heparin is effective in reducing the frequency of leg scan detected venous thrombosis in these patients (Handley et al, 1972)).

Cerebrovascular accidents

Approximately 60 per cent of all patients who sustain a paralytic stroke develop leg scan detected venous thrombosis (McCarthy et al, 1977). Although not definitively established, it is likely that either external pneumatic compression (turpie et al, 1977) or low-dose heparin would be effective in preventing serious venous thromboembolism in this patient group. External pneumatic compression is the prophylactic method of choice in patients with intracerebral haemorrhage.

DIAGNOSIS OF PULMONARY EMBOLISM

The clinical diagnosis of pulmonary embolism is unreliable because the symptoms and signs are all non-specific (McNeil & Bettman, 1982; Hull et al, 1983b). Although dyspnoea, tachypnoea and pleuritic chest pain occur in a majority of patients with angiographically demonstrated emboli, these clinical features are non-specific and cannot reliably distinguish between patients with pulmonary embolism and those with other cardiopulmonary disorders. This is particularly true in elderly patients who have an underlying cardiopulmonary disorder (e.g. chronic obstructive lung disease, congestive cardiac failure) which may mask some of the manifestations of pulmonary embolism.

Historically, a number of laboratory investigations have been used either as screening tests or as definitive diagnostic tests in patients with clinically suspected pulmonary embolism (Hirsh et al, 1981c). These investigations which include serum enzymes and bilirubin, level of fibrin split products, arterial blood gas analysis, chest X-ray and electrocardiographic findings, have all been shown to lack sensitivity and specificity and, therefore, cannot be used either to confirm or rule to out pulmonary embolism. The chest X-ray and E.C.G. are important investigations to rule out other disorders which may simulate pulmonary embolism but cannot be used to diagnose pulmonary emblism.

The diagnostic approach to pulmonary embolism is not as clearcut as the diagnostic approach to venous thrombosis because the diagnostic standard, pulmonary angiography, cannot be peformed in all centres and the non-invasive tests, particularly lung scanning, which are used as a substitute for pulmonary angiography, have not been as carefully evaluated as the non-invasive tests for venous thrombosis (Hirsh, 1982).

Lung scan

Perfusion scintigraphy with technicium-99m is widely used as a screening test in patients with clinically suspected pulmonary embolism (McNeil & Bettman, 1982). This technique detects occluded vessels more than 3mm in diameter and is virtually 100 per cent sensitive in its ability to detect clinically significant pulmonary emboli. This test also has a high negative predictive value, since a normal perfusion scan excludes a diagnosis of pulmonary embolism (Hull et al, 1983b). When this test was first introduced in the late 1960s, it became rapidly accepted as a valid test for the diagnosis of pulmonary embolism, and it was believed that most patients with clinically suspected pulmonary embolism who had an abnormal perfusion lung scan and a normal chest X-ray had pulmonary embolism. However, it was soon realised that the perfusion lung scan was non-specific, since it could not distinguish between pulmonary embolism and a number of non-embolic pathological processes which also affect pulmonary blood flow (McNeil & Bettman, 1982).

With the advent of ventilation scanning in the late 1970s, a new diagnostic concept was developed to improve the specificity of the perfusion lung scan. This concept was based on the premise that patients with pulmonary emboli have an abnormal perfusion scan and a normal ventilation scan (a so-called ventilation/perfusion mismatch), while patients with a primary ventilation defect have a matching abnormality on the perfusion and ventilation scan. When studies comparing the results of pulmonary angiography with ventilation and perfusion scans were performed in patients with clinically suspected pulmonary embolism, it became evident that the mismatch concept was an oversimplification. These studies demonstrated that the probability of pulmonary embolism is 80 per cent or greater when the perfusion scan shows a very large defect (segmental or larger) with a normal ventilation scan (Hull et al, 1983b; Hirsh et al, 1981d; McNeil, 1976; Neumann et al, 1980). On the other hand, patients with smaller perfusion defects (subsegemental or smaller) often do not have pulmonary embolism even though they have a normal ventilation scan, while patients with abnormal perfusion and ventilation lung scans sometimes have pulmonary embolism demonstrated by pulmonary angiography (Hull et al, 1983b).

In summary, therefore, it can be concluded that: (a) perfusion scintigraphy is a very sensitive screening test for patients with clinically suspected pulmonary embolism, (b) a normal perfusion lung scan rules out pulmonary embolism, (c) the ventilation scan is a useful addition to the diagnostic process in patients with large (segmental or larger) perfusion defects if the ventilation scan is normal, since 80 per cent or more of these patients have pulmonary embolism documented by pulmonary angiography, (d) ventilation–perfusion scanning is not useful for making management decisions in patients with small defects (subsegmental or smaller) or in patients with large matched defects, since it is not possible to confirm or rule out pulmonary embolism in patients with these patterns of perfusion–ventilation scan abnormalities.

Pulmonary angiography

Pulmonary angiography is the most definitive means of making the diagnosis of pulmonary embolism and it is the reference method (hull et al, 1983b). Technical improvements in recent years have made this method more accurate and safer (Mills et al, 1980) to perform even in elderly patients. Pulmonary angiography is performed by passing a catheter through the right heart and then injecting dye selectively into each of the main pulmonary artery branches. With selective filling of the artery, accuracy is markedly improved and much less dye needs to be injected. The most reliable criterion for the diagnosis of pulmonary embolism is the presence of an intraluminal filling defect. (Fig. 10.9) A sharp vessel cut-off is an indirect sign and is not diagnostic of pulmonary embolism. When indicated, pulmonary angiography should be performed as soon as possible after a provisional diagnosis of pulmonary embolism has been made by lung scan because thrombi fragment after a few days and false-negative results may occur (McNeil & Bettman, 1982).

A suggested approach to the diagnosis of pulmonary embolism

On the basis of our studies and other reports in the literature, we have

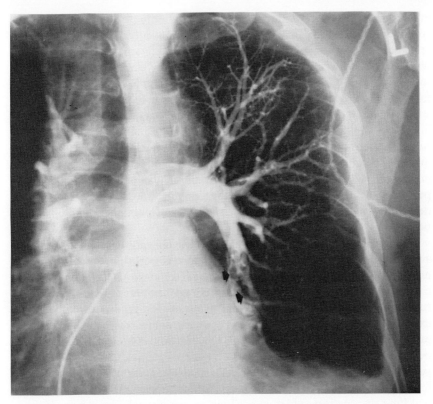

Fig. 10.9 Selective pulmonary angiogram: a constant intraluminal filling defect at the first bifurcation of the left lower lobe main pulmonary artery establishes a definitive diagnosis of pulmonary embolism

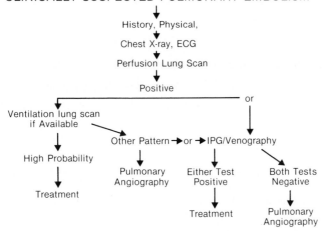

Fig. 10.10 Diagnostic algorithm for patients with clinically suspected pulmonary embolism and abnormal lung scan

evolved an approach to the diagnosis of pulmonary embolism which is summarised in Figure 10.10. Three investigations are key to this diagnostic approach: ventilation–perfusion lung scanning, pulmonary angiography and objective tests for deep-vein thrombosis. There are a number of components to this algorithm. All patients should have a chest X-ray and E.C.G. performed to rule out other conditions which may mimic pulmonary embolism, such as pneumothorax, myocardial infarction, pnemonia etc. A perfusion lung scan should be performed and, if this is normal, clinically significant pulmonary embolism can be excluded and no further investigation is required. If the perfusion lung scan is abnormal and the defect is segmental or greater in size, then a ventilation scan should be performed, and if the perfusion–ventilation scan pattern shows one or more segmental or greater defect(s) which ventilate normally, a diagnosis of pulmonary embolism can be made.

Pulmonary angiography is the most definitive means to diagnose pulmonary embolism in patients who have an abnormal perfusion scan which does not fall into the category of high probability (see above), since none of these patterns has sufficiently high or low predictive power either to confirm or rule out pulmonary embolism. Objective tests for venous thrombosis are extremely useful, since a positive IPG or venogram increases the likelihood of pulmonary embolism (Hull et al, 1983b) and, in patients with an abnormal perfusion scan, a decision to treat with anticoagulants can be made without performing a pulmonary angiogram. Pulmonary angiography should be performed in patients with clinically suspected pulmonary embolism and abnormal lung scan pattern which is not high probability who have normal venograms or in patients where the nature of the underlying pulmonary abnormality needs to be clarified, e.g. investigations of a pulmonary infiltrate, pleural effusion. Plumonary angiography is also indicated before initiating thrombolytic therapy in patients with massive pulmonary embolism.

TREATMENT OF VENOUS THROMBOEMBOLISM

Proximal deep-vein thrombosis and/or pulmonary embolism

The main objectives of the treatment of venous thromboembolism are: (a) to prevent death from pulmonary embolism, (b) to reduce morbidity from the acute event, and (c) to achieve these objectives with a minimum of side-effects. In most patients, these objectives can be achieved with anticoagulants but, because they are not free from side-effects, it is important to ensure that the diagnosis of venous thrombo-embolism is confirmed by objective tests before initiating treatment (Hirsh, 1982).

Heparin is the treatment of choice in patients with proximal deep-vein thrombosis and/or pulmonary embolism because it is effective in both preventing extension of venous thrombi and fatal pulmonary embolism (Hirsh et al, 1981e). The standard approach is to administer an intial bolus of heparin followed by either a continuous infusion or by four-hourly intermittent injections. For most patients, an initial loading dose of 5000 units of heparin is sufficient, but patients with extensive proximal vein thrombosis or pulmonary embolism usually require a higher dose (7000–10 000 units of heparin), whereas very old and frail patients should receive a lower dose (approximately 3000 units). The continuous infusion of heparin is administered in a dosage of 24 000 units per 24 hours, and the dose is adjusted according to results of the monitoring test.

The activated partial thromboplastin time (APTT) is one of the most commonly used methods to monitor the anticoagulant effect of heparin in North America (Hirsh et al, 1981e). When the continous infusion method is used, the aim is to maintain the test result at approximately 1½ times control. When intermittent intravenous heparin is used, the aim is to maintain the APTT atapproximately 1½ times control before the next injection is due. It may be useful to obtain a heparin level in patients who fail to demonstrate adequate prolongation of the activated partial thromboplastin time despite treatment with what appear to be adequate doses of heparin. In these patients, the failure to prolong the APPT may be associated with either low levels of circulating heparin or 'therapeutic' levels of circulating heparin (0.3–0.5 units per ml) (Chiu et al, 1977). If the heparin level is low, the dose of heparin should be increased. If, however, the heparin level is within the therapeutic range (0.3–0.5 units per ml) then we would recommended that the dose should not be increased further. The reason why the APTT-remains relatively short in the presence of adequate heparin levels is not always clear, but in many cases it is due to very levels of coagulation factors (particularly factor VIII) which artificially shorten the APTT.

Intermittent intravenous injection of heparin can be used as an alternative to full-dose continuous intravenous heparin infusion. This appproach has been reported to produce a greater frequency of bleeding in patients who have high risk of haemorrhage (Hirsh et al, 1981f). It should be noted, however, that in these studies higher doses of heparin were used in the group given intravenous heparin, so that the increased rate of bleeding could have been related to the dose rather than the method of administration. Intermittent injection of heparin should be administered every four hours in a dose of 4000–7000 units per injection. Although it is recommended that the dose be adjusted to produce an activated partial thromboplastin time of approximately 1½ times control immediately before the next injection is due, in practice careful laboratory monitoring with intermittent heparin is difficult. Subcutaneous heparin given in full therapeutic doses has been reported to be another effective method of heparin administration, and preliminary studies suggest that it may cause less bleeding. However, this method has not been properly evaluated.

In patients with proximal deep-vein thrombosis or pulmonary embolism, the treatment with intravenous heparin is followed by oral anticoagulants for a period of twelve weeks (Hirsh et al, 1981q) Oral anticoagulants are given to prevent the late recurrence of venous thrombembolism. In patients with an underlying risk factor e.g. lower-limb fracture, paralytic stroke, it is sensible to continue therapy until the risk factor is reversed. Oral anticoagulants should be started four to five days before heparin is stopped, since the full antithrombotic effect of oral anticoagulants may be delayed.

The administration of vitamin K antagonists monitored by conventional levels of anticoagulant controls is associated with an appreciable risk of bleeding (5 per cent major bleeding episodes). Recently we have conducted a series of clinical trials designed to answer the question of whether protection against late recurrence of venous thromboembolism can be achieved without exposing patients to a substantial risk of haemorrhage. In these studies, three anti-coagulant regimens for the long-term treatment of proximal deep-vein thrombosis were successfully explored. These are:

1. Adjusted intermediate dose of subcutaneous heparin (Hull et al, 1982a).
2. Conventional oral anticoagulant therapy using sodium warfarin with prothrombin time (using Simplastin) maintained at $1\frac{1}{2}$ to 2 times control (Hull et al, 1979a).
3. A less intense anticoagulant approach using sodium warfarin with a prothrombin time (using Simplastin maintained at approximately $1\frac{1}{4}$ times control (Hull et al, 1982b).

In the first of these studies, conventional sodium warfarin therapy was compared with an adjusted dose of subcutaneous heparin which we predicted might be associated with a lower risk of haemorrhage without loss of effectiveness in preventing recurrent venous thromboembolism. The dose in the subcutaneous heparin group was adjusted to maintain the mid-interval activated partial thromboplastin time (determined six hours after injection) at $1\frac{1}{2}$ times the control value. The dose was then fixed after the initial three days, and no further anticoagulant monitoring was performed throughout the three months of long-term therapy. Adjusted-dose subcutaneous heparin regimen proved effective in preventing recurrent venous thrombemoblism, and its use was associated with a significantly lower risk of bleeding (less than 2 per cent) than conventional sodium warfarin therapy.

The next study was designed with the premise that a less intense anticoagulant regimen using sodium warfarin might also be effective in preventing recurrence of venous thromboembolism and that it might be associated with a lower risk of bleeding, therefore conventional oral anticoagulant therapy was compared with a less intense regimen using sodium warfarin. The patients randomised into the less intense oral anticoagulant group had their warfarin therapy monitored to maintain the prothrombin time using human-brain thromboplastin (Manchester Comparative Reagent) at twice the control values. This is comparable to a prothrombin time using Simplastin of approximately 15 seconds (or $1\frac{1}{4}$ times the control). This study demonstrated that sodium warfarin administered to provide a less intense anticoagulant effect retained its effectiveness against recurrent venous thromboembolism (the frequency of recurrence was less than 2 per cent) with a greatly reduced frequency of bleeding (less than 5 per cent compared to a frequency of 20 per cent in the conventional sodium warfarin group).

The findings of these randomised trials indicate that the haemorrhagic risk of long-term therapy for venous thrombosis can be substantially reduced by either using an adjusted dose of subcutaneous heparin regimen or a less intense oral warfarin sodium regimen. The adjusted-dose subcutaneous regime can be used in patients who cannot take oral medication, but it should be used with caution in elderly patients, in view of the risk of osteoporosis associated with long-term administration of heparin. A less intense oral anticoagulant regimen can be achieved either by maintaining prothrombin time using Simplastin at approximately 1¼ times control, or by using a more sensitive human-brain thromboplastin (e.g. Manchester Comparative Reagent, which is widely available in Europe) maintained between 24 and 28 seconds (control of 12–13 seconds).

Calf deep-vein thrombosis

Patients with isolated calf-vein thrombosis are usually treated in hospital with heparin for seven days, followed by either oral anticoagulants or by subcutaneous heparin at the dose of 5000 units every twelve hours for six weeks (Hull et al, 1979a).

Major pulmonary embolism

In some patients the clinical manifestations of pulmonary embolism are accompanied by haemodynamic impairment as manifested by hypotension and/or acute cor pulmonale. These very ill patients are at risk of dying over the next 12–24 hours as a reesult of pulmonary vascular obstruction, severe hypoxaemia, arrhythmia, acideamia or even a small recurrent embolism. This clinical picture is seen in patients with massive embolism or with pre-existing cardiac or pulmonary disease. The first step is the management of this condition is to confirm pulmonary embolism by objective testing. The differential diagnosis includes other conditions which may simulate massive pulmonary embolism, such as acute myocardial infarction, dissecting aneurysm of ascending aorta, pericardial tamponade, tension pneumothorax, haemorrhage and septic shock. Although the indication for thrombolytic therapy in patients with acute pulmonary embolism has not been definitely established, rapid lysis of emboli in these critically ill patients is desirable (Verstraete, 1978). In this situation, pulmonary embolism should be confirmed by pulmonary angiogram, and thrombolyttic therapy should be started as soon as possible and continued for 12 to 24 hours; it should be followed by heparin and then oral anticoagulants.

Recurrent venous thromboembolism

The first step in the management of acute recurrent deep-vein thrombosis is to confirm the diagnosis by using objective tests. Patients with acute recurrent deep-vein thrombosis are treated with continuous heparin for a period of seven to ten days, followed by oral anticoagulants for at least a year in view of the high recurrence rate (20 per cent in the following year) in patients who received only three months of oral anticoagulants (Hull et al, 1983a). In addition, life-long anticoagulation should be considered: (a) in patients with more than two episodes of well-documented venous thromboembolism, (b) after a first episode of pulmonary embolism in patients who have a severe underlying cardiopulmonary condition in whom a small or moderate-size pulmonary embolism could be fatal, and (c) in patients with a constitutional abnormality with a tendency to venous thrombembolism (e.g protein C deficiency, antithrombin III deficiency).

TREATMENT OF THE POST-PHLEBITIC SYNDROME

The underlying venous pathology of the post-phlebitic syndrome is irreversible so that these patients cannot be cured either by surgical or medical means (Browse, 1982; Owens, 1978). However, the morbidity of the condition can be reduced by increasing venous return and preventing stasis. These objectives can be best achieved by periodic leg elevation and by the use of custom-fitted graduated-compression stockings (Jones et al, 1980). These stockings help to control venous reflux during standing and exercise and diminish the long-term manifestations of venous hypertension. Most patients experience subjective relief from compression stockings, and there is a strong clinical impression that the application of these stockings at the first sign of post-phlebitic symptoms prevents venous ulceration. We prescribe graduated-compression stockings to all patients with proximal venous thrombosis at the first symptoms of chronic leg swelling or ache.

TREATMENT OF THROMBONEUROSIS

The treatment of thromboneurosis is difficult and prolonged, but with persistence and encouragement a successful outcome can be reached in the majority of patients. Treatment is directed at proving to the patient that symptoms are not caused by a potentially fatal illness and that it is safe to withdraw anticoagulants. This usually requires demonstrating to the patient and to the referring physician that the venogram is normal and that the recurrent episodes of leg symptoms occur in the pressence of normal non-invasive test findings. Sometimes a second venogram is required to convince both patient and referring physician that symptoms are not due to venous thromboembolic disease. We advise thee patient to return gradually to normal physical activity and then develop an exercise programme depending on the patient's preference, consisting of either cycling, jogging or swimming. This acts as a positive reinforcement and helps to focus the patient's attention away from his or her legs.

It should be emphasised that the most effective way of treating thromboneurosis is to prevent it. Prevention is best achieved by investigating patients with suspected venous thrombosis with objective tests and unequivocally ruling out the disorder when the tests are negative. The practice of treating patients for 7–10 days on the basis of clinical diagnosis or equivocal results with objective tests is unacceptable, because patients will attribute further leg symptoms to thromboembolic disease, and a cycle of leg pain and treatment will be established.

REFERENCES

Barnes R W 1982 Doppler ultrasonic diagnosis of venous diseases. In Bernstein E F (ed) Noninvasive diagnostic techniques in vascular disease, p.452. Mosby, St Louis.

Barnes R W et al 1972 Non-invasive quantitation of maximum venous outflow in acute thrombophlebitis. Surgery 72: 971

Bauer G 1950 Patho-physiology and treatment of the lower leg stasis syndrome. Angiology 1: 1

Bell W R, Simon T L 1982 Current status of pulmonary thromboembolic disease: pathophysiology, diagnosis, prevention and treatment. American Heart Journal 102: 239

Browes N L 1982 Venous insufficiency: non operative management. In: Bang N, Glover J, Holden R, Triplett D(eds) Thrombosis and atherosclerosis, p. 275. Year Book Medical Publishers, Chicago.

Burnand K G et al 1977 The relative importance of incompetent communicating veins in the production of varicose and venous ulcers. Surgery 82: 9

Burnand K G et al 1979 The relationship between the number of capillaries in the skin of the venous ulcer-bearing areas of the lower leg and the fall in foot vein pressure during exercise. British Journal of Surgery 68: 297

Chiu H M et al 1977 Relationship between the anticoagulant and antithrombotic effects of heparin in experimental venous thrombosis. Blood 49: 171

Circulation 1977 Special report: prevention of venous thromboembolism in surgical patients by low-dose heparin. Circulation 55: 423A

Clagett G P, Salzman E W 1975 Prevention of venous thromboembolism. Progress in Cardiovascular Diseases 17: 345

Coe N P et al 1978 Prevention of deep vein thrombosis in urological patients: a controlled randomized trial of low-dose heparin and external pneumatic compression boots. Surgery 83: 230

Coon W W, Cooler F A 1959 Some epidemiologic consideration of thromboembolism. Surgery, Gynecology and Obstetrics 109: 487

Coventry M B, Nolan D R, Beckenbaught R D 1973 Delayed prophylactic anticoagulation. A study of results and complications in 2012 total hip arthroplasties. Journal of Bone and Joint Surgery 55A: 1487

DeCamp P T, Ward J A, Ochsner A 1951 Ambulatory venous pressure studies in post-phlebitic and other disease states. Surgery 29: 42

Eskeland G, Solheim K, Skjorten F 1966 Anticoagulant prophylaxis, thromboembolism and mortality in elderly patients with hip fractures. A controlled clinical trial. ACTA Chirurgica Scandinavica 131: 16

Evans D A 1971 The early diagnosis of thromboembolism by ultrasound. Annals of the Royal College of Surgeons of England 49: 225

Gallus A S et al 1976 Prevention of venous thrombosis with small, subcutaneous doses of heparin. Journal of the American Medical Association 235: 1980

Gruber U F et al 1980 Incidence of fatal postoperative pulmonary embolism after prophylaxis with dextran 70 and low-dose heparin. An international multicentre study. British Medical Journal 280: 69

Habersberger P G, Pitt A, Anderson S T 1973 Benous thrombosis in myocardial infarction. Comparison in heparin dosage. British Heart Journal 2: 436

Hampson W G et al 1974 Failure of low-dose heparin to prevent deep-vein thrombosis after hip replacement arthroplasty. Lancet ii: 795

Handley A J, Emerson P A, Fleming P R 1972 Heparin in the prevention of deep venous thrombosis after myocardial infarction. British Medical Journal 2: 436

Hirsh J 1982 Noninvasive tests for thromboembolic disease. Hospital Practice 17: 77

Hirsh J, Hull R 1978 Comparative value of tests for the diagnosis of venous thrombosis. World Journal of Surgery 2: 27

Hirsh J, Salzman E W 1982 Prevention of venous thromboembolism. In: Coleman R W, Hirsh J, Marder V, Slazman E W (eds) Thrombosis and hemostasis: basic principles and clinical practice. Lippincott, Philadelphia

Hirsh J, Genton E, Hull R 1981a Venous thromboembolism. Grune and Stratton, New York

Hirsh J, Genton E, Hull R 1981b Risk factors in thrombosis. In: Hirsh J, Genton E, Hull R (eds) Venous thromboembolism. Grune & Stratton, New York

Hirsh J, Genton, E, Hull R 1981c Venous thrombosis. In Hirsh J, Genton E, Hull R (eds) Venous thromboembolism. An:p. nost Grune & Stratton, New York

Hirsh J, Genton E, Hull R 1981d Diagnosis of pulmonary embolism. In: Hirsh J, Genton E, Hull R (eds) Venous thromboembolism. Grune & Stratton, New York

Hirsh J, Genton E, Hull R 1981e Treatment of venous thromboembolism. In: Hirsh J, Genton E, Hull R (eds) Venous thromboembolism, pp122–144. Grune & Stratton, New York

Hirsh J, Genton E, Hull R 1981f Heparin. In: Hirsh J, Genton E, Hull R (eds) Venous thromboembolism, pp 155–183. Grune & Stratton, New York

Hirsh J, Genton E, Hull R 1981g Vitamin K antagonists (oral anticoagulants) In: Hirsh J, Genton E, Hull R (eds) Venous thromboembolism, pp184–197. Grune & Stratton, New York

Hojemsgard I C, Sturp H 1950 Venous pressure in primary and post-thrombotic varicose veins. ACTA Chirurgica Scandinavica 99: 133

Holmes M C G 1973 Deep venous thrombosis of the lower limbs diagnosed by ultrasound. Medical Journal of Australia 1: 427

Hull R 1981 Venous thromboembolism: applying epidemiology to controversies. Vascular Diagnosis and Therapy An: Vol & p nos

Hull R et al 1976 Impedance plethysmography using the occlusive cuff technique in the diagnosis of venous thrombosis. Circulation 53: 696

Hull R et al 1977 Combined use of leg scanning and impedance lethysmography in suspected venous thrombosis, an alternative to venography. New England Journal of Medicine 296: 1497

Hull R et al 1979a Warfarin-sodium versus low-dose heparin in the long term treatment of venous thrombosis. New England Journal of Medicine 301: 855–858

Hull R et al 1979b Effectiveness of intermittent pulsatile elastic stockings for the prevention of calf and thigh vein thrombosis in patients undergoing elective knee surgery. Thrombosis Research 16: 37

Hull R et al 1979c The value of adding impedance plethysography to ^{125}I-fibrinogen leg scanning for the detection of deep vein thrombosis in high risk surgical patients: a comparative study between patients undergoing general surgery and hip surgery Thrombosis Research 15: 227

Hull R et al 1981a Clinical validity of a negative venogram in patients with clinically suspected venous thrombosis. Circulation 64: 622

Hull R et al 1981b Replacement of venography in suspected venous thrombosis by impedance plethysmography and ^{125}I-fibrinogen leg scanning. Annals of Internal Medicine 94: 12

Hull R et al 1982a Adjusted subcutaneous heparin venous warfarin sodium in the long-term treatment of venous thrombosis. New England Journal of Medicine 3076: 189

Hull R et al 1982b Differential intensities of oral anticoagulant therapy in the treatment of proximal vein thrombosis. New England Journal of Medicine 307: 1976

Hull R et al 1983a The diagnosis of acute recurrent, deep-vein thrombosis: a diagnostic challenge. Circulation 67: 901

Hull R D et al 1983b Pulmonary angiography, ventilation lung scanning and venography for clinically suspected pulmonary embolism with abnormal perfusion lung scan. Annals of Internal Meeicine 98: 891

Johnson G 1980 Chronic venous insufficiency of the lower extremity: an overview. In: Foley W (ed) Advances of the atherosclerotic plaque, p. 195. Year Book Medical Publishers, Chicago p.195.

Jones M A G et al 1980 A physiological study of elastic compression stockings in venous disorders of the leg. British Journal of Surgery 67: 569

Kakkar V V 1972 The diagnosis of deep-vein thrombosis using the ^{125}I-fibrinogen test. Archives of Surgery 104: 152

Kakkar V V et al 1972[125]I-labelled fibrinogen test adapted for routine screening for deep-vein thrombois. Lancet i: 540

Kakkar V V et al 1979 Prophylaxis for postoperative deep-vein thrombosis. Journal of the American Medical Association 241: 39

Lancet 1975 An international multicentre trial: prevention of fatal post-operative pulmonary embolism by low doses of heparin. Lancet ii: 45

LeClerc J R, Hull R D, Hirsh J 1985 The management of the post phlebitic syndrome and its differentiation from recurrent deep vein thrombosis. Wright, New York

McCarthy S T et al 1977 Low-dose heparin as a prophylaxis against deep-vein thrombosis after acute stroke. Lancet ii: 800

McNeil B J, Bettman M A 1982 The diagnosis of pulmonary embolism. In: Colman R W, Hirsh J, Marder V J, Salzman E W (eds) Hemostasis and thrombosis, p. 844. Lippincott, Philadelphia

Mills S R et al 1980 The incidence, etiologies and avoidance of complications of pulmonary angiography in a large series. Radiology 136: 295

Negus D 1968 Calf pain in the post thrombotic syndrome. British Medical Journal 2: 156

Negus D 1970 The post thrombotic syndrome. Annals of the Royal College of Surgeons of England 47: 92

Owens J C 1978 The post-phlebitic syndrome: management of conservative means. In: Bergan J J, Yao J S T (eds) Venous problems, p. 369. Year Book Medical Publishers, Chicago

Roberts V C, Cotton L T 1974 Prevention of postoperative deep-vein thrombosis in patients with malignant disease. British Medical Journal I: 358

Rosenberg L, Evans M, Pollack A V 1975 Prophylaxis of postoperative leg vein thrombosis by low dose subcutaneous heparin or perioperative calf muscle stimulation: a controlled clinical trial. British Medical Journal I: 649

Salzman E W et al 1980 Intraoperative external pneumatic calf compression to afford long-term prophylaxis against deep-vein thrombosis in urological patients. Surgery 87: 239

Shull K C et al 1979 Significance of opoliteal reflux in relation to ambulatory venous pressure and ulceration. Archives of Surgery 114: 1304

Sigel B et al 1972 Diagnosis of lower limb venous thrombosis by Doppler ultrasound technique. Archives of Surgery 104: 174

Skillman J J, Collins R E, Coe N P 1978 Prevention of deep-vein thrombosis in neurosurgical patients: controlled randomized trial of external pneumatic compression boots. Surgery 83: 354

Strandness D E, Summer D S 1972 Ultrasonic velocity detector in the diagnosis of thrombophlebitis. Archives of Surgery 104: 180

Taylor D W et al 1980 Simplification of the sequential impedance plethysmograph technique without loss of accuracy. Thrombosis Research 17: 561

Tripolitis A J et al 1980 The physiology of venous claudication. American Journal of Surgery 139: 447

Turpie A G G et al 1972 Prevention of venous thrombosis in patients with intracranial disease by intermittent pneumatic compression of the calf. Neurology 27: 435

Verstraete M 1978 Biochemical and clinical aspects of thrombolysis. Seminars in Hematology 15: 35

Vieweg W V R et al 1970 Complications of intravvenous administration of heparin in elderly women. Journal of the American Medical Association 213: 1303

The leukaemias

DEFINITION, CLASSIFICATION AND INCIDENCE

The general concept of leukaemia as a group of malignant neoplastic disorders arising among cells of the haemopoietic system and including both acute and chronic forms, with either myeloid or lymphoid characterisation, applies to elderly patients as to younger ones. There are some differences in distribution of subtypes that call for comment, and borderline leukaemic conditions such as preleukaemias, smouldering leukaemias or myelodysplastic states are especially common in the elderly. The area of semantic overlap between primary lymphoid leukaemias and secondary leukaemic phases of non-Hodgkin's lymphoma (NHL) is also more prominent in older patients, since NHL is chiefly a disease of the older age groups.

The conditions which are normally included under the heading of leukaemia are listed in Table 11.1 and the abbreviations subsequently used are also given in that table, together with a summary of the main diagnostic laboratory features or other distinguishing characteristics. A few of the conditions listed in Table 11.1, notably APL and the AMyL subset with t(8;21), are seen especially in younger patients, but so far as the four broad groups of AML, ALL, CML and CLL are concerned, all show a rising incidence with advancing age until around 80 years. The point is illustrated in Table 11.2, which shows features generally confirmed for both sexes and among many populations (apart from the virtual absence of CLL in Japanese). Clearly the chronic leukaemias become increasingly common over the age of 60, while acute leukaemias remain predominantly myeloid, as at all ages over 20.

The statistics of incidence of leukaemia in Britain and in most other Western countries showed an overall increase in the middle years of this century, at least between 1920 and 1970, of the order of three- to five-fold, but it seems likely that much of that increase is apparent rather than real, being due to better medical facilities and improved diagnosis. Nevertheless there may well have been some real increase in both AML and CML and in CLL in middle-aged and elderly patients. The data are reviewed and discussed by Doll (1965, 1972).

Table 11.1 Classification and major cytological features of leukaemias

1. Acute leukaemias
Predominantly primitive cells of stem cell to early differentiated blastic and intermediate forms. Generally reflect a stage of normal early differentiation, within either the myeloid (marrow-derived) series, or the lymphoid series of cells. Mixed myeloid-lymphoid cases are probably rare.
(a) Acute lymphoblastic leukaemias (ALL)
  Cases frequently show at least some and often many cells with coarse Periodic acid-Schiff (PAS) positivity — granules or blocks — against a negative background. Sudan black (SB) and peroxidase reactions are negative. Most cases show terminal transferase (Tdt) positivity. Null cell (stem cell, non B non T) — Ph^1 chromosome, t(9;22), positive in about a third of cases.
  Common ALL — probably all early B-cell cases, showing cALL surface marker and equivalent monoclonal reactivity; some with cytoplasmic immunoglobulin (Ig).
  B-ALL — uncommon cases with surface membrane Ig (SmIg).
  T-ALL — cells react with various specific T-cell monoclonal antibodies (McAbs). Acid phosphatase positivity is often strongly localised.
  Mixed types of ALL occur rarely if at all. Chromosome anomalies such as t(4;11), t(8;14), 8q−, 14q+ and 6q− and hyperdiploidy or pseudodiploidy do not show specific links with ALL subvariants.

(b) Acute myeloid leukaemia (AML)
  Myeloblastic; myeloblastic/myelocytic (AMyL) — localised SB/peroxidase positivity, chloroacetate esterase (CE)+, PAS weak, react with specific myeloid McAbs. A subset shows t(8;21).
  Promyelocytic (APL) — frequent Auer rods; bilobed nuclei, may have coarse granules. SB/peroxidase positivity strong. CE++. PAS+. Often show t(15;17).
  Myelomonocytic (AMML) — some twisted nuclei. Mixed localised and scattered SB, mixed CE and butyrate esterase (BE) reactions in the respective granulocyte and monocyte components. May show 11q−.
  Monoblastic (AMonL) — BE reaction usually predominant. SB shows scattered granules. Acid phosphatase may be strong. PAS ranges from negative to coarse granules. May show 11q−.
  Erythroleukaemia (AEL) — SB/peroxidase negative. PAS usually strongly positive; localised acid phosphatase, moderate BE or CE reactions or mixture. Gross aneuploidy and major karyotypic anomalies common. Cells react with antiglycophorin antibodies.
  Megakaryocytic (AMegL) — SB negative, platelet peroxidase reaction positive at EM level. PAS usually strongly positive; CE and BE negative but AE positive. 5'-nucleotidase positive. Cells react with an anti-platelet antibody.
  Mixed myeloid leukaemias are common: the presence of any PAS positivity in erythroblasts probably indicates involvement of the red cell series and is associated with poorer prognosis. Common chromosome abnormalities, not associated with specific subtypes of AML, include trisomy 8, monosomy 7 or 7q−. Defects of 7 and 5q− are very common in AML developing secondary to earlier treatment with ionising radiation and/or alkylating agents. Some 20 per cent of cases show Tdt positivity.

(c) Blastic transformation of chronic myeloid leukaemia (CML–B1) — may show any of the variants listed above except APL or t(8;21). Ph^1, t(9;22), common.

2. Preleukaemic states
These conditions tend to transform sooner or later into acute myeloid leukaemias; they are usually associated with pancytopenia in the peripheral blood and with striking cytological dysplasia involving various myeloid cell lines on marrow examination. The picture may show chiefly erythroid dysplasia as in sideroblastic anaemia or the di Guglielmo's syndrome, but more commonly shows some left shift in granulocytic and megakaryocytic series, with blast cells increased from around 5 to 25 per cent, sometimes showing Auer rods. There may be a relative or absolute monocytosis in both blood and marrow, with raised lysozyme production, a preleukaemic variant sometimes called chronic myelomonocytic leukaemia. Chromosome anomalies in all these myelodysplastic states are generally similar to those in AML except for the t(8;21), t(15;17) and t(9;22) which are not found. A 5q− refractory anaemia with little excess of

blasts but with frequent megakaryocytic anomalies, and male-to-female ratio of 1:5 is especially notable in elderly patients, as are refractory anaemia with excess of blasts (RAEB) or smouldering leukaemia.

3. Chronic leukaemias
Predominance of more mature cells of either myeloid or lymphoid series.
(a) Chronic myeloid leukaemia (CML) — Ph[1] chromosome t(9;22) present in 85 per cent of cases: LAP score very low.
(b) Chronic lymphocytic leukaemia (CLL) —
     B-cell variant — usual; shows monoclonal SmIg and Fc and C3 receptors.
     T-cell variant — uncommon; reacts with T-cell monoclonals. Usually suppressor subset.
(c) Hairy-cell leukaemia (HCL) — an uncommon disease with typical 'hairy' mononuclear cells of uncertain origin; they show tartrate-resistant acid phosphatase and are probably B-cell derived.
(d) Prolymphocytic leukaemia (PLL) — a variant of CLL with larger more primitive cells, often nucleolated.
     B-cell variant — usual.
     T-cell variant — uncommon; perhaps more often of helper than suppressor subset.
(e) Sezary syndrome (SS) — leukaemic phase of mycosis fungoides (MF) — T-cell origin.
(f) Adult T-cell leukaemias (ATL) — an endemic disease in South-West Japan with demonstrated viral aetiology. A possible parallel has been reported in patients of African origin.

Table 11.2 Leukaemia mortality (annual rate per million) among males in England and Wales 1974–78 by five-year age groups and type of leukaemia

Age group	ALL	CLL	AML	CML
0–4	18.6	0	5.4	1.4
5–14	20.6	0	4.8	0.4
15–24	9.6	0	8.6	1.6
25–34	4.2	0	9.8	4.6
35–44	2.6	0.8	13.8	6.0
45–54	3.0	7.2	23.6	13.0
55–64	5.8	29.4	44.8	18.4
65–74	11.4	81.0	82.4	42.2
75–84	23.0	158.2	136.8	79.4
85+	27.4	297.8	165.2	134.2

BIOLOGICAL FEATURES OF LEUKAEMIAS IN ELDERLY PATIENTS

Leukaemias are neoplastic proliferations of haemopoietic cells, that population being one of those which normally continue in active mitotic replication throughout life. Obvious mitotic inadequacy in the maintenance of the haemic cell population is not a generally recognised feature of advancing age, even in the oldest age groups, but there is probably a progressive depletion of the stem cell compartments both numerically and functionally (Andrew, 1971). Studies with cultured human fibroblasts from donors of different ages show that the replicative lifespan of the cultures is inversely proportional to the age of the tissue donor (Goldstein et al, 1983), and probably the same would be true for normal haemic cell precursors. The consequence of this in relation to treatment may well be a reduced capacity for residual normal bone marrow and lymphoid tissue stem cells to recover after cytotoxic drugs have been used to ablate the leukaemic cells. Such an effect might be expected to occur following either short aggressive courses and combination therapy as commonly used in AML, especially when several courses are required, or more prolonged treatment with alkylating agents which may gradually produce further depletion of stem cell stocks on long continued use as in CML or CLL. Growth patterns of leukaemic cells themselves, when observed in short-term cultures, do not seem to differ between older and younger patients, except perhaps for some increase in the failure rate in the elderly (Moore et al, 1974).

Other manifestations of ageing with repercussions in relation to all forms of leukaemia include depressed immune responses and heightened liability to infection, and secondary effects of chronic degenerative diseases, cardiovascular, renal, respiratory or neurological, which may exacerbate the systemic effects of infiltrating leukaemia or restrict the use of cytotoxic agents. As we have seen, AML is much the more common form of acute leukaemia in the elderly, and patients over 60 years figure prominently in several large scale therapeutic trials. In the recent MRC 8th AML trial for example a preliminary analysis of 637 marrow specimens included 168 (26.4 per cent) from patients over the age of 60, and these have been analysed in terms of the incidence of subvarieties of AML. Comparison with the distribution of subtypes in the younger adult age groups of 15–39 and 40–59 show no significant changes in the pattern of incidence so far as the main groups of AMyL, AMML, and AMoL are concerned, but APL is notably less frequent and AEL notably more frequent among the over 60s. Chromosomal abnormalities are somewhat more common in elderly patients with AML. A recent study of 82 patients (Li et al, 1983) showed 49 per cent of 38 patients over 60 to have abnormal karyotypes as compared with 41 per cent of 44 patients under 60.

Preleukaemic or smouldering leukaemic states are especially common in the elderly, and the frequency and type of chromosomal anomalies in these conditions are generally similar to those in florid AML, except that the specific translocations seem not to occur. Secondary leukaemias, following the use of ionising radiation or alkylating agents in, for example, Hodgkin's disease, may occur in elderly as in younger patients, and the associated frequent chromosome abnormalities appear to be similarly distributed regardless of age. It is, of course, just possible that the increased incidence of chromosome anomalies in the elderly may reflect a greater proportion of 'secondary' cases, not obviously recognisable as such from the history, but perhaps due to prolonged exposure to some undetermined leukaemogenic agent in the environment.

Another biological feature of AML in the elderly, having some parallels with the smouldering leukaemic patterns, is the relative frequency of cases with substantially less than 90 per cent of leukaemic blast cells in marrow aspirates and indeed of so-called 'oligoleukaemia' with only 50 per cent or less of myeloblasts and promyelocytes in the marrow. These features occur at least twice as commonly in patients over 60 as in younger patients (Rai et al, 1983; Keating et al, 1981). There are no obvious growth characteristics of leukaemic cells from elderly patients, however, which might explain this tendency to indolent development. Techniques such as labelling with tritiated thymidine to determine the proportion of leukaemic cells actively synthesising DNA in the S-phase of the cell cycle show no correlation between labelling index and age (Hart et al, 1977), a finding confirmed by flow cytometric analysis (Dosik et al, 1980).

CLINICAL FEATURES AT DIAGNOSIS

Acute leukaemias

Elderly patients have long been noted to manifest an indolent clinical course, at least in AML, more often than younger patients do. This is partly because of the frequent pre-existence of haematological disorders of the broad 'pre-leukaemic' categories mentioned earlier, present in as much as a third of all elderly patients (Keating et al, 1981). A history of even minor symptoms of anaemia, infection or haemorrhage during the weeks or months preceding diagnosis of AML may indicate that a preleukaemic state could have been present, even if laboratory confirmation of abnormal counts at that time is not available. Such prior symptoms are undoubtedly more common in elderly patients than in young ones, but once the leukaemia is established neither anaemia nor thrombocytopenia, nor elevated white count appear more conspicuous in the old, and although there is some disagreement in reported studies (Bloomfield & Theologides, 1973; Rai et al, 1981) fever, infection and haemorrhage do not seem to be notably more frequent at diagnosis in the elderly, although once infection develops it may be more difficult to control. Similarly with splenomegaly, hepatomegaly and lymphadenopathy: no significant differences between older and younger patients emerge in the frequency of organ involvement.

Attempts have been made to achieve a more general assessment of patient capacity to withstand both the disease and the side-effects of toxic drugs used in treatment, by using various measurements of performance status — the capacity of the patient to carry out the normal physical activities of day-to-day life. One such study of 54 patients with AML (Kansal et al, 1976) showed that 42 per cent of patients over 50 years of age had a poor performance status at diagnosis, as compared to 14 per cent of patients less than 50 years old. In this relatively small study the performance status correlated more closely with response to treatment and survival duration than did any other variable, including age per se. This observation is very much in accord with our own clinical impression, that what might be called biological age — age assessed from fitness and activity — is more important prognostically than actual temporal age. A fit 70-year-old patient is far more likely to tolerate anti-leukaemic treatment and to achieve remission and perhaps long-term survival than a 60-year-old patient with poor basic physiological functions and associated chronic illness.

Chronic leukaemias

These are all essentially diseases of the older age groups, and the kinds of comparison made in relation to acute leukaemia as between younger and older patients do not apply here. A brief synopsis of features at presentation not already included in Table 10.1 follows.

CML

The sexes are affected equally. Usual symptoms are of weight loss, malaise, awareness of splenic enlargement and occasionally of anaemia. Splenomegaly is usual and may be marked. Blood picture is diagnostic, with high leucocyte count and presence of precursor granulocytes, metamyelocytes, myelocytes, promyelocytes and an occasional blast cell. Haemoglobin is generally only moderately reduced at diagnosis.

CLL

Male-to-female ratio is 2:1. This is the most common leukaemia in the elderly. The onset is usually insidious with anaemia and lymphadenopathy; the disease is frequently detected at blood test for other purposes. About a third of patients have substantial splenomegaly. An internationally agreed staging system (International Workshop on CLL, 1981) has prognostic significance.

Stage A: No anaemia or thrombocytopenia and less than three areas of 'lymphoid' enlargement from among the five areas: liver, spleen, neck, axillae and groins. Unilateral or bilateral nodes at any of the last three sites count as one.

Stage B: No anaemia or thrombocytopenia, but with three or more involved areas of lymphoid enlargement.

Stage C: Anaemia (Hb $\leq$ 10 g/dl) and/or thrombocytopenia ($\leq$ 100 $\times$ 10^9/l) regardless of the number of areas of lymphoid enlargement.

The blood picture is generally diagnostic, with lymphocytes greater than 10 $\times$ 10^9/l, often greater than 50 $\times$ 10^9/l, usually with B-cell features. Smear cells are common. Marrow infiltration is usually marked. Auto-immune haemolytic anaemia (AIHA) is present in some degree in 10–20 per cent of cases and is severe in about 5 per cent. A third of cases show immune paresis at some stage, but this is not common at diagnosis. The rare T-cell variants (less than 5 per cent) are usually of suppressor-cell lineage and show cytoplasmic granulation. High leucocyte counts, gross splenomegaly and skin infiltration may occur.

HCL

This disease is uncommon — perhaps one case might be seen to ten of CLL — and has a male-to-female incidence ratio of 4:1. The unusual nature of the involved neoplastic hairy cells has excited much interest and controversy (Cawley et al, 1980). Peak incidence is in the 40 to 60 age range, but cases continue to present into the 80s. Symptoms include weakness, weight loss, dyspnoea, with infection and purpura or epistaxis less frequent. Over 80 per cent of patients have palpable splenomegaly, but hepatomegaly is only half as frequent and palpable lymphadenopathy is uncommon, although abnormal abdominal nodes can often be demonstrated on CT scanning.

Anaemia, leucopenia and thrombocytopenia are characteristic, the marrow is difficult to aspirate, but trephine specimens show extensive diffuse or focal infiltration with hairy cells and increase in reticulin fibrosis.

PLL

This is an uncommon disorder related to CLL but with larger lymphoid cells with moderate nuclear/cytoplasmic ratio, usually showing a prominent nucleolus, although the nuclear chromatin is moderately coarsely condensed unlike the leptochromatic nuclei of lymphoblasts. Cases are mostly of B-cell origin, with strong SmIg, but curiously may show positivity to the J5 monoclonal or cALL antibody (Berebi et al, 1983). Some T-cell cases occur, more commonly of the helper subset than in CLL.

Symptoms are much as in CLL, but the peripheral lymphocyte count tends to be very high ($>50 \times 10^9$/l), and massive splenomegaly is usual, with little lymphadenopathy.

Sezary syndrome (SS)

This disease, and mycosis fungoides of which SS is the leukaemic phase, is of T-cell origin, chiefly of the helper subset, with the cells bearing receptors for the Fc of IgM and showing localised acid phosphatase and butyrate or acetate esterase positivity. It occurs in the middle-aged and elderly, with male-to-female ratio of around 1.5:1. A generalised scaly erythroderma is shown, with lymphadenopathy and a leukaemic blood picture, with typical large mononuclear cells with 'cerebriform' folded nuclei (best appreciated on electron microscopy). These 'Sezary cells' are diagnostic, but skin biopsy also shows a characteristic infiltrate with nodular accumulations of neoplastic T-cells —

Pautrier's pseudoabscesses. The bone marrow, on the other hand, usually shows little or no infiltration.

Adult T-cell leukaemia (ATL)

This disorder, recently recognised as an endemic disease in South-West Japan, induced by a retrovirus (ATLV), has unique characteristics reviewed in all aspects in a recent monograph (Hanaoka et al, 1982). It has some similarities to SS but the suppressor T-cell subset is chiefly involved, the skin lesions have a more papular and less generalised distribution, the disease has a more acute onset, clonal cytogenetic abnormalities, including especially trisomy 7, are frequent, and antiviral antibodies are present in all ATL patients and in 25 per cent of healthy adults in the endemic area, but absent in SS. The age range is wide, but the peak incidence is between 40 and 60 years.

Predominant physical findings include lymphadenopathy, hepatomegaly and splenomegaly, present in over 50 per cent of cases and skin lesions in around 50 per cent. Anaemia is usually mild, WBC ranges from minor to marked increase (up to $500 \times 10^9/l$) with the leukaemic cells showing indented and lobulated nuclei, with relatively coarse chromatin and scanty cytoplasm, not unlike Sezary cells but generally somewhat smaller. The marrow is infiltrated but less markedly than in most leukaemias. Hypercalcaemia has been a clinical feature in around 25 to 40 per cent of patients.

A similar clinical syndrome, probably also virus-induced but with less certain endemic distribution, has been observed in black patients from the West Indies (Catovsky et al, 1982), and it now seems likely that other blacks of African origin, whether in Africa, the USA or elsewhere, may be affected (Fleming et al, 1983; Bunn et al, 1983). Whether the Japanese and African disease viruses are identical remains to be established.

TREATMENT

Acute leukaemias

The principles in the treatment of acute leukaemia in general have always been coupled in the older patient with philosophical questions of whether it is in the patient's best interests to embark on a course of aggressive chemotherapy which will, in the large majority of cases, produce more discomfort, distress and malaise than the patient was suffering at the time of presentation. An excellent and comprehensive discussion of the biology and treatment of acute leukaemias in the elderly has recently been provided by Peterson (1982). As recently as the late 1970s, many physicians caring for elderly patients with this disease felt that the price was too high and a policy of more palliative, supportive care was widely practised. The appearance of reports documenting more favourable results in AML (Rees et al, 1977; Gale &

Cline, 1977; Foon et al, 1981) has accompanied a change in attitude towards the management of such cases.

Nevertheless, there is ample evidence that the process of ageing produces changes in the pharmacokinetics of some drugs, and more care is needed in prescribing antibiotics, analgesics, hypnotics, digoxin and ß-blockers as well as cytotoxic drugs in order to avoid clinical disasters which may have no intrinsic relationship to the disease being treated.

The important clinical pharmacokinetic factors which should be considered in the management of a patient with leukaemia are shown below, modified from Richey & Bender (1977) (see also Vestal, 1978; Lancet Editorial, 1983).

1. Variations in absorption of cytotoxic drugs occur in all ages (Zimm et al, 1983), but in some older patients changes in gastric emptying and intestinal perfusion produce less reliable plasma levels of orally administered drugs.
2. Drug metabolism is often dependent on adequate liver function which may be impaired in the elderly.
3. Renal impairment may also contribute to raised and sustained plasma cytotoxic levels which are inappropriate.
4. Low plasma binding of drugs will produce higher 'free' drug concentrations and greater toxicity.

The mechanism of metabolism of some cytotoxic drugs is shown in Table 11.3.

Table 11.3

Cytotoxic drug	Metabolism	Excretion
Daunorubicin	Liver	Bile (no entero-hepatic recycling) Kidneys (14–23% after 5–7 days)
Adriamycin	Liver	Bile — 40% of dose in 7 days Kidneys (5% after 5 days)
If bilirubin level 20–50 μmol/l, decrease initial dose by 50%. If bilirubin level > 50 μmol/l, decrease initial dose by 75%. If bilirubin is normal, follow transaminase levels. If SGPT 2–3 times normal, decrease initial dose by 25%. If SGPT >3 times normal, decrease initial dose by 50%.		
Cytosine arabinoside	Liver	Kidneys 90% in 24 hours Bile 5%
Long half-life in CSF because of absence of cytidine deaminase.		
6-thioguanine	Liver	Kidneys (85% of drug and metabolites in 24 hours)
Allopurinol has no effect on metabolism.		
6-mercaptopurine	Liver	Kidney as metabolites
Allopurinol blocks 6-MP metabolism to 6-thiouric acid.		
Vincristine	Liver	Bile (65% in 72 hours) Kidney (12% in 72 hours)
Patients with obstructive jaundice should have modified doses.		

m-amsa	High plasma protein binding. Liver conjugation with glutathione.	Bile Kidneys — mild renal impairment does not extend half-life.

Half-life markedly prolonged in presence of hepatic dysfunction.

5-azacytidine	Liver	Kidney 70–90% in 24 hours

The drug is quite seriously hepatotoxic.

Asparaginase	Enhanced plasma clearance during hypersensitivity reaction.	Liver excretion ⎫ Very Small Kidney excretion ⎭ Liver sequestration by RE system possibly main method

Apparently no correlation between asparaginase disposition and age, body mass or renal or hepatic function.

Epipodophyllotoxin (VP-16)	High albumin-binding	Kidney 44% at 4 days (70% unmetabolised) Bile (up to 50%–5% intact remainder metabolites).
Busulphan	Extensive metabolism short plasma half-life	Kidney — 95% as inactive metabolites
Chlorambucil	Extensive metabolism in liver. High binding to gammaglobulins. Some drug storage in fat may occur.	Kidneys 60% in 24 hours as metabolites. Faeces — nil.
Cyclophosphamide	Absorption variable Liver metabolism by microsomal enzymes to active metabolites	Exclusively by kidney — 15% unchanged, rest as metabolites.

Significantly prolonged retention of active metabolites in presence of renal failure.

Methotrexate	Liver with appreciable entero-hepatic circulation	Majority by kidney — unchanged (90%). Bile — minimal

Methotrexate and the 7-hydroxymethotrexate metabolite share the responsibility for the renal toxicity of high dose methotrexate.

The most underlying principle in the management of acute laukaemia at any age, but particularly in the elderly, is that great attention be paid to detail. The side-effects of drugs remain one of the most difficult problems to negotiate, and a greater familiarity with the particular needs of the elderly will improve the outlook for this group of patients.

Before a physician decides to treat a patient with intensive chemotherapy, consideration will have been taken of the wishes of the patient and the availability of adequate supportive care during the early difficult period.

Cytotoxic drugs for acute leukaemia

ALL is relatively uncommon and refractory to treatment in the elderly and may well be best managed by similar regimes to those used in AML, an example of which is given here. For ALL patients, the initial induction regime may start with vincristine and prednisone alone or incorporate these agents. The pattern of cytotoxic drug combination may be expected to change with advancing knowledge, but the combination of an anthracycline (daunorubicin, or adriamycin) cytosine arabinoside and 6-thioguanine has proved especially valuable in recent years.

An example of a combination of these drugs (the DAT regime) has recently been used in the Eighth MRC AML Trial involving more than 1100 patients following pilot studies (Rees et al, 1977).

Schedule: Daunorubicin   50mg/m^2 i.v. day 1
           Cytosine arabinoside 100 mg/m^2 12-hourly i.v. days 1–5
           6-thioguanine   100mg/m^2 12-hourly orally days 1–5

In the first course of therapy, each drug was given at half-dose for all patients over 65 years of age. The doses selected for second and subsequent courses were modified according to the response to the first course and it was frequently necessary to increase the therapy to full doses after two or three courses separated at intervals of 10–14 days. This policy of modifying the doses according to the needs of an individual patient is attractive, but the median interval to remission in this large study was long and, whereas the remission rate for patients under 60 years of age was over 70 per cent, only 47 per cent of patients over 60 years of age achieved remission. The results for each five-year age group over 60 are shown in Table 11.4.

Some pilot studies suggest that more aggressive treatment may be justified even in the elderly. Foon et al (1981) used the TAD regime (7 days Ara-C and 6-TG 12-hourly with daunorubicin on days 5, 6 and 7) initially developed at Los Angeles by Gale & Cline (1977), in the treatment of 107 patients ranging in age from 15 to 82 years. No modification to the doses of the drugs for older patients was made in this study. The remission rate for 33 patients over 60 years of age was 76 per cent and identical to that obtained in 74 patients under 60. The median durations of remission and survival were 14 months and 22 months respectively in the older age group.

The importance of supportive care

General considerations. Although the patient's mobility and capacity to deal with normal activities is important, the true extent of infirmity is more influenced by the mental attitude to a situation in the elderly than in the younger patient.

Table 11.4 Analysis of 240 patients over age of 60 in a multicentre trial (MRC AML 8)

Age group	61–65	66–70	71–75	76–80	80+
No. of patients	92	93	44	10	2
Remission rate (%)	53	47	32	27	0

The presence of other concurrent diseases such as chronic respiratory infections, cardiovascular or renal disease or diabetes adds substantially to the potential problems which can be anticipated in the management of a patient with acute leukaemia. The treatment is toxic, highly myelosuppressive, and a galaxy of other side-effects produce a formidable challenge to the physician's clinical acumen and therapeutic skills.

It is important nevertheless to attempt to establish some order in what might otherwise become a confused picture by asking why some patients fail to enter remission. It is necessary to distinguish between ineffective cytotoxic therapy and inadequate supportive care because it has tacitly been held from time to time that poor remission rates require changes in the type of presentation of the remission-induction drugs.

Priesler (1978) tried to determine the reasons why cytotoxic treatment in acute leukaemia was unsuccessful. He concluded that most patients failed to enter remission because of inadequate supportive care. A similar approach has been adopted in the recent British MRC Trial (Eighth).

Each patient who failed to achieve a complete remission was assigned to one of the categories of failure listed in Table 11.5. The overall remission rate in this study was 65 per cent. The analysis was therefore drawn up from the 35 per cent of failures among the patients who were entered into the Trial in a five-year period. The two age groups (above and below 60 years of age) showed very similar reasons for failing to enter remission. Although the remission rate in patients over 60 was only 47 per cent and therefore more were failing to enter complete remission, the clear impression was that in older patients, as in the young, the reason for failure chiefly related to inefficacy of adequate supportive care. There appear to be extenuating circumstances in the elderly because a high percentage of patients have a low performance status at the time of diagnosis, but better supportive care would certainly help to improve the results of treatment of this disorder.

Table 11.5 Reasons for failure to enter remission in 254 non-remitting cases, 112 over 60 years, 142 under 60 years.
Data from MRC AML 8 trial

	Age	
	60+ (%)	<60 (%)
A. Inadequate trial. Patient dies during or within seven days of completing the first course of chemotherapy.	29	30
B. Bone marrow hypoplasia achieved but regeneration occurs predominantly with blast cells.	3.5	10.5
C. Marrow hypocellularity with no peripheral blood blasts but patient dies in hypoplastic phase from haemorrhage or infection.	21	20.5
D. Partial remission. Blast cell population in bone marrow falls to 10–15%.	9	8.5
E. Failure of therapy to achieve any or significant effect on the marrow blast cell population.	34	30
F. Other causes (e.g. patient refused further treatment, accidental death, etc.).	3.5	1.5

Essential requirements for good supportive care include:
1. A well-informed, enthusiastic and optimistic group of senior and junior staff — the latter possibly more important than the former.
2. A close liaison with the Department of Microbiology, preferably with the microbiologist attending ward rounds.
3. Easy access to blood products. Platelet concentrates have generally replaced platelet-rich plasma in most areas. Fresh donor platelets are a luxury few can provide. White cell transfusions are required in less than 5 per cent of cases during remission induction, and many good centres manage without such facilities.
4. A nursing team which understands the important points in the plan of management and shares the enthusiasm of the medical staff.

Treatment of pyrexial episodes. It can sometimes be difficult to decide whether an episode of pyrexia indicates a life-threatening infection. When fever over 38°C is recorded in a neutropenic patient on two occasions four hours apart, it is prudent to assume that a potentially fulminating infection is developing. If this situation develops while a patient is receiving a blood transfusion, proper weight must be given to the patient's previous history of transfusion reactions, but a diagnosis of a transfusion-induced fever is always one that should be made only after a thorough clinical examination has failed to demonstrate a focus of infection and a blood culture has been taken as a precaution. Stopping the transfusion of the suspect unit of blood or platelets coupled with the administration of chlorpheniramine or similar antihistamine may resolve the matter within an hour or two.

The method of taking blood cultures in a patient with fever is important. Hall et al (1976) showed that the success rate in obtaining a positive result from a blood culture was enhanced by taking 45 ml divided equally among three bottles (two aerobic, one anaerobic), and this practice is recommended. Pending the results of microbiology, an antibiotic regime must be instituted with a combination such as gentamycin and cefotaxime, or if pseudomonas infections are frequent, gentamycin and piperacillin. Positive cultures and sensitivities allow for appropriate change in antibiotics. If fever persists, unresponsive to antibiotics for more than five days, an antifungal agent such as amphotericin B should be considered.

Platelet transfusions. The principles upon which platelet transfusions are provided for patients undergoing remission-induction therapy are very loosely interpreted. In a recent review of supportive care methods in 70 hospitals in Britain, carried out in relation to the MRC Eighth AML trial, opinions were fairly evenly divided between those who provided platelets (usually six units of concentrate) when the patient's platelet count fell below 10 or 20 $\times$ $10^9/l$ and the remainder who waited for the first sign of bleeding before requesting them. An exception to the rule in the latter method was made for patients who were thrombocytopenic and pyrexial when the risk of haemorrhage is substantially increased.

No firm recommendations can be made on the timing of platelet therapy for older patients, because on the one hand a patient may not be able to tolerate the extra load on the circulation each day without careful attention to fluid balance and on the other hand the older patient usually tolerates blood loss less well and may have moderately advanced cardiovascular disease which potentiates the risk of haemorrhage. In these circumstances a rigid policy may be less valuable than an individual assessment of a patient's case.

Other aspects of support. The former aspects of supportive care by appropriate transfusions and the treatment of infections are only part of the clinical management of these patients. Scrupulous attention to fluid an electrolyte balance is particularly important in the elderly. Continued nausea and vomiting may produce dehydration and very low levels of calcium, sodium and potassium. The plasma potassium levels may be further depressed by increased loss from the kidney in association with antibiotic and diuretic therapy. A wide range of anti-emetic agents are now available, but some caution is necessary in their use as a wide range of side-effects from respiratory suppression to psychotic behaviour can quickly complicate an already serious clinical problem. Allopurinol should be prescribed soon after the diagnosis is made, and it may be good clinical practice to stabilise the patient's condition for a few days before cytotoxic chemotherapy begins.

Therapy following remission

While there is some degree of accord regarding the choice of cytotoxic agents in the remission-induction phase of treatment, there is less agreement on the policy to follow when remissions have been achieved. Mayer et al (1982) have recently reviewed the question of consolidation therapy and were able to show convincingly that early intensive therapy after remission prolongs the duration of remission and survival. Nevertheless, there is a semantic debate about what constitutes consolidation therapy, i.e. intensive early remission therapy as distinct from maintenance therapy, which is usually less intensive.

In the elderly patient particular care is necessary as the accumulated dose of anthracycline approaches the recommended 550 mg m^2, and a protocol which relies on the contribution of these agents to maintain remission must be viewed with particular caution. Very few controlled trials on the value of post-remission therapy have been reported, and these are rather small. Recent studies of the Cancer and Acute Leukaemia Group B (Ellison & Glidewell, 1979) and SouthWestern Oncology Group (Coltman et al, 1979) on the treatment of AML show substantial advantage in both remission and survival time when AraC and anthracycline antibiotics were continued in remission maintenance regimes.

The principal criterion by which the value of a therapeutic programme is judged is its success in achieving long-term survivals. The results obtained in recent studies are shown in Table 11.6.

The alternative option of a bone marrow transplant in remission is not

Table 11.6   Duration of survival in patients over 60 with AML

	No. of patients	% surviving				Median (months)
		1 yr	2 yrs	3 yrs	4 yrs	
All cases						
AML 8	240	41	21	15	15	13
Peterson et al (1977)	27	—	—	—	—	2
Reiffers et al (1980)	29	32	21	—	—	6
Remitters only						
AML 8	113	76	50	33	33	22
Foon et al (1981)	25	70	48	38	18	22
Reiffers et al (1980)	18	53	35	—	—	22
CALGB (Rai et al 1981)	28	—	—	—	—	19
Peterson et al (1977) (age 61–70)	8	100	34	0	0	14+

— = accurate value not given

open to physicians treating older patients even if a histocompatible donor is available. In the majority of transplantation centres the upper age limit is set at 40 years for the recipient, as problems with graft versus host disease and pneumonitis are poorly tolerated in patients above 40.

An alternative method of attempting remission induction has recently been reported by Housset et al (1982) using very low doses of cytosine arabinoside (10 mg/m^2 12-hourly s.c.). The treatment makes clinical use of the fact that several substances, including cytosine arabinoside, can induce differentiation in myeloid leukaemic cells (Lotem & Sachs, 1974). One of the cases described by Housset was a 74-year-old man with moderately differentiated myeloblastic leukaemia whose marrow returned to normal after 20 days' treatment. It seems very improbable that low-dose Ara-C is inducing remissions by any activity other than a cytotoxic one.

Treatment of relapse

The outlook for patients relapsing from remission of AML is dependent to a large degree on whether relapse occurred while on or off treatment. In the latter case, a return to the initial successful induction regime may prove effective. However, the consideration which once again plays a very significant part in the decision on what therapy to offer is the quality of life. This is particularly important in the elderly at all stages of treatment, but its importance is amplified when a physician is faced with the responsibility of recommending a course of action to a patient who has relapsed. There is no single solution, but even for the patient who relapses on treatment alternative and effective chemotherapy regimes are available. These usually are combinations of drugs including m-amsa, epipodophyllotoxin or high-dose Ara C (Arlin et al, 1981; Willemze et al, 1982).

Treatment of smouldering leukaemia and preleukaemic states

One of the difficulties in deciding when to begin chemotherapy for patients with subacute disease is that it is not possible to say how long the chronic phase will continue. No treatment may be the better approach initially while the course of the disease is monitored carefully, but when the patient begins to have accelerated symptoms or signs this policy will need to be reviewed. Orthodox remission induction therapy may be tried, and low-dose cytosine arabinoside has also been found valuable by Housset (1982).

Keating et al (1978) obtained a remission rate of 25 per cent of patients treated intensively from the time of diagnosis, but for a comparative group who did not receive such treatment the median survival time was nine months and the median interval to the accelerated phase was six months.

CML

The natural history of this condition falls into two periods — the chronic phase which is the stage at which the majority of patients present, and the phase following metamorphosis into either an accelerated proliferation resistant to chemotherapy or the so-called 'blast transformation' which is usually to an AML variant but in about 30 per cent of cases is to a form of ALL.

The chronic phase has a median duration of little more than three years. The standard form of chemotherapy for thirty years has been busulphan. The metabolites of busulphan are excreted slowly from the body and the myelosuppressive effects of the drug continue for approximately two weeks after the drug has been discontinued. There is also some delay in its effect on peripheral white counts at the start of therapy. Those unfamiliar with its use may be tempted to increase the dosage too early and thereby run the risk of producing severe marrow suppression. A suitable starting dose is 4 mg/24h along with allopurinol 100 mg b.d. A MRC Trial is comparing the value of 4 mg busulphan with 2 mg of busulphan and 80 mg 6-thioguanine orally. The doses are modified by altering the number of days per week on which chemotherapy is taken. An attempt is made to maintain the WBC between 5 and 10×10^9/l. The rationale of adding 6-TG is an attempt to obtain more consistent control of the white count with lower doses of busulphan. Unfortunately the value of busulphan in prolonging the chronic phase is far from convincing. The most common side-effect of busulphan is skin pigmentation which appears in approximately one-third of patients after two years of treatment. A more serious complication is pulmonary fibrosis. Fortunately it is very uncommon, but lung function studies are advised for patients starting what may be long-term therapy with this drug. Patients who require increasing doses of busulphan to control the white count may respond to hydroxyurea at a dose of 500–1000 mg/day.

The management of the acute phase of the disease presents a sharp contrast to the relatively straightforward therapy of the chronic phase. Acute myeloid transformation is rarely responsive to currently available therapy even in young patients and the highly intensive therapy cannot be enthusiastically recommended at the present time. It is important, however, to establish the nature of the cell line, as acute lymphoblastic transformation may respond for a time to a vincristine–prednisone combination.

Autologous grafts using stored buffy coat cells taken during the chronic phase have been performed at the time of metamorphosis and have been very successful in some cases of CML, but the procedure is currently reserved for the younger patient.

CLL

In a large percentage of cases with disease at stage A no therapy is necessary at the time of diagnosis.

Indications for treatment include:
1. Evidence of bone marrow failure — anaemia, neutropenia or thrombocytopenia.
2. Development of auto-immune haemolytic anaemia or idiopathic thrombocytopenic purpura.
3. Presence of splenomegaly that is causing symptoms or accompanied by hypersplenism.
4. Symptomatic involvement of lymph nodes, skin or other tissues.

The standard drug is chlorambucil at a dose of 0.1–0.2 mg/kg body weight. It is highly effective in reducing the white count in 70–75 per cent of patients, and it may be possible to maintain good control of the disease for many years while the doses of chlorambucil are altered or the drug discontinued. Steroids may be added if auto-immune haemolytic anaemia or thrombocytopenia develops or when there is evidence of marrow failure. Steroids are by no means always effective in improving marrow function, but a trial of three or four weeks is worth while.

More intensive therapy is sometimes indicated for aggressive disease, and combinations such as pentaCOP (cyclophosphamide 125 mg/m² orally for five days, Oncovin 1.4 mg/m² i.v. day 1, prednisolone 40 mg/m² orally daily for five days has recently been compared with short courses of high-dose chlorambucil 1.5 mg/kg given over three days for progressive disease among patients entering the First MRC CLL trial.

The principal clinical problems in the care of patients with CLL are produced by the results of immunosuppression. Bacterial infections affecting the upper and lower respiratory tract become increasingly common because of the marked degree of neutropenia and hypogammaglobulinaemia in more advanced disease. Replacement therapy with regular injections of pooled human gammaglobulin can be useful, but prophylactic antibiotic therapy is sometimes warranted, particularly in the winter months. Immunisation against respiratory viruses is rarely of any value. The frequency of herpes zoster also increases as immune competence becomes more severely impaired and, although it usually remains localised, it is often very painful. Early treatment with Acyclovir may ablate or modify an infection.

The natural history of CLL is of a transition to a less responsive and more widespread stage of the disease. The rate at which this develops is very variable.

Blast cell crisis is very rare in CLL, although intermediate forms with a mixture of mature and immature lymphoid cells have been described. This 'prolymphocytoid' transformation may respond to a combination of cyclophosphamide, hydroxydaunorubicin, Oncovin and prednisone — CHOP. The improvement is short, however, and the development of this haematological picture carries a very poor prognosis.

The incidence of secondary tumours is higher in patients with CLL than in a control normal population in the same age group. The most common sites are the skin and lower gastrointestinal tract.

PLL

The prognosis is much worse than in CLL, partly because advanced disease is frequently present at diagnosis. Several combinations of cytotoxic agents have been tried, but none has been successful in controlling the disease. The most valuable combination was CHOP. Splenic irradiation (1000 cGy) alone sometimes produces remissions. For patients over 60 it is recommended as the initial treatment of choice.

HCL

The condition is not very amenable to therapy, and the prognosis is closely related to the degree of pancytopenia. Patients having a large spleen and significant cytopenia sometimes benefit from splenectomy and this would be the treatment of choice for the majority requiring treatment. Recently however exciting results have followed the use of alpha interferon (Quesada et al, 1984). Although the original group of patients were all under the age of 60, the treatment has been extended in several collaborative studies to include older patients. Those entering a British study have either failed to respond to splenectomy or have small spleens. Three million units of alpha interferon are given subcutaneously daily for up to four months. A long trial of treatment is necessary because some patients have been found to respond slowly. The drug is given in the evening to minimise the distress caused by 'flu-like symptoms which many experience. The side effects may be controlled by paracetamol and the patient usually finds the treatment more acceptable when the injection is given at the end of the day (Abrams et al, 1985).

ATL

Clinical remissions may often be induced by aggressive combination of chemotherapy with regimes such as CHOP, but they are usually of short duration, and opportunistic infections and metabolic disturbances are frequent and difficult to control (Hanaoka et al, 1982; Bunn et al, 1983).

REFERENCES

Abrams P G et al 1985 Evening administration of alpha interferon, New England Journal of Medicine 312: 443–444

Andrew W 1971 The anatomy of aging in man and animals. Grune & Stratton, New York

Arlin Z et al 1981 Treatment of acute leukemia in relapse with 4'(9-acridinylamino)methane sulphon-M-anisidide (AMSA) in combination with cytosine arabinoside and thioguanine. Cancer Clinical Trials 4: 317–321

Berebi A, Talmor M, Galili N 1983 J5 in prolymphocytic leukaemia. Blood

Bloomfield C D, Theologides A 1973 Acute granulocytic leukaemia in elderly patients. Journal of the Americal Medical Association 226: 1190–1193

Bunn P A et al 1983 Clinical course of retrovirus-associated adult T-cell lymphoma in the United States. New England Journal of Medicine 309: 267–264

Catovsky D et al 1982 Adult T-cell lymphoma-leukaemia in blacks from the West Indies. Lancet 1: 639–643

Cawley J C, Burns G F, Hayhoe F G J 1980 Hairy-cell leukemia. Springer, Berlin.

Coltman C A, Savage R A, Genan E A 1979 Long-term survival of adults with acute leukaemia. Proceedings of the American Society for Clinical Oncology 30: 389

Doll R 1965 The epidemiological picture. In: Hayhoe F G J (ed) Current research in leukaemia. Cambridge University Press, p 280–299

Doll R 1972 The epidemiology of leukaemia. Leukaemia Research Fund, London

Dosik G M et al 1980 Pretreatment flow cytometry of DNA content in adult acute leukemia. Blood 55: 474–482

Editorial 1983 Pharmacokinetics in the elderly. Lancet 1: 568–569

Ellison R R, Glidewell O 1979 Improved survival in adults with acute myelocytic leukemia (AML) Proceedings of the American Association of Clinical Research 20: 161

Fleming A F, Yamamoto N, Bhusnurmath S R, Maharajan R, Schneider J, Hunsman G 1983 Antibodies to ATLV(HTLV) in Nigerian blood donors and patients with chronic lymphatic leukaemia or lymphoma. Lancet 2: 334–335

Foon K A, Zighelboim J, Yale C, Gale R P 1981 Intensive chemotherapy is the treatment of choice for elderly patients with acute myelogenous leukemia. Blood 58: 467–476

Gale R P, Cline M J 1977 High remission-induction rate in acute myeloid leukaemia. Lancet 1: 497–499

Goldstein S, Harley C B, Moerman E J 1983 Some aspects of cellular aging. Journal of Chronic Diseases 36: 103–116

Hall M M, Ilstrup D M, Washington J A 1976 Effect of volume of blood cultured on detection of bacteria. Journal of Clinical Microbiology 3: 643–645

Hanaoka M, Takatsui K, Shimoyama M 1982 Adult T-cell leukaemia and related diseases. Plenum Press, New York

Hart J S, George S L, Frei E III, Bodey G P, Nickerson R C, Freireich E J 1977 Prognostic significance of pretreatment proliferative activity in adult acute leukemia. Cancer 39: 1603–1617

Housset M, Daniel M T, Degos L 1982 Small doses of Ara-C in the treatment of acute myeloid leukaemia: differentiation of myeloid leukaemia cells. British Journal of Haematology 51: 125–129

International Workshop on CLL 1981 Chronic lymphocytic leukaemia: proposals for a revised prognostic staging system. British Journal of Haematology 48: 365–367

Kansal V, Omura G A, Soong S-J 1976 Prognosis in adult acute myelogenous leukemia related to performance status and other factors. Cancer 38: 329–334

Keating M J, McCredie K, Freireich E J 1978 Prediction of progression and survival of untreated acute leukaemia. Proceedings of the American Association of Cancer Research and American Society of Clinical Oncology 19: 340

Keating M J et al 1981 Treatment of patients over 50 years of age with acute leukemia with a combination of rubidazone and cytosine arabinoside, vincristine and prednisone (ROAP). Blood 58: 584–591

Lotem J, Sachs L 1974 Different blocks in the differentiation of myeloid leukemic cells. Proceedings of the National Academy of Sciences 71: 3507–3511

Mayer R J, Weinstein H J, Coral F S, Rosenthal D S, Frei E 1982 The role of intensive post-induction chemotherapy in the management of patients with acute myelogenous leukaemia. Cancer Treatment Reports 66: 1455–1462

Medical Research Council 1983 MRC trials in poor-risk ALL 1972–1980 (In preparation)

Moore MAS, Spitzer G, Williams N, Metcalf D, Buckley J 1974 Agar culture studies in 127 cases of untreated acute leukemia: the prognostic value of reclassification of leukemia according to *in vitro* growth characteristics. Blood 44: 1–18

Peterson B A 1982 Acute nonlymphocytic leukaemia in the elderly: biology and treatment. In: Bloomfield, C. D. (Ed) Adult leukaemias 1. Martinus Nijhoff, p 199–235

Preisler H D 1978 Failure of remission induction during the treatment of acute leukaemia. Medical and Pediatric Oncology (New York) 4: 275–276

Quesada J G et al 1984 Alpha interferon for induction of remission in hairy-cell leukaemia. New England Journal of Medicine 310: 15–18

Preisler H D 1978 Failure of remission induction during the treatment of acute leukaemia.

Rai K R et al 1981 Treatment of acute myelocytic leukemia: a study by cancer and leukemia Group B. Blood 58: 1203–1212

Rees J K H, Sandler R M, Challener J, Hayhoe F G J 1977 Treatment of acute myeloid leukaemia with a triple cytotoxic regime: DAT. British Journal of Cancer 36: 770–776

Richey D P, Bender A D 1977 Pharmacokinetic consequences of aging. Annual Review of Pharmacology and Toxicology 17: 49–65

Willemze R, Zwaan F E, Colpin G, Keunig J J 1982 High dose cytosine arabinoside in the management of refractory acute leukaemia. Scandinavian Journal of Haematology 29: 141–146

Vestal R E 1978 Drug use in the elderly: a review of problems and special considerations. Drugs 16: 358–382

Zimm S et al 1983 Variable bioavailability of oral mercaptopurine: is maintenance therapy in acute lymphoblastic leukemia being optimally delivered? New England Journal of Medicine 308: 1005–1009

Plasma cell disorders

The first description of what was probably multiple myeloma is usually accorded to Henry Bence-Jones and William MacIntyre. These two London physicians reported the case of Mr Thomas McBean who died in 1846 from a disease characterised by bone pain and oedema. They noted the presence of a peculiar urinary protein that first precipitated and then redissolved on heating and the involvement of the bone marrow was recorded by John Dalrymple, the surgeon who performed the autopsy. Although the term multiple myeloma was coined by Rustizky in 1873, the association with plasma cells was only pointed out by Wright in 1900.

Electrophoretic techniques used after 1940 showed an association between a serum monoclonal protein and the plasma cell malignancy. The analysis of monoclonal immunoglobulin in myeloma has been an important factor in developing our understanding of the molecular structure and functions of immunoglobins generally. These and related studies with tissue culture and *in vivo* cell labelling have all contributed to a greater understanding of the origin and kinetics of myeloma cells.

Although chemo-radiotherapy has made an impact on the length and quality of survival in myeloma, the pace of advance in treatment has lagged behind that of other haemopoietic malignancies. Nevertheless, the disease and the efficient management of the very wide range of complications remain a challenging field for physicians and pathologists alike.

The majority of patients are elderly and suffer from chronic pain and debility. The ability of the spouse or of family to care for the patient at home is often limited, and community help is then at a premium. In these circumstances, the experienced help of the geriatrician in long-term management is invaluable.

INCIDENCE

Multiple myeloma is a disease of the elderly and, apart from chronic lymphatic leukaemia, shows the strongest age-dependence of any neoplasm. The mean age at diagnosis is 62 years, but incidence rates increase steadily to the eighth decade (Blattner, 1980). Only 2 per cent of all cases are below the age of 40 years and there is a tenfold increase in incidence from the ages of 50 to 80 years. Although an overall population incidence of 3 per 100 000 has been estimated, this rises to 37 per 100 00 at 80 years. A slight preponderance of males has been noted (61 per cent), and the disease has been found to be twice as common in the black population in the United States as in the white (McPhedron et al, 1972). Amongst the black population myeloma is the commonest haemopoietic malignancy (33 per cent) and amongst whites it is the third commonest (14 per cent). It has been suggested that there may have been a true increase in disease incidence in recent years (Osserman, 1982).

AETIOLOGY AND PATHOGENESIS

Multiple myeloma results from a malignant proliferation of plasma cells primarily in the bone marrow but sometimes also in extramedullary sites. Although plasma cell malignancies in a number of animal models have both a genetic and an environmental basis, neither factor has yet been shown to operate in humans. The BALB/c and NZB mouse strains are susceptible to such tumours induced with certain chemical agents (Potter, 1973). This does not occur in other strains of mice subjected to the same procedures.

Despite occasional reports of family clusters of myeloma cases, good evidence for a genetic predisposition in humans is lacking. The 'two-hit' hypothesis (Salmon & Seligmann, 1974) postulates a double environmental insult in the causation of myeloma. The condition of benign monoclonal gammopathy is quite common in the elderly and results from a monoclonal proliferation of plasma cells all secreting an immunoglobulin of a single idiotype. The number of cells (probably less than 10^{11}) remains static, and progression to an overt malignancy occurs only in a minority of cases. In some patients with myeloma the paraprotein has been shown to have definite antigen specificity (e.g. for strepolysin or gammaglobulin). Salmon & Seligmann (1974) have suggested that in myeloma, as in the mouse model, the initial event is the emergence of a benign clone of B-cells in response to a defined antigenic stimulus (benign gammopathy). Later, in response to an oncogenic stimulus, possibly viral, the clone may undergo malignant transformation with clinically recognisable disease when cell numbers reach 10^{11} to 10^{12} (myeloma).

Although the underlying cause of myeloma remains speculative, much is now known both about its cellular origins and the kinetics of the tumour's growth. The maturation of normal B-lymphocytes and their evolution into antibody-secreting plasma cells can now be followed with the aid of antibodies for either heavy or light chain components of the immunoglobulin molecule (Fig. 12.1). Fluorescent conjugates, or immunoperoxidase techniques identify the early pre-B-cell containing cytoplasmic IgM. Further maturation of these cells results in loss of the cytoplasmic immunoglobulin and acquisition of surface-bound membrane immunoglobulin (IgM and IgD), and these 'virgin' B-cells are capable of response to specific antigens.

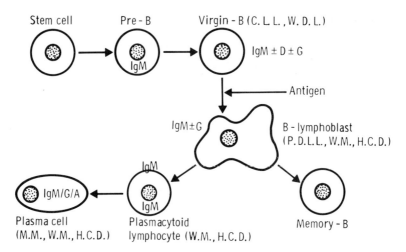

Fig. 12.1 Schematic representation of B-cell maturation and presumed target cells in the B-lymphoproliferative disorders. CLL = chronic lymphatic leukaemia, WDL = well differentiated lymphocytic lymphoma, PDLL = poorly differentiated lymphocytic lymphoma, HCD = heavy chain disease, WM = Waldenström's macroglobulinaemia, MM = multiple myeloma.

Exposure to such antigens results in maturation to lymphoblasts with increased synthesis of surface Ig and then to plasmacytoid lymphocytes capable of cytoplasmic Ig synthesis. Finally these cells develop into fully mature plasma cells losing all surface immunoglobulin but capable of secreting Ig of the appropriate subclass into extracellular fluid.

Using these techniques for identification of cell markers, a wide spectrum of malignancies can be recognised to be of B-cell derivation. Chronic lymphatic leukaemia (B-CLL) is due to a proliferation of cells at the 'virgin' B-lymphocyte stage, whereas most of the non-Hodgkin lymphomas probably derive either from these cells (well differentiated lymphoma, WDLL), or from cells at the lymphoblast stage of maturation (poorly differentiated lymphomas, PDLL). In macroglobulinaemia, plasmacytoid lymphocytes predominate (together with plasma cells) and the clonal expansion of cells at this stage results in secretion of IgM that can be readily identified in serum. In myeloma, plasma cells are involved exclusively, and the clonal nature of the proliferation ensures that both the serum paraprotein and the cytoplasmic immunoglobulin are of a single heavy chain (γ or α) and light chain (κ or λ) type.

The ability to identify the cellular phenotype is of considerable diagnostic importance. Cells in tissue sections can be stained with these antibodies conjugated to peroxidases, and such immunoperoxidase stains for heavy or light chains are of help in determining whether a plasma cell infiltrate is reactive (polyclonal) or malignant (monoclonal).

Myeloma cell kinetics

Most plasma cells in the marrow in myeloma are not in cell cycle, and probably do not represent the true target cell in this malignancy. The ability to study clonogenic stem cells (MCFU-c) that give rise to colonies of plasma cells in culture has permitted a detailed study of cell kinetics in myeloma. Paraprotein synthesis and the sensitivity of myeloma cells to chemotherapeutic agents can also be studied using these techniques (Durie, 1982: Salmon, 1982).

The techniques of labelling and cell-killing with pulsed exposure to tritiated thymidine have brought about a change in the views of tumour growth in myeloma. The proportion of plasma cells in cell cycle (S-phase) at clinical presentation is less than 3 per cent. However, growth of the tumour early in the disease is probably exponential, with a doubling time of two-to-three days, and this is similar to the growth rate of clonogenic cells studied in culture. As tumour size approaches levels at which it can be recognised clinically, the growth fraction falls, reaching a plateau — so-called Gompertzian kinetics.

The inability to achieve a cure in myeloma results from two properties of these malignant cells. Firstly, cells may be present at presentation that are resistant to chemotherapy, and, secondly, even rapid tumour regression frequently tails off into a plateau phase. Although following the initiation of induction therapy the growth fraction increases sharply (with an increased sensitivity to cycle active drugs), about half of all patients plateau at six months and the proportion of S-phase cells falls to pre-treatment levels. Although this is associated with a clinically stable 'remission' phase, all patients eventually relapse, usually with drug-resistant tumour cells. Other patients do not show a stable quiescent phase, the growth fraction remains high and their remission and survival are short (Durie et al, 1980).

CLINICAL FEATURES

Multiple myeloma presents a challenging spectrum of disease to the clinician. The management of acute life-threatening complications which may occur at presentation or later in the disease contrasts with a chronic battle against pain, the palliation of which often becomes of primary concern in later resistant disease.

The clinical manifestations of the disease fall into two main categories: those due to local expansion of the tumour (medullary or extramedullary) and those due to the remote effects of plasma cell products. These latter are both metabolic and also relate to the specific product of these cells i.e. the monoclonal immunoglobulin.

In a review of presenting symptoms in 869 patients at the Mayo Clinic (Kyle, 1975), bone pain was a feature in 70 per cent of cases. The pain may be localised and of acute onset, and often is related by the patient to mild trauma even in the absence of fractures.

Chronic migratory pain is common, but is not usually troublesome at night except on changing position. The most usual sites of pain are chest wall and back, although lesions in the pelvis and the long bones are also common. Joint pain usually implies amyloid involvement.

Anaemia occurs almost invariably at some stage of the disease. Its occurrence at presentation is responsible for the complaints of weakness and easy fatigability. Other general manifestations of the disease, weight loss or fever, are uncommon, in contrast to the lymphomas. However, weight loss may be a feature in advanced disease, and fever results from infections.

Bleeding occurred in only 7 per cent of Kyle's series but commonly complicates advanced disease. Hypercalcaemia is not uncommon at presentation, causing vomiting, constipation, thirst and polyuria and is accompanied by clouding of the sensorium or even coma. Patients may present in renal failure, which may progress rapidly to oliguria, requiring urgent dialysis.

Physical findings

These may be minimal at presentation. Marrow failure, causing anaemia, may result in pallor and cardiac failure. Localised bone tenderness may be observed over areas of osteolysis and may even be accompanied by palpable or visible bony swelling. Local pressure on nerve roots or spinal cord from vertebral bony lesions or fractures or from extra-osseous deposits may result in sciatic pain, motor weakness, loss of sphincter control and even sudden paraplegia. Hepatosplenomegaly is uncommon and, although minor liver enlargement occurred in 26 per cent of the Mayo Clinic series, greater degrees of hepatomegaly suggest amyloid involvement or the rare IgD variant of myeloma.

Skeletal involvement and radiological findings

Skeletal involvement at presentation is extremely common, and radiological evidence for bony involvement has been reported to be found in 80 per cent of cases (Kyle, 1975; Bataille et al, 1982). Involvement may result in generalised osteoporosis, in single or multiple lytic lesions, in pathological fractures and not uncommonly in local soft tissue extensions of these lesions. Fractures may be related to very minimal trauma, and pathological crush fractures and collapse of vertebral bodies are particularly common. There is no osteoblastic reaction in most cases, so that appearances are of punched-out discrete areas of demineralisation without a sclerotic margin. The skull, pelvis, ribs and vertebral spine, together with the proximal ends of the long bones, are most usually affected, and all these areas should be included in the skeletal survey. In the skull, distinction from venous lakes can be difficult sometimes; the involvement of the vertebral pedicles is said to be uncommon, in contrast to other metastatic bone disease. Mandibular involvement may occur, and fractures may occur while eating.

The relative merits of radiological survey and of bone scintigraphy (with ^{99}Tc pyrophosphate or methylene diphosphonate) in diagnosis have been assessed (Kyle, 1975; Bataille et al, 1982; Ludwig et al, 1982). Radiological assessment was superior in the majority of cases, with 44 per cent showing concordance, 38 per cent positive on radiology alone and only 18 per cent on bone scan alone (Bataille et al, 1982). Nevertheless, resolution of the scan lesions was seen in 90 per cent of patients achieving a remission of their disease. In contrast, radiological lesions rarely improve with treatment, so that although a radiological survey is of much more value at presentation, there may be a place for scintigraphy in the follow-up of resolving bone lesions.

Renal involvement: 'myeloma kidney'

Impairment of renal function is an important and dangerous complication of myeloma. It has been found in half of all patients at presentation and is the second most common cause of death after infection (DeFronzo et al, 1978; Kyle, 1975). In the First M.R.C. Myelomatosis Trial, renal function was found to be the single most important factor determining prognosis, and they reported that the death rate in patients with a blood urea in excess of 12 mmol/l was five times that of patients with a normal urea at presentation (Galton et al, 1973).

Myeloma may cause impaired renal function through a number of different mechanisms, resulting in either acute or chronic failure, nephrotic syndrome (generally with amyloidosis) or rarely Fanconi's syndrome. Emphasis has been placed on readily correctable abnormalities such as hypercalcaemia, hyperuricaemia and hyperviscosity in the pathogenesis of renal disease (Cohen & Rundles, 1975). A raised serum calcium or uric acid may undoubtedly be associated with acute renal failure, and the vomiting and polyuria associated with hypercalcaemia aggravate the water loss caused by a direct effect on tubular water resorption in the kidney. The use of contrast medium for intravenous urography is generally contra-indicated because of the combination of hypertonicity and dehydration, and 50 per cent of reported cases of oliguric renal failure have been attributed to this (Cohen & Rundles, 1975).

The underlying cause of the progressive chronic renal failure so often seen in myeloma is still a contentious issue. A strong association between urinary light-chain excretion and renal function has been reported (DeFronzo et al, 1978), although not by all investigators (Kyle & Elveback, 1976). Of 35 patients studied, all 9 without Bence-Jones proteinuria had creatinine clearances (Ccr) of more than 50 ml per minute. More than half of those with urinary Bence-Jones protein had Ccr of less than 50 ml per minute. The magnitude of light-chain proteinuria correlated with the degree of renal insufficiency (DeFronzo et al, 1978). Most patients with a daily excretion of Bence-Jones protein of over 1 gram had severe renal failure (mean Ccr of 8 ml per minute). A similar relationship was observed in the First MRC study (Galton et al, 1973).

The concept of tubular blockages by Bence-Jones casts now seems less likely, since occasional patients are reported with very high excretion rates of light chains but with normal renal function. Also, histological studies of renal biopsy material have shown that casts, where present, contain albumin, immunoglobulin and mixed κ and λ light chains, and that profound renal dysfunction may occur without any tubular casts (Kyle & Bayrd, 1976). Marked tubular atrophy is the pathological feature that best correlates with the clinical manifestations of 'myeloma kidney'. Light chains are metabolised by tubule cells and may be directly toxic to them (DeFronzo et al, 1978).

Defective acidification of the urine and failure to concentrate the urine may both occur and, rarely, Fanconi's syndrome has been described in myeloma (Maldonado et al, 1975). In all these cases there was Bence-Jones proteinuria, and the proximal tubular dysfunction preceeded the diagnosis of myeloma by a number of years in some cases.

Amyloidosis of the kidney was seen in 7 per cent of one series (Kyle, 1975) and may cause nephrotic syndrome or renal failure. Urinary infection is an uncommon primary cause of renal failure, although it may aggravate an existing renal lesion.

Neurological complications

The nervous system may be affected in myeloma directly through encroachment on spinal cord or nerve roots, or indirectly because of hypercalcaemia or hyperviscosity. A polyneuropathy (with or without amyloidosis) may occur. Either spinal cord compression (SCC) or involvement of the cauda equina has been seen in up to 30 per cent of cases, and the incidence of SCC has been reported to be 6–16 per cent in different series (Brenner et al, 1982; Silverstein & Doniger, 1973; Cohn & Rundles, 1975).

Pressure on nerve roots (radiculopathy) or on the spinal cord usually follows extradural extension of a vertebral body lesion, although compression may occur due to fracture collapse of a vertebra or solitary extramedullary plasmacytoma.

The two most important features in the management of SCC are recognition of premonitory signs and symptoms and urgent treatment of paresis once this occurs. In 80 per cent of such cases back pain precedes paraplegia, and radicular pain may be present in over half the cases (Brenner et al, 1982; Dahlström et al, 1979). Any weakness, numbness or urinary difficulties should be considered to herald imminent paresis and should be the signal to institute urgent investigation to determine the level of cord compression. In many series, the commonest location of the lesion has been in the thoracic spine for reasons that are not clear (Dahlström et al, 1979; Benson et al, 1979; Brenner et al, 1982). Radiological survey and tomograms may suffice to locate the lesion, but contrast myelography is generally needed to confirm this prior to laminectomy.

Surgical relief of compression is considered by most to be essential and should be followed by radiotherapy. If laminectomy is performed within 24 hours of presentation, 50 per cent of patients may be expected to recover function completely and 30 per cent to obtain a partial recovery (Brenner et al, 1982). However, instances of useful recovery of function have been described even when delay in surgery has occurred, and an aggressive approach is still justified in these cases.

There is no association between SCC and other features of the disease (e.g. Ig subclass), and overall survival of those who recover complete function is the same as for those without SCC. Radiotherapy without surgical intervention may be indicated only in those with advanced disease or in whom surgery is contra-indicated for other reasons.

Peripheral neuropathy is not a common occurrence in myeloma. Amyloidosis complicating myeloma may cause a carpal tunnel syndrome through infiltration of the flexor retinaculum, or else a 'stocking-glove' sensori-motor neuropathy may occur with autonomic involvement. Neuropathy without amyloid may also occur, and a special association with solitary or multiple plasmacytomas has been described (Delauche et al, 1981). An association with osteosclerotic lesions and with polycythaemia, skin pigmentation and finger-clubbing was also noted. CSF protein was raised in such cases.

Within the skull, cranial nerve palsies may occur through direct tumour encroachment. Orbital lesions may cause optic nerve or oculomotor involvement, with consequent opthalmoplegia. Intracranial plasmacytomas are usually secondary to skull involvement, but rare instances of tumours unassociated with bony lesions have been reported.

The hyperviscosity syndrome

The increased immunoglobulin content of the serum due to the monoclonal protein leads to an increase in viscosity which, if of sufficient magnitude, causes a variety of clinical problems. The pentameric structure of IgM makes the incidence of the hyperviscosity syndrome (HVS) highest in macroglobulinaemia (see below), the condition in which it was first described by Waldenström. However, it may occur in up to 10 per cent of myeloma patients, more especially those with IgA (25 per cent) or IgG_3 paraprotinaemias (Preston et al, 1978), because of the tendency of the former to polymerise and of the latter to form molecular aggregates.

The viscosity (relative to water) at which symptoms occur is highly variable and may depend on individual factors such as primary disease of the microvasculatur, packed cell volume (PCV) and cardiac status. Thus levels of less than 4 are rarely symptomatic, between 5 and 8 most subjects have symptoms, and over 8 clinical manifestations are almost invariable (Bloch & Maki, 1973).

The most common presenting features of HVS are epistaxis and oozing from the gums. Visual loss may occur, and a retinopathy is a virtually constant feature. The retinopathy is characterised by flame haemorrhages, distended tortuous veins with a 'string of sausages' appearance, and papilloedema and retinal vein thrombosis may occur. Neurological symptoms range from lethargy, headache or vertigo to fits and even coma.

In addition, HVS may aggrevate renal failure and, if the paraprotein has the characteristics of a cryoglobulin, may contribute to Raynaud's phenomenon. The plasma volume is often expanded in these patients and bears a direct relationship to plasma viscosity (Russell & Powles, 1978).

Hypercalcaemia

A raised serum calcium occurs in 10–20 per cent of patients with myeloma (Kyle, 1975). It results from increased bone resorption by osteoclasts and is probably most severe in those with the most osteolytic bone lesions (Durie et al, 1981). It has been demonstrated that osteolytic bone lesions in myeloma are caused by osteoclast activity and that this is induced by factors secreted by plasma cells, so-called osteoclast activating factor, OAF (Mundy et al, 1974). The pathology is distinct from that occurring in other metastatic bone disease in which parathyroid hormone or prostaglandins are involved, and in which osteoblastic activity produces a rise in alkaline phosphatase. In myeloma, hypercalcaemia is not accompanied by a rise in this enzyme (unless healing fractures are present).

The levels of OAF production rather surprisingly do not correlate with hypercalcaemia, though they do parallel the severity of osteolytic lesions (Durie et al, 1981). In causing symptoms it is the level of ionised calcium that is of importance and, since 55 per cent is bound to albumin and levels of the latter may be reduced, it is clearly important to allow for this in evaluating laboratory calcium levels.

In very rare cases, abnormal calcium binding by the paraprotein has been observed. These patients had asymptomatic hypercalcaemia with normal ionised calcium levels.

The earliest symptoms of hypercalcaemia are anorexia, nausea, vomiting and constipation. Later on, confusion and somnolence develop and may procede to coma. Polyuria and polydipsia will cause dehydration, and a progression to acute renal failure may occur due to a combination of calcium deposition in the kidney, hyperviscosity and fluid depletion.

Defects of haemostasis

A bleeding diathesis has been observed in 15 per cent of myeloma patients, and even more commonly in IgA myeloma (Lackner, 1973). Although thrombocytopenia due to marrow failure may be contributory, it is usually not sufficiently severe at presentation to account for bleeding. Hyperviscosity (and accompanying hypervolaemia) may play a part in capillary bleeding, but this is usually of less significance in myeloma than in macroglobulinaemia.

More important are the multiple effects of the paraprotein on platelet function and upon the coagulation pathway. The bleeding time is often prolonged, reflecting abnormal platelet function. Impaired platelet aggregation *in vitro* to ADP and decreased platelet factor III release have been demonstrated, as has impaired platelet adhesiveness, and all these abnormalities can be reproduced in normal platelets by exposing them to myeloma proteins (Lackner, 1973). This suggests surface coating of platelets by paraprotein with resulting defects in platelet membrane properties.

A number of disturbances of the coagulation cascade have been described, the most common being a prolonged thrombin and reptilase time. The paraprotein behaves as an inhibitor of fibrin monomer polymerisation. Factor VIII inhibitors and non-specific inhibition of thromboplastin generation have also been described. Long clotting times due to depressed levels of factors II, V, VII and VIII have been demonstrated and ascribed to complexing *in vivo* of these factors with the paraprotein. Factor X deficiency observed in patients with amyloid complicating myeloma does not respond to infusion of fresh plasma and is also presumably caused by *in vivo* binding to the immunoglobulin.

It is important to remember that actual haemorrhagic problems correlate much better with the bleeding time and with platelet aggregation or adhesion than with any of the clotting abnormalities described.

Infections

The ability of myeloma patients to combat infection may be impaired for a number of reasons. Not only is normal immunoglobulin synthesis depressed, but there is evidence for increased catabolism of IgG, and the response to antigenic stimulation (e.g. pneumococcal vaccine) is often depressed. Cellular immunity is also affected, and impaired synthesis of immunoglobulins *in vitro* by myeloma lymphocytes has been demonstrated (Paglieroni & MacKenzie, 1977). Mononuclear cells from myeloma patients have been shown to suppress response to antigen by normal cells, although the identity of such suppressor cells is not certain. Macrophages may be the source of material that directly inhibits plasma cell antibody synthesis (Ullrich & Zolla-Pazner, 1982).

Recently analysis of lymphocyte subsets in myeloma using panels of monoclonal antibodies has shown a relative increase in suppressor T-lymphocytes (OKT8+) over helper OKT4+ cells (Mills & Cawley, 1983). Thus at least two different pathways of immune suppression may be operating in myeloma.

Approximately half of all patients experience a serious infectious episode in their disease, and this may very often contribute to a fatal outcome (Cohen & Rundles, 1975). Respiratory and urinary infection occur most commonly, and organisms often isolated are the polysaccharide-encapsulated pneumococcus, *H. influenza* and meningococcus, as well as the gram-negative enteric bacteria. *Staphylococcus aureus* infection is not uncommon (Norden, 1980). Herpes viral infections (zoster and simplex) occur frequently in these patients, as they do in other B-cell malignancies, and disseminated H. zoster may occur.

LABORATORY FINDINGS

The blood count

Normochromic, normocytic anaemia is very common in myeloma, although macrocytosis is occasionally seen. Macrocytosis is common in treated patients. Anaemia may be aggravated by red cell dilution by an expanded plasma volume. The presence of the paraprotein may be reflected in a high ESR, marked rouleaux formation by red cells and a bluish background staining on the blood film. Both leucopenia and thrombocytopenia may occur, but a leucoerythroblastic blood picture is uncommon. A few circulating plasma cells may be seen and, more rarely, patients develop frank plasma cell leukaemia (more than $2 \times 10^9/l$).

The bone marrow

The degree to which plasma cells infiltrate the bone marrow is highly variable in myeloma. In many cases the aspirate will reveal sheets of plasma cells virtually replacing normal haemopoietic tissue. In others the increase in plasma cell numbers is less marked, although generally exceeding 10 per cent of nucleated cells. Involvement is often patchy, so that single aspirates may appear normal and further aspirates from other sites, and preferably a trephine biopsy, are useful in revealing irregular distribution of the infiltrate. The identification of plasma cell infiltration may be particularly important in differentiating myeloma from a benign paraproteinaemia when other evidence of clinical disease is lacking.

A reactive increase in bone marrow plasma cells may be seen in malignancy, connective tissue disease, liver disease or chronic infections. In distinguishing between these conditions and myeloma, emphasis has been placed on morphological atypia, but unfortunately no single feature of plasma cell morphology is diagnostic. Nuclear cytoplasmic asynchrony with a large nucleolus, polyploidy, cytoplasmic inclusions (Russell bodies) 'flame' cells with abundant eosinophilic cytoplasm, although all features often seen in myeloma, may also be seen in reactive states.

Probably the most useful histological procedure in differentiating a reactive from a neoplastic plasmacytosis is the immunoperoxidase technique (see above). The demonstration of a single heavy or light chain type in the cytoplasm of plasma cells confirms the clonal (and therefore malignant) nature of these cells, even when numbers fall short of being diagnostic (i.e. less than 30 per cent).

The paraprotein

Except in exceedingly rare cases (less than 1 per cent), a paraprotein is found in serum and/or urine in all patients with myeloma. This is usually accompanied by depressed levels of normal immunoglobulin.

In 80 per cent of patients a serum monoclonal protein is detected (M-protein) and of these 60 per cent are IgG and 20 per cent IgA. Two-thirds of M-proteins are of κ light chain type, the rest being λ. Rarely, IgD M-protein has been found (1 per cent of patients) and because serum levels are usually low, may be mistaken for Bence-Jones myeloma. Of the IgG and IgA myeloma patients 50–70 per cent also excrete free light chains in their urine. In some patients (20 per cent) a serum paraprotein is not detectable despite the presence of free light chains in the urine, so-called Bence-Jones myeloma.

Although an elevated serum globulin often first raises the possibility of myeloma, quantitative Ig levels, zone electrophoresis and immunoelectrophoresis of serum and urine are essential in the confirmation and identification of an M-protein.

Zone electrophoresis

This usually identifies a monoclonal immunoglobulin as a dense band in the gamma or pre-beta region (Fig. 12.2). Loss of the usual diffuse gamma band indicates accompanying immunoparesis. Occasionally a double band is seen due to complexing of the M-protein either with itself (IgA polymers) or with IgG (rheumatoid factor). Rarely this is due to a true biclonal gammopathy. The technique of immune fixation is useful in these circumstances to identify the discrete bands.

Immunoglobulin quantitation

This is performed by densitometric study of the electrophoretic strip (for the M-protein) by radial immune diffusion (Macini) or by laser nephelometry. The latter method is gaining in popularity because of its rapidity.

Immunoelectrophoresis (IEP)

This is the most effective way of proving that an individual has a serum or urine paraprotein and of identifying heavy and light chain type. The serum or urine is applied to wells in agar gel and subjected to electrophoresis (Fig. 12.2). After this procedure, antisera to whole human Ig, and to IgG, IgM and

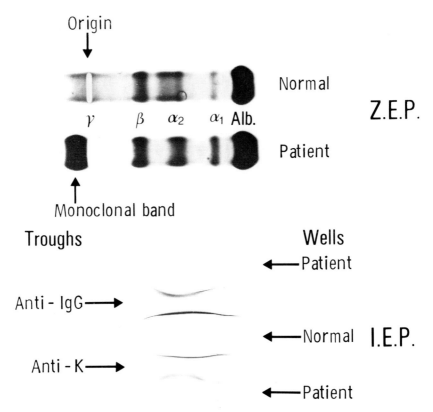

Fig. 12.2 Zone electrophoresis (ZEP) and immunoelectrophoresis (IEP) from a patient with IgG κ multiple myeloma. The paraprotein is seen as a dense cathodal band (above), and as thickened area of precipitation with anti-IgG and anti-κ (below).

IgA as well as to κ or λ light chains, are added to horizontal troughs. Arcs of precipitate form in the gel as these diffuse into the agar and meet the respective Ig zones. Thickening, bowing and kinking of these arcs are diagnostic of a monoclonal protein.

In the case of urine, unless total protein excretion exceeds 1 g/day, 50–100 times concentration of the specimen is necessary to detect light chains. Even if not detected on zone electrophoresis, the IEP may still reveal the presence of monoclonal protein. Since some non-specific leakage of Ig into urine may occur, the use of anti-sera to free κ and λ chains is recommended to confirm Bence-Jones proteinuria.

The other tests for B-J protein (heat precipitation and Bradshaw's Ring test) are insensitive and inferior to the techniques outlined above.

Other laboratory investigations

In addition to the blood count, bone marrow aspirate and the investigation of serum and urine paraprotein, other investigations are important both at presentation and in follow-up. Plasma viscosity (at 37°C) should be determined and the presence of a cryoglobulin and cold agglutinins looked for. Uric acid level may be raised (although clinical gout is unusual), and the calcium, alkaline phosphatase and albumin levels are measured. The level of serum ß2-microglobulin may be of value in assessing tumour burden (see below). Renal function must be evaluated, and glomerular filtration rate and 24-hour urine protein levels estimated. The significance of disturbances in coagulation and bleeding time has been discussed.

CLINICAL STAGING AND PROGNOSTIC FEATURES

The assessment of tumour burden and of risk factors is important in myeloma, as it is in other malignancies. The estimation of prognosis and the proper evaluation of various treatment schedules both derive from the ability to stage patients' disease, although in myeloma there is, as yet, no unanimity as to how this is best done.

A number of clinical features have long been recognised as being of significance in determining length of survival. Thus renal function has been cited as the single most important prognostic determinant, but other factors of importance are the extent of osteolytic lesions, hypercalcaemia, anaemia, performance status, the level and class of paraprotein and light-chain proteinuria.

The influence of immunoglobulin subtype on the prognosis has been assessed (ALGB, 1975; Shustik et al, 1976), and it seems that IgA myeloma patients may fare worse than those with IgG. Patients with Bence-Jones myeloma undeniably have a shorter survival, and patients with λ light chains had a mean survival of only 10 months against 30 months in those with κ light chains (Shustik et al, 1976). This relationship of κ to λ was also found in those with an IgG or IgA serum component.

An attempt has been made to estimate the actual tumour burden in myeloma using the staging system devised by Durie & Salmon (1975). They assessed plasma cell numbers in patients by measuring both *in vitro* production of paraprotein by myeloma cells in culture and *in vivo* synthesis rates. They have stratified patients into three groups according to those clinical features they found correlated best with the tumour load estimated in this way. The features concerned are Hb value, serum calcium, level of paraprotein production (and light-chain excretion), and extent of bony involvement (Table 12.1). The important influence of renal function on prognosis is recognised by subclassifying each of the three groups into A or B according to whether creatinine levels in serum were over 177 μmole/l. A recent application of this staging system to 237 patients at St Bartholomew's Hospital showed the median survival in groups I, II and III to be 62, 32 and 6 months respectively (Woodruff et al, 1979).

Table 12.1   Myeloma staging system of Durie & Salmon (1975)

Stage I: Low myeloma cell mass ($< 0.6 \times 10^{12}$cells/m^2)
Criteria: All of the following:

Hb > 100g/l
Serum calcium (corrected) < 3.0 mmol/l
X-rays: normal bone structure or solitary lesion only
M-component production rates:
(a) IgG value < 50 g/l
(b) IgA value < 30 g/l
(c) Urine light-chain excretion < 4 g/24 h

Stage II: Intermediate myeloma cell mass (0.6–1.2×10^{12}cells/m^2)
Criteria: Fitting neither Stage I nor III

Stage III: High myeloma cell mass ($> 1.2 \times 10^{12}$cells/m^2)
Criteria: Any of the following:

Hb < 85 g/l
Serum calcium (corrected) > 3.0 mmol/l
Advanced lytic bone lesions
M-component production rates:
(a) IgG value > 70 g/l
(b) IgA value > 50 g/l
(c) Urine light-chain excretion > 4 g/24 h

Subclassified: A or B according to the absence or presence of renal impairment

Others have produced staging systems based on empirical observations alone. Merlini et al (1980) studied 173 patients from presentation to death and found that survival in IgG disease could be predicted from serum creatinine, calcium and percentage of plasma cells in the bone marrow. In IgA disease, Hb level, calcium and serum paraprotein levels are predictive features.

Recently published results of the third myelomatosis trial (MRC, 1980c) found the three major determinants of survival were the Hb, the blood urea and the clinical performance status. Their best prognostic group (22 per cent) had a probability of two-year survival of 76 per cent, and their intermediate (56 per cent) and poor (22 per cent) group had two-year survivals of 50 per cent and 9 per cent respectively.

The level of ß2-microglobulin in the serum (SB2M) has very recently been claimed to be a valuable marker for staging myeloma (Bataille et al, 1983). A close correlation was found between myeloma cell mass and SB2M, and between survivals in patients with high or low levels at presentation. Thus patients with SB2M of less than 6μg/ml had a median survival of 52 months from diagnosis, compared to only 26 months in those with levels of more than 6μg/ml. Further confirmation of the prognostic value of this simple test is awaited.

It is clear that, although different staging methods place different emphasis upon various clinical and laboratory features, patients with renal impairment and anaemia at presentation do worst of all. Those with Bence-Jones myeloma form a poor prognostic subgroup, perhaps because the tumour is less differentiated and has a shorter doubling time. Hypoalbuminaemia often considered to be an adverse feature probably reflects a homeostatic response to raised oncotic pressure; and bears a relationship to the paraprotein level in serum (Merlini et al, 1980).

TREATMENT

The introduction of melphalan and later of other chemotherapeutic agents for the treatment of myeloma undoubtedly led to prolongation of survival in this condition. A median survival of only 7 months from diagnosis in the pre-melphalan era has been increased to 24 months (McIntyre, 1979). However, despite much intensive study with a variety of regimes, comparatively little progress has resulted in further extending survival. In particular the use of cycle-active agents which it was thought would dramatically reduce tumour load during induction have made disappointingly little impact on survival duration. The issue of maintenance therapy during remission also remains unsolved.

Melphalan is still the most effective first line treatment in myeloma. Approximately 50 per cent of patients will respond to this drug, and the response rate rises to 75 per cent when prednisone is added (Woodruff, 1981). Although prednisone does not actually reduce plasma cell numbers, it may act both by increasing catabolism of immunoglobulin, thereby reducing the level of paraprotein, and by inhibiting the activity of OAF. Melphalan may be given in continuous low dose daily or by intermittent oral administration. The latter is probably marginally more effective. Most commonly melphalan is given as 10 mg o.d. for seven days together with prednisone 40 mg o.d. also for a week. Direct comparison of this regime repeated at six-weekly intervals with melphalan administered alone, showed no difference in survival (MRC, 1980a). Cyclophosphamide, either orally or parenterally, may be equally effective, and the same MRC trial using cyclophosphamide 150 mg o.d. gave identical survival figures to those in the two melphalan regimes. Intravenous cyclophosphamide (600 mg i.v. every three weeks) has also been evaluated and was not shown to be any more effective (MRC, 1980b). There is no evidence that cyclophosphamide is useful in patients not responding to melphalan, but it may have a place in those unable to tolerate melphalan and is less myelosuppressive.

Combination chemotherapy

A summary is provided in Table 12.2. In the United States, the Southwest Oncology Group (SWOG) have attempted to improve response rates and survival by combining melphalan and prednisone with such agents as vincristine, adriamycin, cyclophosphamide or BCNU (Alexanian et al, 1977). Given as courses at three-weekly intervals, response rates of 67 per cent, have been achieved and median survivals of 32 months.

The cancer and leukaemia group B (CALGB) have compared oral melphalan with prednisone with a multiple regime of intravenous melphalan, BCNU and cyclophosphamide with prednisone (BCMP). They concluded that in good risk cases survival was equal in both groups, but BCMP was more effective in prolonging survival in the poor-risk group (Harley et al, 1979). Case et al (1977) at Sloan-Kettering have used the M-2 protocol and achieved an 83 per cent response rate with a median survival of 50 months. These excellent results are coupled with a 60 per cent response rate in patients resistant to melphalan with a 20-month survival in this group.

Recently McElwain & Powles (1983) have treated patients with high-dose melphalan (HDM). They achieved complete remission in three patients with disappearance of the paraprotein and clearing of marrow plasma cells. It is possible that such high doses of chemotherapy (with attendant severe myelo-suppression) may be indicated in younger patients if prolonged survival can be demonstrated.

Table 12.2 Combination chemotherapy for previously untreated patients with myeloma

Reference	Regime	Response (%)	Median survival (months)
Alexanian et al (1977) SWOG	MCPV (3-weekly) Melphalan 5 mg/m²/day × 4 p.o. Cyclophosphamide 100 mg/m²/day p.o. × 4 Prednisone 60 mg/m²/day × 4 Vincristine 1 mg i.v. day 1	60	32
	CAPV (3-weekly) Cyclophosphamide 100 mg/m²/day p.o. × 4 Adriamycin 25 mg/m² i.v. day 1 Prednisone 60 mg/m²/day × 4 Vincristine 1 mg i.v. day 1	67	30
	VBAP (3 weekly) Vincristine 1 mg i.v. day 1 BCNU 25 mg/m² i.v. day 1 Adriamycin 25 mg/m² i.v. day 1 Prednisone 60 mg/m²/day × 4	65	32
Harley et al (1979) CALGB	BCMP (6-weekly) BCNU 100 mg/m² i.v. day 1 Cyclophosphamide 300 mg/m² i.v. day 1 Melphalan 8 mg/m² i.v. day 1 Prednisone 1–2 mg/kg/day × 7	68	25
Case et al (1977)	M-2 (5-weekly) Melphalan 0.01–0.25 mg/kg/day × 4–7 p.o. Cyclophosphamide 10 mg/kg i.v. day 1 BCNU 0.5–1.0 mg/kg i.v. day 1 Vincristine 0.03 mg/kg i.v. day 1 Prednisone 0.5–1.0 mg/kg × 14	83	50

Maintenance therapy

Since successful induction therapy does not result in eradication of the disease, it has generally been the practice to continue with therapy even in remission. The logic of this approach has been challenged recently in view of the 'quiescent' state of the tumour cells in plateau phase (Durie et al, 1980). It seems that if pre-treatment features are consistent with a low tumour mass and therapy results in disappearance of the serum paraprotein, then continuation of treatment beyond one year is not beneficial (Alexanian et al, 1978). Apparently the likelihood of response to first line treatment when such patients do eventually relapse is greater if maintenance is withheld.

Treatment of refractory disease

A summary is provided in Table 12.3. Patients who are resistant to melphalan or who have relapsed on such treatment may respond to adriamycin and BCNU (Alberts et al, 1976). Half of patients responded, but in only 2 of 13 patients did remission exceed 12 months. The addition of adriamycin has been found to be effective in relapsed patients by a number of groups. Kyle et al (1982) obtained a 20 per cent response rate in melphalan-resistant cases with BCNU, adriamycin and prednisone (BAP), and Bonnet et al (1982) achieved 30 per cent response in a similar regime with added vincristine (VBAP). Alexanian et al (1983) found that 47 per cent of their refractory patients responded to pulses of prednisone, vincristine and adriamycin, with

Table 12.3 Treatment of melphalan-resistant and relapsing patients

Reference	Regime	Response (%)	Median survival (months)
Alberts et al (1976)	AB (4-weekly) Adriamycin 30 mg/m^2 i.v. day 1 BCNU 30 mg/m^2 i.v. day 1	54	—
Case et al (1977)	M2 (see above)	50	22
Kyle et al (1982)	BAP (6 weekly) BCNU 75 mg/m^2 i.v. day 1 Adriamycin 30 mg/m^2 i.v. day 1 + 22 Prednisone 0.6 mg/m^2 day 1–7, 21–28	22	8
Bonnet et al (1982)	VBAP (3-weekly) Vincristine 1 mg i.v. day 1 BCNU 30 mg/m^2 i.v. day 1 Adriamycin 30 mg/m^2 i.v. day 1 Prednisone 100 mg × 4	25	8
Alexanian et al (1983)	Vincristine 1.5 mg i.v. day 1 Adriamycin 35 mg/m^2 i.v. day 1 Prednisone 45 mg/m^2/day on days 1–5, 9–13, 17–21 (every 25 days)	47	—

median survival duration of 16 months in responders. Unfortunately, patients who are *primarily* unresponsive to melphalan are less likely to respond to alternative regimes than are relapsing patients who previously showed a satisfactory response to such therapy.

Acute leukaemia

There is an increased incidence of acute leukaemia in myeloma, and the frequency has been estimated at 6 per cent after two years, and 17 per cent at 50 months (Woodruff, 1981). It is not yet clear to what extent this is treatment related, and occasional cases of simultaneous presentation of the two diseases have been reported. The likely relationship to alkylating agents strengthens the argument for discontinuation of chemotherapy wherever possible.

Management of complications in myeloma

The successful treatment of myeloma depends as much upon the efficient management of the many complications outlined above as upon selecting appropriate chemotherapy. This subject has been well reviewed by Cohen & Rundles (1975), Early et al (1981) and Woodruff (1981).

Renal failure

Correction of dehydration, hypercalcaemia and hyperuricaemia (with allopurinol) are essential and may forestall the onset of acute oliguric renal failure. Alkalinisation of urine may be helpful by increasing the solubility of urates and of Bence-Jones protein. In severe cases, haemodialysis may be indicated, and if hyperviscosity (more than 4.0) is present, plasmapheresis can be considered adjuvant treatment.

In many patients with renal impairment at presentation a marked improvement in function will be seen once the acute problems have been overcome and chemotherapy started. The progression of chronic renal failure is also frequently halted or slowed by effective chemotherapy, although complete restoration of normal renal function is unusual. Renal amyloidosis, if present, is not responsive to existing treatments.

Hypercalcaemia

The first rule in management is to ensure adequate rehydration of patients who may be dehydrated as a direct result of their hypercalcaemia. A urine output of 3–4 litres per day should be achieved, and this usually requires the intravenous administration of saline. The addition of frusemide, itself a calciuric diuretic, will augment calcium excretion. Steroids should be given (50–100 mg prednisone daily) and, where possible, definitive chemotherapy should be started, since long-term control of the hypercalcaemia depends upon reduction of the tumour mass.

In some cases these measures will be found to be ineffective or too slow to reverse potentially dangerous coma or renal failure. Mithramycin in a dose of 15 μg/kg daily for up to four days acts rapidly to reverse hypercalcaemia through a direct action on osteoclasts (Stamp et al, 1975). Although myelo-suppressive, these doses of mithramycin do not generally cause severe or prolonged cytopenia. An alternative to mithramycin is calcitonin given 4–8 units/kg per day, but the action may be short-lived (Delamore, 1982).

The use of phosphate intravenously is potentially hazardous and, although oral phosphate may be an adjuvant to therapy, gastrointestinal disturbance often follows.

Recently the diphosphonates (EHDP or Cl_2MDP) have been used for long-term control of hypercalcaemia. Since they seem to act directly to prevent bone resorption, they may provide hope for bone-sparing therapy in a variety of malignant conditions (Siris et al, 1980).

Radiotherapy

The use of radiotherapy in multiple myeloma is entirely palliative. The tumour is very radiosensitive, and 20 Gy to local areas of pain generally result in notable relief. Much higher doses are used for solitary plasmacytomas (40–50 Gy), but even in these cases radiographic evidence of bone healing is rarely seen. It is important to ensure that palliative radiotherapy does not compromise definitive chemotherapy because of its additional myelosuppressive effect.

Plasma exchange

Because hyperviscosity problems are uncommon in myeloma, the need for plasmapheresis arises comparatively rarely. It may be an adjuvant to the treatment of acute renal failure (by improving renal perfusion). Since half of the total IgG or IgA is extravascular, apheresis on alternate days is required to maintain a fall in paraprotein level, and it must be accompanied by effective chemotherapy in order to maintain clinical improvement.

Infections

Because of the immunoparesis, infections frequently progress rapidly even in the presence of a normal neutrophil count. Prompt institution of parenteral antibiotics in full dosage is vital and, as in all immunocompromised patients, cannot always await the identification of the pathogen. In these circumstances an aggressive approach is essential, and the choice of antibiotic should be guided by the likely source of infection and supplemented by a broad-spectrum agent such as gentamycin or piperacillin, or one of the newer cephalosporins (cefuroxime, cefotaxime). The administration of immunoglobulin is usually ineffective.

MONOCLONAL GAMMOPATHIES OF UNCERTAIN SIGNIFICANCE (MGUS) AND INDOLENT DISEASE

The incidental finding of a serum paraprotein unsupported by other evidence of myeloma was formerly termed benign monoclonal gammopathy. However since a small number eventually develop a plasma cell malignancy, the expression MGUS is preferable. Kyle (1982) has described the course of 241 such individuals over ten years, and found that only 11 per cent actually developed myeloma at five years. Paraprotein levels remained unchanged in 57 per cent, and 9 per cent showed an increase. He concluded that paraprotein levels of over 20 g/l (IgG, IgM) or over 10 g/l (IgA) were more likely to reflect an underlying malignancy and that Ig levels over 30 g/l were almost invariably due to malignancy. The overall incidence of MGUS over the age of 70 years was 3 per cent.

The distinction between myeloma and MGUS is important and can often be quite difficult. Kyle (1982) found that immunoparesis and even Bence-Jones proteinuria occasionally occurred in these individuals, although the latter did not exceed 1 g/24 hours. A negative bone marrow aspirate does not exclude myeloma, since distribution of the infiltrate is often patchy. He found that neither the level of paraprotein nor the presence of Bence-Jones protein predicted development of myeloma, and concluded that the only reliable indication of developing myeloma was an increasing level of Ig on serial estimations.

Patients who are clinically well but in whom a diagnosis of myeloma can be made confidently on the grounds of a high paraprotein level with Bence-Jones protein and marrow plasmacytosis may occasionally present a problem in management. If anaemia is not present, and there is no evidence of renal or metabolic disorder, such patients should not be treated initially. They should be followed intensively, and if Ig levels rise or other manifestations of disease become apparent, chemotherapy should be instituted. In this manner some patients with indolent or 'smouldering' myeloma are spared unnecessary chemotherapy with its attendant inconvenience and long-term hazards. The diagnostic criteria of the South-West Oncology Group (Durie & Salmon, 1977) provide useful guidelines in evaluating clinical and laboratory findings in these cases (Table 12.4).

SOLITARY PLASMACYTOMA

Isolated plasma cell tumours constitute 10 per cent of all plasma cell malignancies. They may occur in bone or as extra-osseous deposits, the latter most commonly in the head and neck (Bataille, 1982; Fudenberg & Virella, 1980). Approximately one-quarter of these cases are accompanied by a serum para-

Table 12.4 Diagnostic criteria for multiple myeloma (Durie & Salmon, 1977)

Major criteria
I.   Plasmacytomata on tissue biopsy.
II. Bone marrow > 30% plasma cells.
III. Monoclonal globulin on serum electrophoresis. IgG >35 g/l; IgA >20 g/l; κ or λ chain
     excretion >1 g day with no evidence of other proteinuria on urine electrophoresis.

Minor criteria
a. Bone marrow 10–30% plasma cells.
b. Monoclonal globulin but less than levels defined above.
c. Lytic bone lesions.
d. Reduction in any or all physiological immunoglobulins, IgG <6 g/l; IgA <1 g/l; IgM <0.5 g/l

Diagnosis confirmed in symptomatic patients
1. I + b, I + c, I + d.
2. II + b, II + c, II + d.
3. III
4. a + b + c, a + b + d.

protein which may disappear following surgery or radiotherapy. Persistence of the paraprotein suggests disseminated disease.

Progression to multiple myeloma (often after many years) occurs in 50 per cent of bone plasmacytomas, but recurrence or multiple myeloma is less common in adequately treated extra-osseous lesions (15 per cent). Treatment is by surgical excision and/or radiotherapy. If paraproteinaemia is detected at presentation, its persistence some months after treatment should be an indication for systemic chemotherapy. Regular follow-up is required in all cases because of late dissemination in many patients despite adequate treatment.

WALDENSTRÖM'S MACROGLOBULINAEMIA

This condition, which was first described by Waldenström in 1944, is defined as a slow-growing malignant lymphoproliferative disorder with a monoclonal IgM paraprotein in the serum. The average age of presentation is 60 years, and cases under the age of 40 years are rare.

Fatigue and weakness are prominent presenting symptoms, and the hyperviscosity syndrome accounts for a range of clinical problems in as many as 50 per cent of cases (MacKenzie & Fudenberg, 1972). Bleeding manifestations are common (40 per cent), especially recurrent epistaxis and purpura, and can be attributed to a combination of factors including hyperviscosity, hypervolaemia and a haemostatic defect. Neurological disturbance may occur in 25 per cent of patients, ranging from confusion, or even coma, to a polyneuropathy of similar type to that observed in myeloma. Milder symptoms of headache, tinnitus and dizziness are common, and blurring of vision occurs in 10 per cent of cases. Splenomegaly is common. Liver enlargement and lymphadenopathy are frequent.

The visual disturbance is due to a distinctive retinopathy with tortuous congested retinal veins, progressing to typical 'sausage'-like venous constrictions and retinal haemorrhages. In the patients in whom the paraprotein has the properties of a cryoglobulin, Raynaud's syndrome or cold urticaria may occur.

In contrast to myeloma, bone lesions are rare. Renal failure may occur, though it is less common and less severe than in myeloma. The mechanism is usually IgM deposition in the glomerular basement membrane, although in a number of cases amyloid deposition results in nephrotic syndrome.

The disease results from a malignant clonal expansion of a plasma cell precursor secreting IgM, and unlike myeloma is characterised by abnormal proliferation in liver, spleen and lymph nodes as well as in the marrow. The cellular infiltrate is pleomorphic with a variable admixture of plasmacytoid lymphocytes and mature plasma cells, often with a prominent increase in mast cells. The lymph node architecture is preserved with a similar pleomorphic infiltrate of plasma cells and lymphocytes, some of which show PAS-positive nuclear inclusions. An excess of mast cells and the monoclonality of the infiltrate for cytoplasmic IgM help to differentiate this from other lymphoproliferative disorders.

Macroglobulinaemia is not difficult to diagnose in the elderly patient with hepatosplenomegaly, lymphadenopathy and a prominent IgM paraprotein band (more than 20 g/l). However, in many cases the diagnosis may have to be made with more slender evidence, and the distinction between a benign IgM paraproteinaemia and the early manifestations of Waldenström's disease is often subtle.

Laboratory findings

In addition to the serum paraprotein, urinary free light chains are sometimes found (25 per cent of cases). The majority of the IgM paraproteins (80 per cent) are of κ light chain type. The marrow aspirate generally shows the aforementioned pleomorphic infiltrate of cells, with varying proportions of lymphocytes, plasmacytoid lymphocytes and plasma cells.

An estimate of plasma viscosity is essential since symptoms can be expected when this rises above 4. Cryoglobulin, cold agglutinins, inhibitors of coagulation and of platelet aggregation are looked for. Anaemia is very common, and is usually normochronic and normocytic in type; red cell mass and plasma volume, if evaluated, will often show the latter to be increased, thereby contributing to the lowered PCV. Thrombocytopenia may occur, but is usually only moderate and is rarely responsible for the commonly observed bleeding episodes.

Treatment

As in the case of IgG and IgA paraproteinaemia, an IgM paraprotein in the absence of symptoms and without organ or marrow infiltrates does not require active treatment. Levels of IgM over 20 g/l are rarely benign, and indications for intervention include a rising IgM level or increasing anaemia. Patients who are symptomatic or who have obvious organ involvement require treatment.

If hyperviscosity is a problem, this may be managed effectively by plasmapheresis. Exchange of 2–3 litres of plasma should be performed at daily or alternate day intervals until viscosity is below 4. At the same time chemotherapy should be started, the first choice being chlorambucil at a dose of 4–8 mg daily, decreasing to 2–4 mg daily. The blood count should be monitored regularly at first (two-weekly), as should IgM and viscosity levels. Cyclophosphamide (50–150 mg daily) is an alternative to chlorambucil, but with either drug only 50 per cent of patients can be expected to respond. Recently improved response rates have been claimed for the M_2 protocol (see above) with a 100 per cent response rate (Case, 1982).

Prognosis

There has been considerable variation in estimates of prognosis in this very elderly group of patients. Mean survival of 34 months from diagnosis has been quoted, but survivals of 75 months in patients with nodular as opposed to diffuse marrow infiltrates have been claimed (Chelazzi et al, 1979). Data on patients treated with more aggressive regimes are still awaited. It should be emphasised that many patients have very indolent disease and may require little or no chemotherapy at all.

REFERENCES

Alberts D S, Durie B G M, Salmon S E 1976 Doxorubicin/BCNU chemotherapy for multiple myeloma in relapse. Lancet 1: 926–928
Alexanian R, Salmon S, Bonnet J, Gehan E, Hant A, Weick J 1977 Combination therapy for multiple myeloma. Cancer 40: 2765–2771
Alexanian R, Gehan E, Hant A, Saiki J, Weick J 1978 Unmaintained remissions in multiple myeloma. Blood 51: 1005–1011
Alexanian R, Yap B S, Bodey G P 1983 Prednisone pulse therapy for refractory myeloma. Blood 62: 572–577
ALGB 1975 Correlation of abnormal immunoglobulin with clinical features of myeloma. Archives of Internal Medicine 135: 46–52
Bataille R 1982 Localised plasmacyotoma. In: Clinics in haematology 11:1. Saunders, London ch 6, p 113–122
Bataille R, Chevalier J, Rossi M, Sany J 1982 Bone scintigraphy in plasma-cell myeloma. Radiology 145: 801–804
Bataille R, Durie B G, Grenier J 1983 Serum beta₂ microglobulin and survival duration in myeloma: a simple reliable marker for staging. British Journal of Haematology 55: 439–447
Benson W J, Scarffe J H, Todd I D H, Palmer M, Crowther D 1979 Spinal cord compression in myeloma. British Medical Journal: 1541–1544
Blattner W A 1980 Epidemiology of multiple myeloma and related plasma cell disorders: an analytical review. In: Potter M(ed) Progress in myeloma. Elsevier, New York, ch 1, p 1–67
Bloch K J, Maki D G 1973 Hyperviscosity syndromes associated with immunoglobulin abnormalities. Seminars in Haematology 10 (2): 113–124
Bonnet et al 1982 VBAP combination in the treatment of relapsing or resistent multiple myeloma: a South-West Oncology Group Study. Cancer Treatment Reports 66: 1267–1271

Brenner B, Carter E, Tatarsky I, Gruszkiewicz J, Peyser E 1982 Incidence, prognostic significance and therapeutic modalities of central nervous system involvement in multiple myeloma. Acta Haematologica 68: 77–83

Case D C 1982 Combination chemotherapy (M2) protocol (BCNU, cyclophosphamide, vincristine, melphalan and prednisone) for Waldenström's macroglobulinaemia: preliminary report. Blood 59: 934–937

Case D C, Lee B, Clarkson B D 1977 Improved survival times in multiple myeloma treated with melphalan, prednisone, cyclophosphamide, vincristine and BCNU: M2 protocol. American Journal of Medicine 63: 897–903

Chellazzi G, Bettini R, Pinotti G 1979 Bone marrow patterns and survival in Waldenström's macroglobulinaemia. Lancet ii: 965–966

Cohen H J, Rundles R W 1975 Managing the complications of plasma cell myeloma. Archives of Internal Medicine 135: 177–184

Dahlström U, Järpe S, Lindström F D 1979 Paraplegia in myelomatosis — a study of 20 cases. Acta Medica Scandinavica 205: 173–178

DeFronzo R A, Cooke R, Wright J, Humphrey R L 1978 Renal function in patients with multiple myeloma. Medicine 57: 151–166

Delamore I W 1982 Hypercalcaemia and myeloma. British Journal of Haematology 51: 507–509

Delauche M C, Clauvel J P, Seligmann M 1981 Peripheral neuropathy and plasma cell neoplasia: a report of 10 cases. British Journal of Haematology 48: 383–392

Durie B G M 1982 Staging and kinetics of multiple myeloma. In: Clinics in haematology 11:1. Saunders, London, ch I, p 3–18

Durie B G M, Salmon S E 1975 Clinical staging system for multiple myeloma — correlation of measured myeloma cell mass with presenting clinical features. Response to treatment and survival. Cancer 36: 842–854

Durie B G M, Salmon S E 1977 Multiple myeloma, macroglobulinaemia and monoclonal gammapathies. In: Hoffbrand A V, Brain M C, Hirsch J. Recent advances in haematology, Churchill Livingstone, Edinburgh, p 243–261

Durie B G M, Russell D H, Salmon S E 1980 Reappraisal of plateau phase in myeloma. Lancet 2: 65–68

Durie B G M, Salmon S E, Mundy G R 1981 Relation of osteoclast activating factor production to extent of bone disease in multiple myeloma. British Journal of Haematology 47: 21–30

Early A P, Ozer H, Henderson E S 1981 Multiple myeloma. New York State Journal of Medicine 81(6): 883–893

Fudenberg H H, Virella G 1980 Multiple myeloma and Waldenström macroglobulinaemia: unusual presentations. Seminars in Haematology 17: 63–79

Galton D A G et al 1973 Report on the first myelomatosis trial: part I. Analysis of presenting features of prognostic importance. British Journal of Haematology 24: 123–129

Harley J B et al 1979 Improved survival of increased risk myeloma patients on combined triple alkylating agent therapy: a study of the CALBG. Blood 54: 13–21

Kyle R A 1975 Multiple myeloma. Review of 869 cases. Mayo Clinic Proceedings 50: 29–40

Kyle R A 1982 Monoclonal gammopathy of undetermined significance (MGUS): a review. In: Clinics in haematology 11:1. Saunders, London, ch 7, p 123–150

Kyle R A, Bayrd E D 1976 The monoclonal gammopathies. Thomas, Springfield

Kyle R A, Elveback L R 1976 Management and prognosis of multiple myeloma. Mayo Clinic Proceedings 51: 751–760

Kyle et al 1982 Multiple myeloma resistant to melphalan: treatment with doxorubicin, cyclophosphamide, carmustine (BCNU) and prednisone. Cancer Treatment Reports 66: 451–456

Lackner H 1973 Hemostatic abnormalities associated with dysproteinemias. Seminars in Hematology 10(2): 125–133

Ludwig H, Kumpan W, Sinzinger H 1982 Radiography and bone scintigraphy in myeloma: a comparative analysis. British Journal of Radiology 55: 173–181

MacKenzie M R, Fudenberg H H 1972 Macroglobulinaemia: an analysis of forty patients. Blood 39: 874

Maldonado J E, Velosa J A, Kyle R A, Wagoner R D, Holley K E, Salassa R M 1975 Fanconi syndrome in adults. A manifestation of a latent form of myeloma. American Journal of Medicine 58: 354–364

McElwain T J, Powles R L 1983 High dose intravenous melphalan for plasma cell leukaemia and myeloma. Lancet ii: 822–824

McIntyre O R 1979 Current concepts in cancer. Multiple myeloma. New England Journal of Medicine 301: 193–196

Medical Research Council 1980a Report on the second myelomatosis trial after five years of follow up. British Journal of Cancer 42: 813–822

Medical Research Council 1980b Treatment comparisons in the third MRC myelomatosis trial. British Journal of Cancer 42: 823–830

Medical Research Council 1980c Prognostic features in the 3rd MRC myelomatosis trial. British Journal of Cancer 42: 831–840

Merlini G, Waldenström J G, Jayakar S D 1980 A new improved clinical staging system for multiple myeloma based on analysis of 123 treated patients. Blood 55: 1011–1019

McPhedran P, Heath C W, Garcia J 1972 Multiple myeloma incidence in metropolitan Atlanta, Georgia: racial and seasonal variations. Blood 39: 866–873

Mills K H G, Cawley J C 1983 Abnormal monoclonal antibody-defined helper/suppressor T-cell subpopulations in multiple myeloma: relationships to treatment and clinical stage. British Journal of Haematology 53: 271–275

Mundy G R, Cooper L G, Schechter R A, Salmon S E 1974 Evidence for the secretion of an osteoclast stimulating factor in myeloma. New England Journal of Medicine 291: 1041–1046

Norden C W 1980 Infections in patients with multiple myeloma. Archives of Internal Medicine 140: 1150–1151

Osserman E F 1982 Plasma cell dyscrasias: a current perspective. Acta Haematologica 68: 167–168

Paglieroni T, MacKenzie M R 1977 Studies on the pathogenesis of an immune defect in multiple myeloma. Journal of Clinical Investigation 59: 1120–1133

Potter M 1973 The developmental history of the neoplastic plasma cell in mice: a brief review of recent developments. Seminars in haematology 10(1): 19–32

Preston F E, Cooke K B, Foster M E, Winfield D A, Lee D 1978 Myelomatosis and the hyperviscosity syndrome. British Journal of Haematology 38: 517–530

Russell J A, Powles R L 1978 The relationship between serum viscosity, hypervolaemia and clinical manifestations associated with circulating paraprotein. British Journal of Haematology 39: 163–175

Salmon S E 1982 Cloning and sensitivity of myeloma stem cells. In: Clinics in haematology 11:1. Saunders, London, ch 3, p 47–63

Salmon S E, Seligmann M 1974 B-cell neoplasia in man. Lancet ii: 1230–1233

Shustik C, Bergsagel D E, Pruzanski W 1976 κ and λ light chain disease: survival rates and clinical manifestations. Blood 48: 41–51

Silverstein A, Doniger D E 1973 Neurological complications of myelomatosis. Archives of Neurology 9: 534–544

Siris E S, Sherman W H, Baquirin D C, Schlatterer J P, Osman E F, Canfield R E 1980 Effects of dichloromethylene diphosphonate on skeletal calcium in multiple myeloma. New England Journal of Medicine 302: 310–314

Stamp T C B, Child J A, Walker P G 1975 Treatment of osteolytic myelomatosis with mithramycin. Lancet i: 719–722

Ullrich S E, Zolla-Pazner S 1982 Immuno-regulatory circuits in myeloma. In: Clinics in haematology 11:1. Saunders, London, ch 5, p 87–112

Woodruff R 1981 Treatment of multiple myeloma. Cancer Treatment Reviews 8: 225–270

Woodruff R K, Wadsworth J, Malpas J S, Tobias J S 1979 Clinical staging in multiple myeloma. British Journal of Haematology 42: 199–205

Polycythaemia and myelofibrosis

POLYCYTHAEMIA

Polycythaemia, first recognised at the beginning of the nineteenth century, is characterised by an increase in the red blood cell count, haemoglobin or packed cell volume (PCV). There are two main causes — true and relative polycyathaemias (Table 13.1). Only in the true polycythaemias is the red cell mass increased. This is found in two situations: primary polycythaemia rubra vera and the secondary polycythaemia. The latter usually results from increased erythropoietin activity, due either to an appropriate physiological response to decreased blood oxygen saturation, or to an inappropriate production of the hormones. In relative polycythaemias the red cell mass is within the normal range and the raised packed cell volume is due either to an abnormal reduction of plasma volume or to the combination of a high normal red cell mass or a low normal plasma volume.

Polycythaemia vera

Polycythaemia vera is a chronic, progressive myeloproliferative disorder, in which there is an absolute increase in the red cell mass associated in two-thirds of patients with increased white cell and platelet counts.

Table 13.1 Classification of polycythaemias

True polycythaemia
  1 Primary
      Polycythaemia rubra vera

  2 Secondary
      Chronic lung disease
      Renal disease   e.g. tumours, cysts (single or multiple)
                    hydronephrosis
      Tumours   e.g. cerebellar haemangioma, uterine fibroids
      Others   e.g. altitude, abnormal haemoglobins, heavy smoking

Relative polycythaemia (also called spurious, stress or pseudopolycythaemia and Gaisbock's syndrome)

Aetiology

The disease is a disorder arising from a mutation of the pluripotent stem cell. *In vitro* marrow studies and work on glucose-6-phosphate dehydrogenase variants in females with polycythaemia vera indicate the presence of two populations of erythroid precursor cells. One is autonomous and proliferates, even in the absence of erythropoietin, while the other behaves normally and is erythropoietin-dependent. The first population is therefore likely to represent an autonomous mutant clone (Adamson, 1976; Golde, 1977).

Patients with polycythaemia rubra vera have normal, low or absent erythropoietin levels in the urine and plasma, and show an appropriate rise after venesection. The low erythropoietin levels are due to the normal feedback inhibition by the increased red cell mass.

Incidence

Polycythaemia vera is an uncommon disorder. An American study found the annual incidence rate was four to five new cases per million population. (Modan, 1965). It affects the middle-aged and elderly, with the peak incidence between 50 and 60 years. The mean age of onset has gradually increased over the last 60 years from 44 in 1912 to 60 in 1964. There is a slightly higher incidence in men than in women, the ratio being approximately 1.5:1. The influence of racial factors is conflicting. Modan (1965) found a greater than expected incidence in Jews, and a low incidence among blacks, but these findings have not been confirmed.

Clinical features

The signs and symptoms of the disease result partly from the overproduction of red cells and platelets — which leads to increased viscosity and possible vascular thrombosis — and partly from the increased blood volume, which causes engorgement of various organs.

The onset is insidious, so insidious indeed that the diagnosis may be an accidental finding when an unrelated disorder is investigated. The symptoms are often vague, e.g. headache, dizziness, tinnitus, inability to concentrate, irritability and blurred vision, and may all too easily be attributed to old age or more commonly occurring conditions seen in the elderly. However, the diagnosis will be suggested by the patient's clinical appearance — red colour of the skin and mucous membranes which may have a cyanotic tinge in cold weather, telangiectasia on the face, and congested vessels of the conjunctivae and retinae. The spleen is usually moderately enlarged in most cases, whilst the liver is only slightly enlarged. Sternal tenderness may be found.

The main features of the disease occur when, more commonly, thrombosis or, less frequently, haemorrhage occurs. The circulation of the central nervous system is most often involved, resulting in transient ischaemic attacks, cerebrovascular accidents and visual disturbances, such as scotomata, diplopia and temporary blindness. When the cardiovascular system is involved, a patient may develop dyspnoea on effort, angina or myocardial infarction. Peripheral vascular involvement can cause erythromelgia, arterial and venous thromboses, Raynaud's phenomenon and even gangrene. When the blood supply to the gastrointestinal tract is affected, indigestion and flatulence can results, with about 1 in 10 patients having peptic ulceration. Thrombosis of the portal venous system can cause portal hypertension and bleeding oesophageal varices.

Approximately 1 in 10 patients, usually male, have clinical features of gout, although one-third have hyperuricaemia, which results from increased synthesis and degradation of nucleoprotein. The incidence rises with the duration of the disease. Renal stones and tophi may develop. A family history of gout is not common.

Troublesome generalised pruritis, perhaps due to histamine release from basophil granulocytes, occurs in about two-thirds of patients. The symptom is often worse in the hands and feet, and is aggravated on bathing or getting into a warm bed.

Laboratory findings

The red blood count is raised to 6.5–$7.5 \times 10^{12}/l$. The haemoglobin is increased to 18–24 g/dl. The PCV is usually greater than 0.52. Since the red cell mass cannot be accurately deduced from the haemoglobin, PCV and red cell count, it must always be measured directly, using an isotopic label. Red cell mass exceeding 36 ml/kg in men and 32 ml/kg in women indicates polycythaemia.

The peripheral blood film shows normal red cell morphology, but, as iron deficiency is common, either from repeated venesection or a bleeding tendency, microcytosis may be seen. The white cell count is raised in about two-thirds of patients to values of 12–$30 \times 10^9/l$, but higher values occur in the later stages of the disease. There is sometimes a slight shift to the left in the granulocytic series, and occasionally metamyelocytes, myelocytes or even earlier forms may be seen in the peripheral blood.

The leucocyte alkaline phosphatase (LAP) score is increased. In 70–90 per cent of patients the score is 100–350, but in some cases, especially in the early stages of the disease, the score is within the normal range.

The platelet count is raised in 65 per cent of patients at the time of presentation and is usually in the region of 400–$800 \times 10^9/l$. Very occasionally, considerably higher counts are seen. Sometimes there are abnormalities of morphology and function. The platelets may be abnormally large and bizarre in shape. Fragments of megakaryocytes may also be seen. The defective platelet function is probably the major cause of haemorrhagic complications seen in this disease. The serum vitamin B_{12} and B_{12} binding capacity is often high.

The bone marrow shows hypercellularity. Erythropoiesis is normoblastic, and the normoblasts may have the ragged vacuolated cytoplasm of iron deficiency, especially if the patient has been treated with venesection. There may be no free stainable iron present. Granulocyte precursors may also show hyperplasia, and megakaryocytes may be increased in number. The main haematological findings are summarised in Table 13.2.

Chromosomal abnormalities in patients with polycythaemia vera have been described, but are unusual, and many have received myelosuppressive treatment, making it difficult to determine to what extent the abnormalities are due to treatment or related to the disease itself.

Course and prognosis

The natural history of the disease shows there are three phases of development. Initially, patients with polycythaemia have few, if any, symptoms for a period of several years. In the next, erythraemic phase, the classical symptoms, signs and major complications develop. It is during this period, which can also last several years, that most fatalities occur. Ultimately, the third phase occurs, with the development of myelosclerosis and less commonly, leukaemia. The incidence of leukaemic change is greater in those treated with alkylating agents and possibly in those receiving ^{32}P as well.

Survival times in adequately treated patients have lengthened considerably, especially in younger patients. The mean is 13 years from time to diagnosis. However, the major cause of death remains that of vascular complications. Irrespective of the type of therapy used, the prognosis is worst in the elderly and those who develop major complications.

Treatment

The objective of treatment is to reduce the likelihood of vascular complications by reducing the packed cell volume and maintaining it at an optimal level, and treating the thrombocythaemia when present. The methods by which this is best achieved are still controversial, and will remain so until the uncertainties surrounding what is the natural history of the disease, as opposed to what is the consequence of previous treatment, have been resolved.

Table 13.2 Haematological findings in polycythaemia vera

	Men	Women
Haemoglobin	>18.0 g/dl	>17.0 g/dl
PCV	>0.55	>0.52
RBC	>6.5 × 10^{12}/l	>6.0 × 10^{12}/l
WBC	12–30 × 10^9/l	12–30 × 10^9/l
Platelets	400–800 × 10^9/l	400–800 × 10^9/l
Red cell mass	>36 ml/kg	>32 ml/kg

Immediate symptomatic relief is obtained by venesection. This should be carried out cautiously in the elderly, who frequently have pre-existing cerebrovascular and cardiovascular disease. The recommended regime is removal of 200–300 ml of blood twice weekly until the PCV has fallen to within the desired range. There is evidence of continuing risk of vascular lesions when the PCV is only slightly raised and the PCV should therefore be reduced to 0.45. Where reduction in blood volume is considered hazardous, the volume withdrawn can be replaced with high-molecular-weight dextran. Following the initial treatment, the rate of rise of the PCV should be observed. If it is low, and the patient only requires venesection infrequently, then no further treatment is necessary, so long as thrombocythaemia is not a problem. It should be borne in mind that this procedure produces iron-deficiency anaemia, and this in itself produces symptoms and a rise in platelets.

Since venesection does not depress bone marrow cell production, it may fail to control the situation. At this stage myelosuppressive therapy will be needed. Unfortunately, drug therapy in the elderly can present considerable logistic problems of follow-up and compliance. Therefore it is usually preferable to commence with ^{32}P in an intravenous dose of 5–7 millicuries. This will take two to three months to achieve maximal effect, so venesection may need to be carried out in the interim. Sometimes a second, smaller dose of ^{32}P is required after three months to bring the disease under complete control. Treatment with ^{32}P gives satisfactory control in over three-quarters of patients, and remission can last two years or even longer.

Although radioactive phosphorus is the treatment of choice for the elderly, alkylating agents can be used for continuing-care patients, where compliance and follow-up present less problems. Many drugs are used, e.g. busulphan chlorambucil and cyclophosphamide, but chlorambucil is the treatment of choice, since it has fewer side-effects. Busulphan has a potent action on platelets which makes it valuable for those patients with marked thrombocytosis. It is given in doses of 4–6 mg/day until the white cell count and/or platelet count falls by 50 per cent. The dose should then be reduced by 50 per cent and the drug then stopped altogether when the platelet count falls below $250 \times 10^9/l$ or the white blood count falls below $10 \times 10^9/l$. The PCV takes longer to fall, so regular venesection is necessary at the beginning of the treatment. Busulphan can produce irreversible damage to stem cells and long-lasting severe thrombocytopenia and neutropenia, hence considerable care is required in its use. The mortality due to its use is significant. Remission, once obtained, can last for months or even years. Busulphan should not be used for extended periods of time, since irreversible pancytopenia, skin pigmentation and pulmonary fibrosis can result. When melphalan is used, the initial dose is 4–8 mg for five days, reducing to 2 mg three times a week for four weeks. If, after a month of treatment, the white cell count and platelet count are still high, a further month's therapy should be given, and this regime should continue until the platelet count and white cell count are normal. Relapse often occurs within five to six months: a considerably shorter time compared with busulphan. Chlorambucil is used at a dose of 2–4 mg daily until the count has fallen to appropriate levels.

Allopurinol, given in doses of 300 mg/day, should be given to patients with hyperuricaemia. It should also be given prophylactically to patients who are being treated with ^{32}P or chemotherapy. Acute gout should be treated with non-steroidal anit-inflammatory drugs.

Pruritis is a particularly difficult symptom to treat. Often it improves as the polycythemia comes under control. Antihistamines are not very satisfactory, and the response to other agents such as cholestyramine and cimetidine is variable and rather unsatisfactory. However, if pruritis is a major problem, then it is worthwhile trying these drugs. Avoidance of precipitating factors, such as heat, is recommended.

Symptoms of a transient nature involving the peripheral vasculature often improve dramatically once the disease has come under control, and surgery should be avoided if possible. However, persisting symptoms, in spite of good haematological control, may make surgery necessary.

Secondary polycythaemia

The secondary polycythaemias are usually the result of increased erythropoietin activity, which is either an appropriate response to decreased blood oxygen saturation, or to an inappropriate production of the hormone. There are many causes (Table 13.1), many of which, however, are seldom seen in the elderly.

Chronic lung disease is the commonest cause in the older age groups. However, not all chronic hypoxic patients develop polycythaemia. Many patients with pulmonary disease and abnormal arterial gas tensions have a normal PCV, and most have increased erythropoietin levels. There is no really good explanation for this, but it has been suggested that erythropoiesis is depressed by chronic infection. Splenomegaly is absent. In patients with chronic lung disease who have exceptionally high PCV greater than 0.70, there is now evidence that clinical improvement may follow venesection. Treatment otherwise depends on the cause of the secondary polycythaemia and should be dealt with appropriately. The distinguishing features of polycythaemia, secondary polycythaemia due to hypoxia and relative polycythaemia are shown in Table 13.3.

Familial polycythaemia is rare and is usually due to an abnormal haemoglobin with a high oxygen affinity. The normal P_{50} is 25–27 mm/Hg. In these disorders it is in the region of 12.

Myelofibrosis

Myelofibrosis is a myeloproliferative disorder characterised by moderate to severe anaemia, a very variable peripheral blood picture, fibrosis of the bone marrow and myeloid metaplaisa in the spleen, liver and other organs. It

Table 13.3 Typical findings in PRV; polycythaemia secondary to hypoxia and relative polycythaemia

Findings	PRV	Polycythaemia 2° to hypoxia	Relative polycythaemia
Granulocytosis	Present	Absent	Absent
Thrombocythaemia	Present	Absent	Absent
Splenomegaly	Present	Absent	Absent
LAP	Increased	Normal	Normal
Red cell mass	Increased	Increased	Normal
Plasma volume	Normal or reduced	Normal or reduced	Reduced
Arterial oxygen saturation	Normal	Decreased or normal	Normal
Erythropoietin	Normal or decreased	Increased	Normal

results from a proliferation of a mutant clone involving a stem cell, which has the capacity to differentiate into red cells, granulocytes and platelets (Adamson & Fialkow, 1978). Not uncommonly, there is also an osteoblastic proliferation with new bone formation. It is not known whether the marrow fibrosis is a reaction to the abnormal proliferation or part of it. It used to be considered that the myeloid metaplasia found in the liver, spleen and elsewhere was a compensatory process, but this is probably another feature of the stem cell proliferation.

Clinical features

Myelofibrosis may develop during the course of polycythaemia vera or thrombocythaemia, but usually there is no previous history. Once again, it is a disease of the middle-aged and elderly, with a peak incidence in the 50–70 age group. Both sexes are affected equally.

The disease progresses slowly and, because the onset is insidious, the diagnosis is often made when a patient is being investigated for an unrelated disorder. Symptoms caused by anaemia, such as lethargy, weakness and dyspnoea on effort are common. Sometimes patients present with symptoms related to the size of the spleen, such as abdominal swelling, discomfort after eating, heartburn and even ankle oedema. Splenomegaly is almost invariably present, ranging in size from just palpable to massive, virtually filling the whole abdomen. Splenic infarction causes acute left hypochondrial pain, and a rub can often be heard. Hepatomegaly is often present and portal hypertension may result from splenic vein thrombosis or extramedullary portal tract proliferation or increased portal tract blood flow. Patients with portal hypertension may present with bleeding, oesophageal varices, or ascites.

Gout is not uncommon, and pruritis also occurs which is particularly troublesome after exposure to heat. Patients may also complain of leg cramps, and bone pains — symptoms all too easily attributed to old age.

Platelet function is sometimes abnormal, and the patient may present with spontaneous bruising or bleeding from the gastrointestinal tract. About a third of patients with myelofibrosis have a patchy osteosclerosis, usually involving the axial skeleton and proximal ends of the humerus and femur. Other sites, such as the cranium, are occasionally involved.

Laboratory findings

At the time of presentation anaemia is present in over two-thirds of cases. Although it may be mild or moderately severe initially, it becomes much more marked as the disease progresses. The red cells show marked polychromasia, anisocytosis and poikilocytosis and 'tear drop' cells. Frequently there are both nucleated red cells and immature granulocytes in the peripheral blood. Folate deficiency is relatively common. A low dietary intake and a marked increase in turnover of haemopoietic cells both contribute to this deficiency. Iron deficiency is also sometimes present if there has been blood loss. The white cell count is often elevated, consisting mainly of mature neutrophils, but there are usually some immature forms as well.

The platelet count may be increased or decreased depending on the state of the disease. In the early phases values up to $1000 \times 10^9/l$ may be found. The platelet morphology is abnormal, with giant form and circulating megakaryocyte fragments being seen in the blood film. As the disease progresses, and the spleen enlarges, the platelet count tends to fall.

Bone marrow aspiration is usually unsuccessful (dry tap), but because of the patchiness of the myelofibrotic process, occasionally hypercellular forms are obtained. Trephine biopsy of the iliac crest is essential for accurate diagnosis. The amount of haemopoietic cell activity and marrow fibrosis is variable. Silver staining for reticulin shows and increase in reticulin fibre formation even when hypercellular fragments have been obtained.

Blood uric acid levels are usually high in myelofibrosis.

Course and prognosis

Many patients remain stable for many years with a relatively normal haemoglobin and minimal splenomegaly. In some the course of the disease is less benign with a gradual, general decline, worsening anaemia and increasing splenomegaly. Although the median survivial is about three years from the time of diagnosis, many patients survive longer. Bad prognostic signs are severe anaemia which fails to respond adequately to transfusion, severe leukopenia, spontaneous bleeding and severe weight loss. All these symptoms can be due to folate deficiency. The usual cause of death is progressive anaemia, with approximately 20 per cent of cases terminating in acute myeloblastic leukaemia.

Treatment

There is no specific treatment. Patients with mild symptoms will need only periodic assessment. Anaemia will be the main symptom requiring treatment. Folate deficiency is not uncommon and will respond to folic acid therapy. This is one of the few conditions where long-term folate prophylaxis is reasonable at a dose of 5 mg daily. It is important to ensure that the patient absorbs vitamin B_{12} normally. Androgens are given to many anaemic patients, but not all respond; there who do develop benefit only after some weeks.

When the anaemia is severe enough to cause cardiovascular symptoms, it should be treated with blood transfusion in order to maintain the haemoglobin at values of 9–10 g/dl. However, before embarking on a programme of repeated transfusions, the overall condition of the patient should be carefully evaluated. The rise in haemoglobin after the transfusion is often less than expected, and eventually the rise becomes less and of somewhat shorter duration until benefit lasts only a week or two. This, in fact, may be due to destruction of transfused cells by the spleen.

Splenic pooling of blood is an important factor causing anaemia and should be assessed by ^{51}Cr studies. Busulphan is extremely effective in reducing the size of the spleen, and a short course can be followed by prolonged improvement.

Splenic irradiation has also been used to reduce the size of the spleen, with variable results. Splenectomy is not advisable in the elderly, due to the high operative mortality and morbidity, and some possible rebound increase in platelet count. However, embolisation via an arterial catheter is a less hazardous method of infarcting areas of the spleen.

Patients with hyper-uricaemia should be treated as mentioned earlier.

RELATIVE POLYCYTHAEMIA

This condition is characterised by a raised venous PCV associated with a normal total red cell mass. It occurs in two groups of patients. In the first, the condition is usually acute and secondary to dehydration. However, the cause remains obscure in the second group, which characteristically develops in middle-aged and elderly males. These patients have a chronic increase in venous PCV associated with hypertension, thromboembolic disease, together with increase in serum cholesterol and uric acid concentration (Kaung & Peterson, 1962; Russell & Conley, 1964). They are often plethoric, overweight, and have evidence of strees, anxiety and tension. They may complain of non-specific symptoms of headache, giddiness, dyspnoea, sweating and abdominal pain. The features of polycythaemia rubra vera, such as splenomegaly, thrombocytosis and increased leucocyte alkaline phosphatase activity are absent.

The clinical significance of the raised venous PCV is unclear, and this affects management. Patients who have not been treated, but followed up for long periods, show no evidence that the PCV increases with time, and no features of polycythaemia rubra vera develop. However, some clinicians still treat patients with venesection, although this does not necessarily offer protection from thromboembolism. Of course patients who are overweight, hypertensive, or who smoke, should be given appropriate advice or treatment.

Various names, such as pseudopolycythaemia, stress polycythaemia, Gaisbock's disease and benign erythrocytosis have been given to this condition. Whether these are all distinct entities or are all one and the same disease is debatable (Hall, 1965). Indeed, it has been argued that the features of relative polycythaemia are all essentially independent variables (Fessel, 1965).

ESSENTIAL THROMBOCYTHAEMIA

Characteristically, in this condition there is a marked increase in the number of platelets which often have abnormal functions and morphology, resulting in the clinical features of both thrombosis and bleeding. It occurs most often in the middle-aged and elderly (Gunz 1960). The presentation is variable: it may be an incidental finding in some asymptomatic patients. However, it usually presents as a spontaneous bleeding disorder of variable severity, often affecting the gastrointestinal tract, and often occurring repeatedly over several years. Spontaneous bruising is common. Thrombotic lesions, usually of small vessels, are associated with peripheral ulceration and/or gangrene, chilblains or erythromelalgia. A few patients have splenomegaly which may be quite marked and associated with hepatomegaly. Splenic infarction is not uncommon. Hess' test is usually negative.

Laboratory investigations show an increased platelet count of $1-3 \times 10^{6}/\mu l$, while the platelets themselves often show abnormal morphology and function which may explain the paradoxical presence of both bleeding and thrombosis. The haemoglobin and red cell morphology are usually normal, unless there has been, for example, a recent bleed. The white cell count is normal. The leucocyte alkaline phosphatase is often increased, but the Philadephia chromosome is not found. The bleeding time is often prolonged, but coagulation time is normal. The bone marrow shows a marked increase in number and size of megakaryocytes, with hyperplasia of the erythroid and myeloid series.

The disease tends to run a chronic course with a slow increase in platelet count occurring in untreated patients, and ultimately myelofibrosis can develop. Death may be due to haemorrhage, thromboembolism or unassociated illness.

Treatment aims to reduce the platelet count to normal values, using either ^{32}P or melphalan. A large dose of ^{32}P (10–12 millicurie) is required. Asymptomatic patients should be treated in order to reduce the risk of haemorrhage. Aspirin can be helpful in patients with thrombotic lesions.

REFERENCES

Adamson J W, Fialkow P J, Murphy S, Prohal J F, Steinmann L 1976 Polycythaemia vera: stem
cell and probable clonal origins of the disease. New England Journal of Medicine 295: 913–916
Adamson J W Fialkow P J 1978 The pathogenesis of myeloproliferative syndromes. British
Journal of Haematology 38: 299–303
Fessel W J 1965 Odd men out: individual with extreme values. Archives of Internal Medicine
115: 736–7
Golde D W, Bersch N, Cline M J 1977 Poycythemia vera: hormonal modulation of
erythropoiesis in vitro. Blood 49: 399–405
Gunz F W 1960 Haemorrhagic thrombocytopenia: a critical review: Blood 15: 706–723
Hall C A 1965 Gaisbock's disease: redefinition of an old syndrome. Archives of Internal
Medicine 116: 4–9
Kaung D T, Peterson R E 1962 Relative polycythaemia of pseudopolycythaemia Archives of
Internal Medicine 110: 456–460
Modan B 1965 An epidemiological study of polycythemia vera. Blood 26: 657–665
Russell R P, Conley C L 1964 Benign polycythaemia: Gaisbock's syndrome. Archives of Internal
Medicine 114: 734–740

Lymphomas

INTRODUCTION

The malignant lymphomas are a small but important group of cancers. Hodgkin's disease, for example, accounts for only 1 per cent of all new cancers in the United States of America, but its importance is much greater because it affects the young, and even in its disseminated form is curable. Much attention has been paid to Hodgkin's disease and non-Hodgkin lymphoma for this reason. Considerable progress has resulted from the study of the young and middle-aged (Canellos et al, 1978; Canellos, 1979; Kaplan, 1980; Peckham, 1975). There are differences between young and elderly patients in clinical presentation, pathology, response to therapy, and survival. It is important to be aware of these differences if treatment of the late middle-aged and elderly group of patients is to be correctly managed. It can be shown that the main determinants for survival in Hodgkin's disease are age and stage at presentation (Kaplan, 1980). The survival for three different age groups (15–53, 54–64, and 65–74) is shown in 479 patients attending St Bartholomew's Hospital from 1968 to 1983. The poor survival of the elderly in this series allows no room for complacency (Fig. 14.1). At the present time, some 10 per cent of patients with Hodgkin's disease are over 60 years old, and this percentage can be expected to increase with a steadily ageing population.

EPIDEMIOLOGY OF THE LYMPHOMAS

The age distributions of 234 patients with Hodgkin's disease and 617 patients with non-Hodgkin lymphoma attending St Bartholomew's Hospital between 1968 and 1983, and 1972 and 1983 respectively, are shown in Figure 14.2. It will be seen that patients with Hodgkin's disease are younger. More than 60 per cent present before late middle age, and only 10 per cent are over 65. There is undoubtedly an influence of referral pattern in such figures. Elderly sick patients may well not be referred for active therapy. MacMahon 1966, 1971, Gutensohn & Cole, 1980 and Gutensohn 1982 have commented on the bimodal incidence of Hodgkin's disease and have suggested, from differences

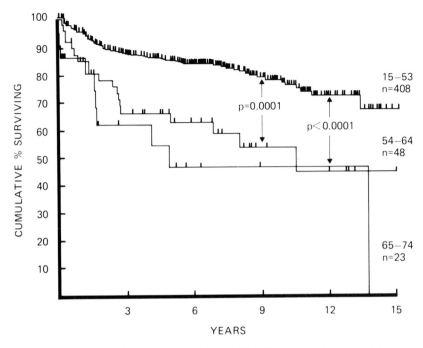

Fig. 14.1 Overall survival of 479 patients with Hodgkin's disease treated at St Bartholomew's Hospital 1968–1983 showing survival for three age groups: 15–53 years, 54–64 years and 65–74 years

in clinical presentation, histology and progression, that there may be two or more 'Hodgkin's diseases'. This hypothesis, of considerable academic interest, cannot deny that both forms, if managed incorrectly, are inevitably fatal.

Study of the curves of incidence and survival in Figure 14.3, derived from statistics produced by the National Institute of Health (Young et al, 1981) shows that a large proportion of the undoubted success in the management of Hodgkin's disease has been due to the effectiveness of treatment in the younger patient. In the figure, based on data collected in the early 1970s, the second peak of incidence is closely paralled by that of mortality. In their account of Hodgkin's disease in the elderly, Lokich et al (1974) commented on the poor survival in 47 patients over 60 years of age. The disease was more advanced in the elderly, and more elderly patients had symptoms, a feature usually associated with an increased tumour burden. In comparing groups of late-stage patients who were comparable, significantly shorter median durations of survival were seen in the elderly compared to the younger patients. It was appreciated that differences in therapeutic approach might be responsible, but the results of more extensive recent studies have increased understanding of this problem.

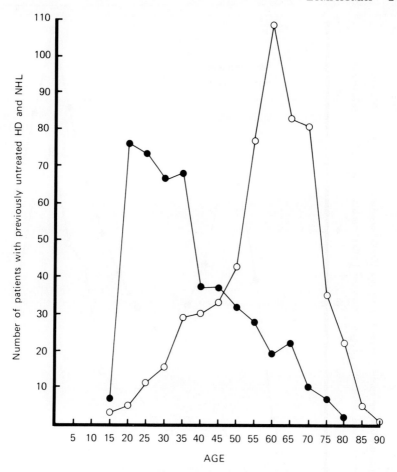

Fig. 14.2 Age at presentation of 234 patients with Hodgkin's disease (closed circles) and 617 patients with non Hodgkin lymphoma (open circles)

DIAGNOSIS AND STAGING

Before discussing these recent findings it may be helpful to outline the principles of diagnosis and staging that have now received general acceptance. The diagnosis of malignant lymphoma can only be made on the basis of a stained section of a lymph node. Occasionally a biopsy of an extranodal mass or a bone marrow biopsy will give the diagnosis. In Hodgkin's disease, review by an experienced pathologist will allow a diagnosis to be made usually, but not always, based on the presence of the Sternberg-Reed cell. The pathologist will also be able to classify the condition on the basis of the Rye classification into 'lymphocyte predominant', 'mixed cellularity', 'lymphocyte depleted' and 'nodular sclerosing' forms (Lukes et al, 1966).

Non-Hodgkin lymphoma can also be diagnosed only on a properly stained

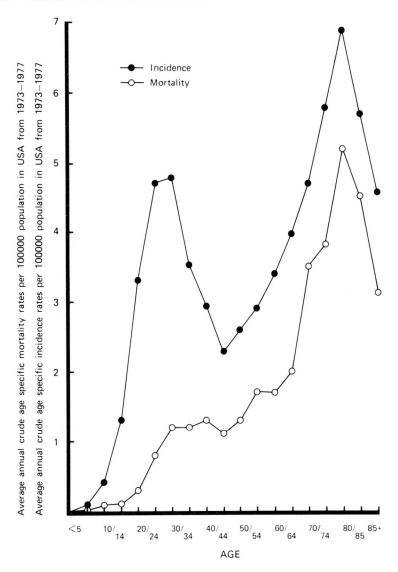

Fig. 14.3   The crude age-specific incidence and mortality for Hodgkin's disease from Surveillance Epidemiology End Results Incidence and Mortality Data 1973–1977. Monograph 57 of National Cancer Institute

lymph node or extranodal tissue biopsy. Here, however, histological classification is far from settled. Many series of patients have now been reported in the literature on the basis of the biologically unsatisfactory classification reported by Rappaport (1966). More coherent classifications are those of Lukes & Collins (1974) and Lennert (1978), but it must be said that there is no general agreement yet on the classification of the non-Hodgkin lymphomas. For the practising physician all current schemes depend on the type of cell, its mitotic activity, blast-like characteristics and arrangements within the lymph node, to subdivide them into either high-grade or low-grade malignancies. These terms used to equate with poor and good prognosis categories, but a strange paradox, by which modern intensive chemotherapy has produced long-term survival and even cure in the high-grade malignant lymphomas, but has not affected the course of the low grade lymphomas, makes it necessary to use categories such as 'good' and 'bad' prognosis with great care.

The histological classifications of Hodgkin's disease and non-Hodgkin lymphomas are set out in Table 14.1

STAGING OF LYMPHOMA

The extent of disease has been shown to be of such importance that this, too, must also be briefly considered. Staging of the lymphoma patient must begin with a full history and complete clinical examination. The presence or absence of symptoms such as sweating, fever, loss of weight are of great importance, both modifying treatment and affecting its outcome. The clinical

Table 14.1 Histological classification of Hodgkin's and non-Hodgkin's lymphoma

Hodgkin's disease
  Lymphocyte proliferative
  Nodular sclerosing
  Mixed cellularity
  Lymphocyte depleted
Non-Hodgkin's lymphoma

Kiel classification	Rappaport equivalent (Lennert, 1978)
Low grade malignancy	
M L lymphocytic (CLL and others)	M L well-differentiated diffuse
M L lymphoplasmacytoid (immunocytic)	⎰ M L lymphocytic type with dysproteinaemia ⎱ Lymphoproliferative diseases with dysproteinaemia
M L centrocytic	M L well ⎱ differentiated ⎰ nodular poorly ⎰ lymphocytic ⎱ diffuse
M L centroblastic/centrocytic follicular follicular and diffuse diffuse	⎰ well and poorly differentiated M L ⎱ lymphocytic histiocytic lymphocytic ⎱ nodular histiocytic ⎰ diffuse
High grade malignancy M L centroblastic	⎰ M L histiocytic nodular or diffuse ⎱ M L undifferentiated nodular or diffuse
M L lymphooblastic Burkitt type convoluted cell type others M L immunoblastic	⎰ M L undifferentiated ⎱ M L poorly differentiated lymphocytic diffuse ⎱ M L histiocytic diffuse

examination will reveal the presence of lymphadenopathy and enlargement of the liver or spleen. A radiograph of the chest will determine the presence of mediastinal or hilar lymphadenopathy in most cases. Investigations such as lymphography, CAT scanning and bone marrow biopsy may be necessary.

Staging laparotomy, in which splenectomy is combined with sampling of coeliac and paraortic lymph nodes and liver biopsy for histology, is now less often done, but is still essential in Hodgkin's disease if the object is to produce long relapse-free survival by use of radiotherapy alone. Most non-Hodgkin's lymphoma patients are now rarely, if ever, subjected to staging laparotomy because of the frequency with which the disease occurs at extra-nodal sites, the sometimes rapid progression of the disease, and its occurr-ence in more elderly patients. It is evident from a number of studies that pathologically staged (PS) patients with Hodgkin's disease (that is, those patients in whom the extent of disease has been defined by laparotomy) have a longer relapse-free interval following diagnosis and treatment than those who are only clinically staged (CS). Although in most series there is evidence that the overall survival of PS and CS patients differs little, relapse is more frequent in the CS patients, and it is possible that the survival in these patients will eventually be shorter. The Ann Arbor staging classification (Carbone et al, 1971) is shown in Table 14.2, and the Stanford nomenclature, in which terms such as 'Clinical stage IIIA' or 'Pathological Stage IIB' are used when appropriate. It will be seen that A and B relate to the absence and presence of symptoms respectively.

CLINICAL MANIFESTATIONS IN THE ELDERLY

Larger series are now being reported in which the clinical manifestations in the late-middle-aged and elderly patients are now being reported in great

Table 14.2   Ann Arbor staging classification*

Stage	Definition
I	Involvement of a single lymph node region (I) or a single extralymphatic organ or site (I_E)
II	Involvement of two or more lymph node regions on the same side of the diaphragm (II) or localised involvement of an extralymphatic organ or site and of one or more lymph node regions on the same side of the diaphragm (II_E)
III	Involvement of lymph node regions on both sides of the diaphragm (III), which may also be accompanied by involvement of the spleen (III_S) or by localised involvement of an extralymphatic organ or site (III_E) or both (III_{SE})
IV	Diffuse or disseminated involvement of one or more extralymphatic organs or tissues, with or without associated lymph node involvement

The absence or presence of fever, night sweats, and/or unexplained loss of 10% or more of body weight in the 6 months preceding admission are to be deemed in all cases by the suffix letters A or B, respectively.

* Adopted at the Workshop on the Staging of Hodgkin's Disease held at Ann Arbor, Michigan, in April 1971 (Carbone et al, 1971).

detail. In a study of therapeutic responses and survival in advanced Hodgkin's disease, Petersen et al (1982) reported the survival of 385 previously
untreated patients with Stage III and IV disease. Of these, 205 patients were
less than 40 years of age, 107 were 40–59, and 73 were over 60. They were all
investigated similarly and treated on identical treatment programmes. There
was no significant difference in the incidence of Stage IIIA, IIIB, IVA and
IVB disease among the three groups. The only significant abnormalities were
firstly in the histological subtype, in which nodular sclerosis was much more
frequent in those under 40 years of age, and secondly, in the clinical presentation, it was found that the older patient was more likely to have an enlarged
liver. The positive findings are shown in Table 14.3.

When these same features are studied in 479 patients diagnosed and treated
at St Bartholomew's Hospital between 1968 and 1983, and where a young
group of patients aged 15–25 are compared with elderly middle-aged patients
of 55–64 and over 64, the same increased frequency of nodular sclerosing
disease is seen in the younger age group (Table 14.3). It was also evident that
there is a tendency with increasing age for advanced disease to be more
prevalent, but again, it is necessary to be cautious, for this may be a result of
referral patterns. Elderly fit patients, with localised disease, may be treated in
local hospitals having facilities for radiotherapy.

Intercurrent disease occurs more frequently in the elderly patient, and may
have a significant effect both on investigation are unlikely to be subjected to
staging procedures, and diabetes, chronic renal disease and gastrointestinal
disorders may do much to modify therapy.

Given that the type of histology is no longer a major determinant of
prognosis, and that there is no major difference in the extent of disease
between the young and the elderly, it may be asked whether elderly patients
with Hodgkin's disease who have been adequately staged and treated are at a
greater risk of dying from their condition than their younger fellow sufferers.

Table 14.3   Pretreatment clinical characteristics of untreated patients with Hodgkin's disease at
St Bartholomew's Hospital 1968–1983

	Age in years		
	13–25	54–64	> 65
No. of patients evaluable	155	47	22
% males	55	76	59
% patients with			
Stage I	18	21	22
II	39	8	18
III	30	30	22
IV	13	41	38
% histological subtype			
lymphocyte predominant	13	25	9
nodular sclerosing	69	40	32
mixed cellularity	15	20	36
lymphocyte depleted	0.6	8	18
other	2.4	7	5

EFFECT OF STAGING AND THERAPY ON THE SURVIVAL OF ELDERLY PATIENTS WITH HODGKIN'S DISEASE

Austin-Seymour and her colleagues (1983, 1984) identified 52 patients over 60 who attended the divisions of Radiation Therapy and Medical Oncology between 1958 and 1981 at Stanford, California. They were assessed for adequacy of investigation and completeness of their therapy. In patients CS I–IIIA, adequate staging was defined as a lymphogram and laparotomy; for CS IIIB, a lymphogram and a bone marrow biopsy. Patients with Stage IV disease required a bone marrow aspiration, a positive liver biopsy, or other evidence of disseminated disease. In Stanford, current appropriate therapy for Stage PS I-IIA is subtotal lymphoid irradiation. Total lymphoid irradiation is used for PS IIB. Patients with IIIA or PS IIISA are treated with total lymphoid irradiation; hepatic irradiation is added if the spleen is found to be involved. Patients with PS IIIB–IV are treated with combination chemotherapy with and without radiotherapy.

In describing their results, the survival of 52 patients aged 60 or over was compared with the survival of 1169 patients of whom 174 were less than 17 years old, 874 were between 17 and 49, and 69 were between 50 and 59. The five-year freedom from relapse was 81 per cent for the youngest patients, 70 per cent for the patients between 17 and 49, and 63 per cent for patients between 50 and 59. In the over-60s the freedom from relapse was 38 per cent. In a multivariate analysis, age was the most significant variable.

In the elderly patients, more than half had advanced disease, and the incidence of nodular sclerosing disease was also high. Nearly half had intercurrent illness, with cardiac problems, hypertension, diabetes mellitus, chronic obstructive airways disease, or peripheral vascular disease. Nevertheless, 88 per cent had a lymphangiogram, and nearly half underwent staging laparotomy. Thirty-nine (75 per cent of patients) completed adequate staging.

Of 32 patients with CS I–IIIA, 19 were considered to be adequately staged and 15 of these were PS I–IIIA. All 15 of these had adequate treatment on the Stanford criteria. Five-year survival and freedom from relapse among these 15 patients were 86 and 79 per cent respectively, a remarkably good result. Eleven of the 15 patients are alive (at the time of writing) with no evidence of disease.

In the 13 patients who did not have a laparotomy and were CS I–IIIA, five died from progressive Hodgkin's disease, four from intercurrent disease, and only four were alive without evidence of Hodgkin's disease. Survival in the clinical stage of some optimally treated patients was therefore 35 per cent. It is important to note that the incidence of intercurrent disease was not significantly different in the two groups, but the age of those subjected to laparotomy was lower than of those who did not undergo the operation.

Elderly patients with advanced disease (i.e. IIIB–IV) did poorly, even when given appropriate therapy. The median survival of the adequately treated patients, 18 in number, was 39 months, while that of the palliatively or inadequately treated patients (6) was 15 months. Of the 12 patients who achieved a complete response after adequate treatment, 9 relapsed and only 3 of these were salvaged. From these results it would appear that if the older patient has PS I-IIIA disease and is adequately treated, he or she may do well, but with more advanced disease, chemotherapy in the elderly is either less effective or there may be problems with its administration.

The results described above are, of course, from one centre that may have a particular type of referral, and naturally has its own policy with regard to treatment. It seemed appropriate, therefore, to examine what might be seen in a similar age group at another centre. At St Bartholomew's Hospital, where the same criteria have been used to describe adequate staging, radiotherapy is restricted to patients with Stage I–IIA disease, chemotherapy and radiotherapy is used for patients with B symptoms, unless they are Stage III or IV, when only chemotherapy is used. The doses of radiotherapy are also lower than those used at Stanford.

In discussing the results at St Bartholomew's, it was decided to consider two groups, the late-middle-aged (54–64) and the elderly (over 65), as this might help to show trends which were particularly related to age. In the 479 patients seen between 1968 and 1983, 48 were over 54 and 23 over 65. Adequate staging in the CS I–IIIA group was considered to be lymphangiography and laparotomy, in the IIIB and later stages, bone marrow biopsy was required, but liver biopsy was not. Other evidence such as pleural effusion or extra nodal masses that were subjected to either cytology or histology were taken as evidence for Stage IV disease.

In late middle age, the number with early (I–III) versus late (IIIB–IV) was approximately equal. In Stage I–IIIA, 13 were PS and 12 CS. All the PS patients received adequate treatment, and 9 are alive with no evidence of disease. Of 12 who were CS, 11 had adequate treatment and 8 of these are alive. There was one patient who was CS and inadequately treated who is also alive without disease, and it can be seen that if the admittedly small numbers are plotted, there is no real significant difference in survival between the two groups (Fig. 14.4). The five-year survival in both groups is over 85 per cent and is comparable to the Stanford results, though it has to be remembered that this is in a slightly younger age group. Comparison of the two age groups for intercurrent disease showed two deaths in the PS group and one in the CS group. It would therefore appear from both studies that, certainly as far as the older patient is concerned, adequate staging and treatment leads to a disease-free survival and overall survival which is comparable to that seen in the young.

Unfortunately, relatively few patients were available in the elderly (over 65) age group treated at St Bartholomew's Hospital. There were 23, 10 of whom were in the early stage of the disease, and 13 with advanced IIIB–IV disease. It can be seen that the overall survival in this group is poor, at only just over 30 per cent (Fig. 14.5). Because of age and infirmity, only two

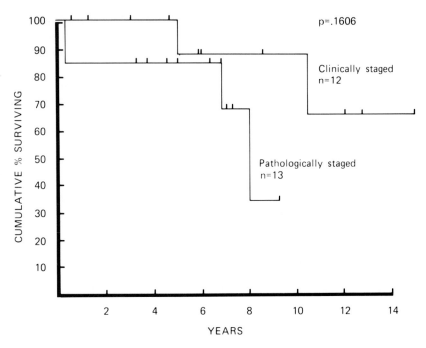

Fig. 14.4. Overall survival of patients with Hodgkin's disease Stage I-IIIA where 13 were pathologically staged and 12 clinically staged

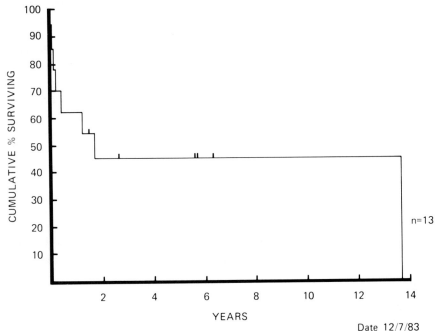

Date 12/7/83

Fig. 14.5 Overall survival of patients over 65 years of age with Stage IIIB to IVB. The poor outlook for these patients is clearly seen

patients were subjected to laparotomy. Of the eight who were CS, five were adequately treated, and of these four are alive. There is one surviving patient in the PS group who was adequately treated. Of the three patients inadequately staged and inadequately treated, only one survives.

In 13 patients with Stage IIIB or IV disease, 10 were adequately staged and 7 adequately treated. In this group the importance of adequate treatment appears unequivocal, with 5 of the 7 patients alive and well. There are no survivors at all in the other groups, which total 6 patients. Four died of Hodgkin's disease, one of a second malignant tumour, and another of bronchopneumonia.

Although the numbers are small, they confirm the clinical impression that if the very elderly patient can be supported and receive adequate treatment for his Hodgkin's disease, he or she will do well, and that policies for investigation may need to be modified if morbidity and mortality are to be reduced.

Why is failure to achieve adequate seen so often in the elderly? The reasons for the differences in ability to administer chemotherapy to old people have been examined by Peterson et al (1982). They studied 385 previously untreated patients with Stage III or IV Hodgkin's disease, and compared the groups who were less than 40 years of age, over 40 but less than 60, and a third group who were over 60. All patients received prednisolone, procarbazine, or a vinca alkaloid, and either nitrogen mustard or BCNU and CCNU. All patients received six courses and then were randomised to either two years or five years of maintenance therapy. The drugs were given every four weeks, but the total quantity administered was modified according to the total white cell and platelet count. The complete response rates according to treatment and age are given in Table 14.4. Complete response (CR) was seen in 63 per cent of the 385 patients. The CRs for patients less than 40 were 70 per cent, 66 per cent in patients in the 40–59 year-groups, and only 40 per

Table 14.4 Complete response rates according to treatment and age (Peterson et al, 1982)

| Treatment | Age in years[+] | | | p[‡] |
	< 40	40–59	≥ 60	
MOPP	40/59 (68%)	22/35 (63%)	12/29 (41%)	0.025
MVPP	26/35 (74%)	17/22 (77%)	5/9 (56%)	0.25
Subtotal	66/94 (70%)	39/57 (68%)	17/38 (45%)	0.008
COPP	23/38 (60%)	10/18 (56%)	6/13 (46%)	0.10
CVPP	31/44 (70%)	11/15 (73%)	3/14 (21%)	0.005
BOPP	23/29 (79%)	11/17 (65%)	3/8 (38%)	0.25
Subtotal	77/111 (69%)	32/50 (64%)	12/35 (34%)	0.0005
Total	143 205 (70%)	71/107 (66%)	29/73 (40%)	< 0.0001

+ Values = No. of complete responses/No. of patients.
‡ CR rate at <60 vs ≥60 yrs.

cent in those over 60 years of age. There appears to be no great advantage for the different regimens, although MVPP does show a trend towards consistently higher percentage response rates in all age groups. If an elderly patient received more than 90 per cent of the scheduled drug dosage, then the CR rate was 50 per cent compared to 48 per cent of those who received less than 90 per cent, and this of course is not significant. This implies that it would be unlikely that simply increasing the dose of chemotherapeutic agents would have an effect on improving response rate in the elderly patient, and would suggest, perhaps, that Hodgkin's disease in this group is a more intractable and aggressive disease.

The incidence of life-threatening toxicity was 14 per cent in patients under the age of 40 years, and was less than half of the 33 per cent seen in those patients over 60 years of age. A feature of this study was the careful analysis of the number of patients who received more than 90 per cent of each of the major agents, either alkylating agents, vinca alkaloids, or procarbazine. The results are shown in Table 14.5. This indicates that, apart from the first one or two courses in the case of alkylating agents and vinca alkaloids, and with the exception of procarbazine, there is a marked difference in tolerance when patients under 60 years of age are compared with those over 60. Leucopenia,

Table 14.5 Patients receiving over 90 per cent of planned drug doses during each course of treatment (Peterson et al, 1982)

Treatment course No.	% of patients			$p^\star$
	< 40 yrs	40–59 yrs	> 60 yrs	
Alkylating agent				
1	90	86	82	0.06
2	66	64	45	0.007
3	70	64	53	0.019
4	62	49	42	0.005
5	47	30	19	< 0.001
6	43	31	31	0.062
Vinca alkaloid				
1	98	86	76	0.031
2	72	64	43	< 0.001
3	65	49	47	0.004
4	58	46	33	0.001
5	52	19	21	< 0.001
6	49	18	25	< 0.001
Procarbazine				
1	90	82	87	0.221
2	62	59	51	0.128
3	65	57	60	0.314
4	54	51	40	0.122
5	42	33	29	0.068
6	42	32	36	0.218

* Significance value is based on a trend test to determine whether there is a correlation between increasing age and decreasing drug dose.

thrombocytopenia and neurological complications are significantly more common in the 60-year-old group. It would appear that not only is the disease more aggressive, but normal haemopoietic cells are more susceptible to the effects of chemotherapy, and this is also true of the nervous tissue, which is also more easily damaged. In Peterson's study, the lower complete remission rate, the shorter duration of complete remission, all contribute to the poor survival in the elderly group of patients. This result contrasts with the finding of De Vita et al (1980) who were unable to show any age-related effect in patients treated at the National Cancer Institute. However, this may well have been due to the fact that there was a predominance of younger patients in the National Cancer Institute study.

Elderly patients with Hodgkin's disease therefore need to be treated with great caution. If their general condition appears to be good, and they have limited disease, then after a careful explanation of what is involved in terms of both investigation and treatment, considerable efforts should be made to stage adequately and treat their condition. It must be remembered that the factors that influence drug administration in the elderly apply just as much to cytotoxic chemotherapy as to any other drugs that are administered at this stage. Caird (1983) has written an admirable review of this subject. The pharmacokinetics of drugs will be affected by the fall in the lean body mass in the elderly patient, the reduction in total body water, the decrease seen in glomerular filtration, and a number of other features which affect drug absorption and excretion in old age. It must also be remembered that there is likely to be an increased failure of compliance, and this may be a major but as yet undocumented factor in some oral chemotherapy regimens. Failure of temperature regulation and a pyrexial response to infection may be a trap for the unwary, and particularly so in the elderly patient whose imunological status and cellular response is compromised by chemotherapy.

Elderly patients with more advanced disease should have limited invasive investigation, and a bone marrow biopsy is probably adequate. The overall survival of this group of patients, whatever combinations of therapy are used, is likely to be poor, varying from 30 to 40 per cent in most series. There may well be a case for exploring alternative multidrug regimens for the elderly patient, with the use of procarbazine and the administration of stem cell sparing drugs such as cyclophosphamide and etoposide.

NON-HODGKIN LYMPHOMA

Non-Hodgkin lymphoma may occur throughout life. In children, these diseases are virtually all of the high-grade variety. Low-grade lymphomas start to make their appearance in early middle age, and subsequently make their contribution to the steadily increasing numbers of patients with non-Hodgkin lymphomas that are seen in the late-middle-aged and elderly population (Elias, 1979). Unlike Hodgkin's disease, no 'double peak' of incidence is seen and, except in the young, long survival and cure rates have not made a great impact on the mortality rates, certainly not of the order seen in Hodgkin's disease (Fig. 14.6).

The current management of patients with non-Hodgkin lymphoma of the low-grade or favourable, and high-grade or unfavourable, histology has recently been reviewed (Lister & Malpas, 1983). In summary, Stage I non-Hodgkin lymphoma of favourable histology (i.e. predominantly follicular lymphoma) responds well to local irradiation. It would be difficult to demonstrate any survival advantage for additional chemotherapy. It has to be remembered that it is quite uncommon for patients to present at this stage, or indeed Stage II. Stage II follicular lymphoma recurs sooner than Stage I, and

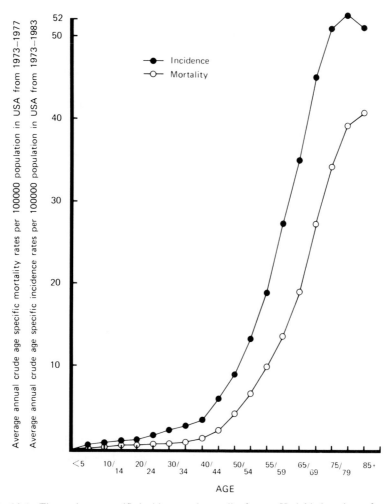

Fig. 14.6 The crude age-specific incidence and mortality for non-Hodgkin lymphoma from Surveillance Epidemiology End Results Incidence and Mortality Data 1973–1977. Monograph 57 of National Cancer Institute

so adjuvant chemotherapy in addition to local radiotherapy is justifiable for these patients.

In generalised lymphoma of favourable histology, several studies have shown that it is possible to induce clinically complete or near complete remission with relatively conservative therapy, or simple alkylating agents, or an alkylating agent with vincristine and prednisolone. Subsequent relapses may be treated with similar therapies and remissions achieved. There is not evidence that intensive chemotherapy makes any difference to survival and, in this case, moderately intensive therapy, with its lack of serious side effects, is entirely justifiable. The survival of 80 patients with low-grade lymphoma, aged 54–64, and 57 patients of over 65 years of age treated at St Bartholomew's Hospital between 1972 and 1983 is shown in Fig. 14.7. The median survival of patients in the late-middle-aged group is five years, whilst in elderly patients it is 3.5 years. Survival in the elderly is shorter, and raises the question why this should be so.

EFFECTS OF STAGING AND TREATMENT IN ELDERLY PATIENTS WITH NON-HODGKIN LYMPHOMAS

The stage of the disease is an important determinant for survival, and in comparison of the late-middle-aged and elderly patients, adequacy of staging

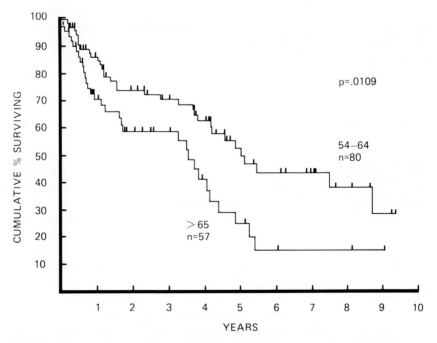

Fig. 14.7   The overall survival of late-middle-aged and elderly patients with non-Hodgkin lymphoma treated at St Bartholomew's Hospital 1972–1983 showing the significantly worse survival in the elderly patient

and the extent of disease in the two groups needs to be known. In the 93 patients with low-grade lymphoma aged 54–64, 91 were completely staged, and 2 were incompletely staged. In 80 patients over the age of 65, with low-grade lymphoma, 70 patients were completely staged and 10 incompletely staged. Very few patients, therefore, were inadequately assessed, and it is therefore reasonable to compare stages in the late-middle-aged and the elderly population. In the age group 54–64, patients with Stage I and II disease were 21 per cent, compared to 16 per cent in the over-65-year-olds. For Stage III and IV disease the figures were 79 and 84 per cent respectively. Consequently, no increased frequency of advanced stage, and therefore potentially poorer prognosis, was seen in the patients over 65.

It would have been expected that intercurrent illness might have been seen more frequently in the very old, but in the patients seen at St Bartholomew's there was no difference in the incidence of haemorrhage, infection, renal, cardiac or pulmonary failure in the two age groups.

The prescribed course of therapy for low-grade non-Hodgkin lymphoma at St Bartholomew's Hospital is a six-week course or chlorambucil 10 mg daily, followed by a two week interval, and then a succession of six courses of a fortnight of chlorambucil at 10 mg a day. If this is accepted as adequate therapy, and anything less is inadequate, then examination of the survival curve for the patients treated in this way at St Bartholomew's shows a significant difference in survival for patients given adequate therapy in the 54–64 and in the 65 and over age groups, compared with inadequate therapy. These are clearly shown in Figures 14.8 and 14.9.

As would be expected, the survival of patients with high-grade malignancies in both the late-middle-aged and elderly groups is very poor. This is shown in Figure 14.0, where the overall survival of 54 patients aged 54–64 is compared to the 22 patients aged over 65. This survival curve includes all stages of the disease, and, as can be seen, there is no significant difference in survival between the two age groups.

The effect of therapy on the elderly patient's survival may be seen more clearly in the homogenous group of Stage III and IV patients, who were given courses of cyclophosphamide, adriamycin, Oncovin (vincristine) and prednisolone (CHOP), or derivatives of this regimen (Table 14.6).

In Table 14.6, the effect on survival of various numbers of courses of these combinations is examined in 99 patients. The survivors are given in brackets in the table. Only two patients survive out of those who only received one to two courses of therapy, whereas in those receiving more than five courses, 20 are alive (at the time of writing). However, whereas 61 per cent of the young patients are achieving five or more courses, only 24 per cent of the elderly do so. Thirteen of the young patients are alive, and only two of the elderly — a difference which is highly significant statistically. Treatment was more frequently modified in the elderly, but if the under-54s are compared with the over-54s, the number surviving (15/46) compared with 14/54 is very little different.

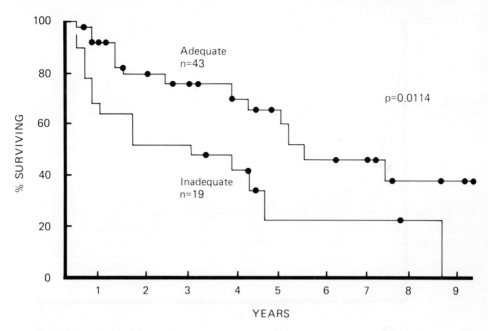

Fig. 14.8   The effect on survival of 'adequate' and 'inadequate' therapy in patients with non-Hodgkin lymphoma aged 54–64

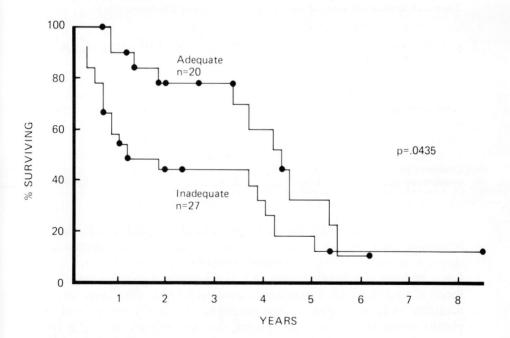

Fig. 14.9   The effect on survival of 'adequate' and 'inadequate' therapy in patients with non-Hodgkin lymphoma over 65 years of age

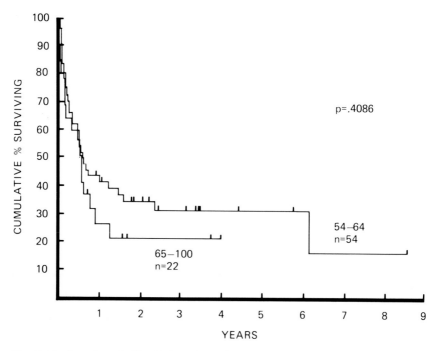

Fig. 14.10 Overall survival in elderly patients with 'high-grade' non-Hodgkin lymphoma. There is no significant difference in survival between patients aged 54–65 and over 65

Table 14.6 High-grade non-Hodgkin's lymphoma Stage III-IV treated at St Bartholomew's Hospital 1972–1983: Age-related tolerance of therapy and outcome

| | Age group (No. in brackets) | | | |
| Cycles of therapy | < 54 (46) | 54–64 (36) | > 65 (17) | p value |
	% completing course (No. alive in brackets)			
1–2	13% (1)	33% (1)	41% (0)	0.03
3–4	26% (1)	28% (1)	35% (5)	
> 5	61% (13)	39% (5)	24% (2)	0.01
Total receiving modified treatment	17%	28%	53%	0.009

It must be concluded that the elderly patient with low grade non-Hodgkin lymphoma does not need extensive staging procedures, and laparotomy should be avoided. If possible, adequate chemotherapy should be given, and this is probably an alkylating agent such as chlorambucil given for sufficient length of time to induce a complete or good partial remission. Great care is necessary to avoid toxicity, or too precipitate falls in the white count or platelet count. If therapy is not optimal, then the patient's survival is not going to be good, but a fairly satisfactory median survival of 3.5 years can be expected, even in the patients over 65 years of age.

In the elderly patient with high-grade lymphoma, the outlook is poor. Treatment is less well tolerated, and if fewer than three courses of combination chemotherapy are given, then the patient is unlikely to live very long. Modification of therapy must be used judiciously, but if these combinations can be given, then results may be as good (or as bad) as those seen in younger patients with extensive high grade lymphoma. It probably does the patient a disservice to temporise and use minimal doses of an alkylating agent such as that used for low-grade lymphoma. It is probably better to make a definite decision to palliate and support the elderly patient with antibiotics, blood transfusions, analgesics and where necessary, local radiotherapy.

Acknowledgements

I am very grateful to Dr H S Dhaliwal for providing data on which most of this chapter was based, and to Ms K Ash and Miss M Faux for its presentation. I am particularly indebted to Dr Saul Rosenberg for the information on the Stanford Experience with elderly patients with Hodgkin's disease and permission to quote from their results. Thanks are due to Mrs Jo Barton for typing the manuscript and for her patience.

REFERENCES

Austin-Seymour M, Hoppe R T, Cox R, Rosenberg S, Kaplan H 1983 Hodgkin's disease in patients older than sixty years. Proceedings of American Society for Clinical Oncology, 2, Abstract C-858, p 219
Austin-Seymour M M, Hoppe R T, Cox R S, Rosenberg S A, Kaplan H S 1984 Hodgkin's disease in patients older than sixty years. To be published.
Caird F I 1983 Medicine in old age. In: Oxford Textbook of Medicine, 1st edn, vol 2. Oxford University Press, Oxford, section 25
Canellos G P, Lister T A, Slarin A T 1978 Chemotherapy of non-Hodgkin lymphoma. Cancer 42: 932–940
Canellos G P (ed) 1979 The lymphomas. Clinics in haematology No. 8, part 3. Saunders, London
Carbone P P, Kaplan H S, Musshof K, Smithers D W, Tubiana M 1971 Report of the Committee on Hodgkin's disease staging classification. Cancer Research 31: 1860–1861
DeVita V T, Simon R A, Hubbard S M, Young R C, Berard C W, Moxley J H et al 1980 Curability of advanced Hodgkin's disease. Long term follow up of MOPP-treated patients at the National Cancer Institute. Annals of Internal Medicine 93: 587–595
Elias L 1979 Difference in age and sex distribution among patients with non-Hodgkin's lymphoma. Cancer 43: 2540–2546
Gutensohn N M 1982 Social class and age at diagnosis of Hodgkin's disease: new epidemiologic evidence for the 'two disease hypothesis'. Cancer Treatment Reports 66: 689–695
Gutensohn N, Cole P 1980 Epidemiology of Hodgkin's disease. Seminars in Oncology 7: 92–102
Kaplan H S 1980 Hodgkin's disease. Harvard University Press, Cambridge, Mass.
Lennert K 1978 Malignant lymphomas other than Hodgkin's disease. Springer, Berlin
Lister T A, Malpas J S 1983 The lymphomas — current management. Postgraduate Medical Journal 59: 219–228
Lokich J J, Pinkus C G, Moloney W C 1974 Hodgkin's disease in the elderly. Oncology 29: 484–500
Lukes R J, Craver L F, Hall T C, Rappaport H 1966 Report of the Nomenclature Committee. Cancer Research 26: 1311
Lukes R J, Collins R D 1974 Immunological characteristics of human malignant lymphomas. Cancer 34: 1488–1503

MacMahon B 1966 Epidemiology of Hodgkin's disease. Cancer Research 26: 1180–1200
MacMahon B 1971 Epidemiological considerations in staging of Hodgkin's disease. Cancer Research 31: 1854–1857
Peckham M J ed. 1975 Symposium on non-Hodgkin's lymphomata. British Journal of Cancer 31: Supplement II
Peterson B A, Pajak T F, Cooper M R, Nissen N I, Glidewell O J, Holland J F et al 1982 Effect of age on therapeutic response and survival in advanced Hodgkin's disease. Cancer Treatment Reports 66: 889–898
Rappaport H 1966 Tumours of the haemopoietic system. In: Atlas of tumour pathology. Armed Forces Institute of Pathology, Washington D C, section III, fascicle 8
Rudders R A, Kaddis M, Delus R A, Casey H 1979 Nodular non-Hodgkin lymphoma (NHL); factors influencing prognosis and indicators for aggressive treatment. Cancer 43: 1643–1651
Young J, Percy C, Asire A, Berg J, Cusaro M, Gloecklen L et al 1981 Surveillance, epidemiology and end results. In: Incidence and mortality. Bethesda National Institue of Health, Monograph no. 57

Drug-induced blood dyscrasias

INTRODUCTION

Adverse drug reactions are diagnosed by clinical features, laboratory tests, other signs of drug sensitivity and the effects of rechallenge, but this is not always a straightforward or simple matter. An association between a drug and a blood dyscrasia may be established from the history by noting the time of onset of the reaction relative to the time of administration, the result of any previous administration, the dosages given, the reactions produced, the effect of stopping the drug and the history of any similar problems in the family. Unfortunately, however, the drug history may be inadequate or complicated by 'over-the-counter' medications. Furthermore, the fact that the drug is known to have an association with a particular blood dyscrasia does not necessarily prove that it is the cause in a particular patient. Laboratory tests, which can assist in diagnosis, vary in their specificity and reliability. Theoretically, rechallenging the patient with the suspected drug has much to recommend it, but ethically this is seldom possible.

Types of drug reaction

Rawlins (1981) has classified adverse reactions into two groups: Group A, where the reaction is part of the drug's normal pharmacological action, and Group B, where the reaction is bizarre (Table 15.1).

Type A reactions occur more frequently in the elderly because pharmacokinetics and pharmacodynamics alter with age, particularly drug elimination.

Table 15.1 Types of adverse drug reactions

Features	Type A	Type B
Pharmacology	Normal but augmented	Novel and bizarre
Predictable	Yes	No
Dose-dependent	Yes	No
Morbidity	High	Low
Mortality	Low	High

Renal function deteriorates steadily with advancing years, which is particularly important for drugs such as digoxin and gentamycin, which are excreted by the kidney. Liver function also deteriorates with age, though to a lesser degree than renal function, and results in less efficient drug metabolism. Consequently, it is not surprising that the elderly are particularly liable to develop reactions when given doses of drugs designed for younger patients. Target organ sensitivity also changes with increasing years — the brain, for example, becoming increasingly sensitive to drugs which act on it. Type B reactions are not related to the drug's normal pharmacology, and can result from substances added to the drug during manufacture, *in vitro* degradation of products, immunological reactions or genetic factors which alter target organ sensitivity, e.g. red blood cell G6PD deficiency.

Incidence of adverse reactions

Adverse drug reactions occur with increasing frequency and severity in the elderly (Seidl et al, 1966; Hurwitz, 1969; Bottiger et al, 1979a). Williamson (1979) has shown, in a multicentre study of 2000 admissions to geriatric departments in the United Kingdom during 1975–76, that about 1:10 were partly or entirely due to drug side-effects. As might be expected, the incidence rose with the number of drugs prescribed. Many patients failed to recover fully after the drug(s) were stopped. The medications most frequently given were diuretics, analgesics, antidepressants, hypnotics, sedatives, digoxin, potassium salts and haematinics, but those causing most side-effects were hypnotics, rigidity controllers, corticosteroids, antidepressants and digoxin.

Timoney (1978), who reviewed adverse reactions in all ages reported to the National Drugs Advisory Board in Ireland during 1968–75, found that adverse reactions to the skin and subcutaneous tissue were most common, while haematological reactions were the least common, forming 5 per cent of the total, which compares with 10 per cent of the total found by Bottiger & Westerholm (1973). Bottiger and colleagues (1979b) found the incidence of drug-induced cytopenias during 1966–75 increased with age, especially in those over 55 years. More women than men were affected. Drugs most frequently implicated were sulphonamides, oxyphenbutazone, chloramphenicol, methyldopa, diuretics and quinine. Drug-induced thrombocytopenias and agranulocytosis were more common than haemolytic and aplastic anaemias.

The impact of mortality due to adverse drug reactions falls mainly on the elderly. Adelstein & Loy (1979) found, during 1968–72 in the United Kingdom, that although the overall death rate due to drugs had fallen, the proportion occurring in the elderly had risen. The drugs implicated were corticosteroids, anticoagulants, phenylbutazone and other analgesics, tranquillisers, and antineoplastic agents. OPCS data for 1980 show that 2422 deaths in the United Kingdom were attributed to drugs with a peak incidence at 45–60 years — analgesics, sedatives, hypnotics and psychotropic drugs caused most deaths. Bottiger and colleagues (1979a), in a survey of fatal reactions due to drugs in Sweden 1965–75, found that, although the incidence of reported adverse reactions increased during the ten-year period, the mortality was fairly constant, with those over 60 years more likely to die. Women were prescribed more drugs than men, developed more reactions, but had a lower mortality. The drugs most associated with fatal reactions were antibiotics, sulphonamides and analgesic drugs, such as indomethacin and phenylbutazone.

Although haematological side-effects are less common than other adverse reactions, they are more likely to have a fatal outcome. Bottiger and colleagues (1979a) found that haematological side-effects cause 40 per cent of drug deaths, while a further 16 per cent were due to bleeding and thromboembolic disease. This compares with 9 per cent of deaths due to liver toxicity and 4 per cent due to skin reactions. In the United Kingdom about one-third of fatal drug reactions between 1964 and 1968 were due to haematological side-effects (Girwood, 1971). The WHO Research Centre for International Monitoring of Adverse Reactions during 1968–72 reported a 17 per cent mortality due to haematological side-effects (Timoney, 1978). The mortality due to aplastic anaemia and agranulocytosis is greater than with haemolytic anaemia and thrombocytopenia.

APLASTIC ANAEMIA

Aplastic anaemia is the least common of the major blood dyscrasias, but one of the most lethal. Its incidence rises sharply in those over 65 years and is more frequent in women than in men (Bottiger et al, 1979b).

Clinical features

The clinical picture is variable. There is usually a delay of four to eight weeks, or sometimes longer, after exposure to the drug before aplasia develops, which usually occurs after a second exposure, suggesting an immunological causation. While the onset in the elderly may be abrupt with bleeding or infection, usually it is insidious, with patients presenting with symptoms of anaemia such as fatigue, tiredness and dyspnoea. Sometimes infections can present as a toxic confusional state. Bleeding manifestations may be slight, but can be severe enough to cause fatal cerebral haemorrhage. Examination of the patient is unremarkable other than signs of anaemia, infection and thrombocytopenia. The slow development of symptoms can make it difficult to obtain an accurate drug history; indeed, a positive drug history is only obtained in about 40 per cent of patients.

Blood and marrow changes

Aplastic anaemia is characterised by a normocytic, or slight to moderate macrocytic anaemia and two of the three following abnormalities in the peripheral blood: a granulocyte count of less than 500 cells/mm^3, a platelet count of less than 20 000/mm^3, or a reticulocyte count of less than 1 per cent. When patients present with gradual onset of symptoms, the haemoglobin is usually less than 7.0g/dl. Neutrophils may show toxic granulations and increased alkaline phosphatase activity. Immature white cells and normoblasts may be seen in the peripheral blood. When the leucopenia is mild, only the neutrophils may be reduced, but in severe cases there is a lymphopenia and monocytopenia. Typically, the bone marrow, when taken by trephine biopsy, shows hypocellularity with patches of normal or increased cellularity. The ESR is raised. ^{59}Fe isotope studies show poor clearance and turnover of iron, poor uptake by the bone marrow, low utilisation and no extrameduallary haemopoiesis. Culture of the bone marrow on agar produces few colonies, but these grow well.

Drug causes

Though many drugs can cause aplastic anaemia, most cases are due to relatively few medications. Bottiger and colleagues (1979b) report a marked change in causative drugs during recent years: between 1966 and 1970, oxyphenbutazone, chloramphenicol and phenylbutazone were most commonly reported, but these were displaced in 1971–5 by sulphonamides, cytostatics and acetazolomide, presumably due to increased knowledge of the side-effects of the first group of drugs. However, Timoney (1978) reported that phenylbutazone and oxyphenbutazone continued to be the most commonly reported drugs to the WHO Research Centre during 1968–75.

The drugs described below have been associated with aplasia, and include examples of those likely to be prescribed to the elderly patient.

Antibacterial drugs

Choramphenicol. This drug has two differing actions on the bone marrow. More commonly there is a dose-related reversible marrow depression, mainly affecting the erythroid cells, but which can involve platelets and granulocytes. Less commonly there is an irreversible, late onset bone marrow aplasia, usually involving all three cell lines, and associated with high mortality.

These dangers have severely curtailed the oral and parenteral use of chloramphenicol. However, aplasia has been reported following the use of chloramphenicol topical spray or eye ointments (Rosenthal & Blackman, 1965; Abrams et al, 1980; Del Giacco et al, 1981). Although none of these patients was elderly, the cases emphasise the need for care in the use of these topical preparations. How the systemic effect is produced is uncertain, but it may result either from absorption through the conjunctival membrane or by drainage down the lacrimal duct with eventual gastrointestinal absorption.

Sulphonamides, penicillins and metronidazole. These drugs occasionally cause aplasia, sometimes in elderly people (White et al, 1980).

Anti-rheumatic drugs

Phenylbutazone and oxyphenbutazone. McCarthy & Chalmers (1964) reviewed the association of phenylbutazone and aplasia and found that the majority of cases occurred in women over the age of 60 years. Most patients were not on other drugs likely to cause aplasia. Fowler (1967), in a further review, considered that phenylbutazone and oxyphenbutazone were likely to cause agranulocytosis in younger patients but aplastic anaemia in the elderly. Mortality increased sharply with increasing age, symptoms often developing after many months of treatment. Inman (1977) reviewed the histories of 269 patients whose death certificates issued during 1975 did not mention a drug as the cause of the aplasia or agranulocytosis. He found that 83 (31 per cent) deaths were probably drug-induced, with 39 cases of aplasia caused by phenylbutazone (28) and oxyphenbutazone (11). Once again, it was clear that mortality rose sharply with age, especially in elderly females. He did not consider this excesss to be due to the greater use of drugs by this age group, or to the fact that women outlive men.

Gold. Kay (1973, 1976) reviewed the relationship between gold and aplasia. The majority of patients developed marrow depression after receiving more than 450 mg of gold, although some cases developed after smaller doses. Eosinophilia, traditionally regarded as a warning sign, was found in only a few cases, but this could be partly explained by infrequent recording of differential white counts. She concluded that aplasia was a serious, but rare, complication of gold therapy, best avoided by regular full blood counts, with reduction of dose when clinical remission is achieved.

Penicillamine. This drug may cause a reduction in red cells, neutrophils or platelets during long-term administration (Dixon et al, 1975). Kay (1979), in a review of ten patients with pancytopenia associated with penicillamine therapy found that the dose range was 250–1000 mg/day with an average of 615 mg. The duration of therapy was 3–60 months, with a mean of 16. The age range of the patients 35–68 years. The role of penicillamine in the causation of aplasia in patients previously treated with gold is disputed. Smith & Swinburn (1980) concluded from their experience that there is no increased incidence of adverse reactions due to penicillamine in patients who have had an adverse reaction to gold, and there was no increased risk if penicillamine is started within six months of stopping gold therapy. However, Kean and colleagues (1980) considered that patients who have had reactions to gold were more likely to develop reactions to D penicillamine.

Other anti-inflammatory drugs which may be associated with aplasia include indomethacin (Canada & Burka, 1968), sulindac (Bennett et al, 1980; Miller, 1980; Sanz et al, 1980) and fenprofen (Ashraf et al, 1982). Some of the patients were over 60 years.

Cytotoxic drugs

These drugs, by their very nature, depress bone marrow function and are therefore usually given intermittently. The group includes alkylating agents such as cyclophosphamide, busulphan and melphalan; anti-metabolites, such as methotrexate and mercaptopurine and the vinca alkaloids, such as vincristine and vinblastine.

Anti-epileptic drugs

The hydantoins are associated with aplasia. Huguley and colleagues (1966) point out that diphenylhydantoin and methylphenylethyl-hydantoin caused 45 cases out of a total of 50 due to anti-epileptic drugs reported to the AMA Registry. Gabriel and colleagues (1966) reviewed 14 cases, together with two of their own, due to hydantoin. The age range was 9–48 years and most patients were male. Their view of cases due to oxazolidines shows a similar age incidence.

The association of carbamazepine with aplasia has been reviewed by Hart & Easton (1981). They concluded the prevalence to be less than 1/50 000. The duration of therapy prior to the onset of aplasia varied from 4 to 330 days. The patients' age and total dose did not appear to be major causative factors. They considered that routine laboratory monitoring was not justified.

Anti-depressants

Mianserin was the subject of a 'Current Problem' report in 1983. The drug has been associated with severe blood dyscrasias, including aplastic anaemia. The reported rate of dycrasias in 1982 was in the order of three reports per 100 000 general practice prescriptions. The median age of the patients was 67 years. The number of reports relating to the elderly was proportionally greater than would be accounted for by the increased usage in that age group. Durrant & Read (1982) report a fatal case in a 65-year-old female.

Anti-thyroid drugs

Because thiouracil causes toxic effects, including aplasia, it is now little used. Carbimazole is less toxic, but some of the reported cases of aplasia occur in the elderly.

Other drugs

Oral antidiabetic drugs, such as chlorpropamide (Harris, 1971; Gill et al, 1980) and tolbutamide (Huguley et al, 1966) may occasionally cause aplasia in middle-aged patients. Aplasia following the use of chlorpropamide occurs either within one month of starting the treatment or after a period of six months to seven years. Cimetidine is more associated with agranulocytosis, but aplastic anaemia has been described in a 49-year-old lady, who was given the drug in addition to a number of other medications, including acetaminophen which can, of itself, cause aplasia (Tonkonow & Hoffman, 1980).

Prognosis

The prognosis for patients with aplastic anaemia is poor. About half the patients die within six months, usually from bleeding or opportunistic infections. However, patients can survive for long periods in a relatively stable state when the neutrophil count remains about 500/mm³. There is poor correlation between the degree of hypocellularity and prognosis. Occasionally, patients with aplastic anaemia develop leukaemia or paroxysmal nocturnal haemoglobinuria.

Treatment

The treatment of aplastic anaemia has four aims. Firstly, any potential toxic drug must be stopped if at all possible, but unfortunately the blood picture may not improve as a result. Secondly, the anaemia will probably require blood transfusions. Thirdly, any infection will need vigorous treatment, and there must be scrupulous skin and mouth care. Fourthly, it may be possible to stimulate the bone marrow to return to normal with anabolic steroids. Corticosteroids may be useful in controlling bleeding manifestations. At present, bone marrow transplants have no place in the treatment of elderly patients.

AGRANULOCYTOSIS

Agranulocytosis is one of the most common haematological adverse drug reactions, with the main impact falling on the elderly (Arneborn & Palmblad, 1978; Bottiger et al, 1979b). The studies show either an equal sex incidence or a predominance of males. The mortality is high, with as many as one-third of patients dying, usually of infection.

Clinical features

The onset of the disease may be acute or subacute with constitutional upset and/or infection. Symptoms may occur within a few days of the last dose of the drug, which may have been taken for long time, or appear almost immediately a new drug is started. Phenothiazines, for example, cause symptoms between 20 and 40 days after starting treatent. Agranulocytosis due to phenylbutazone develops about three months after the drug has been started, often with a preceding rash (Mauer, 1955). Patients complain of fever, headache, nausea, sweating, generalised aches and pains, with marked weakness. Exudative pharyngitis is characteristic, and may be followed by ulceration of the mouth, oesophagus, small and large bowel, vagina and skin. In severe cases septicaemia occurs.

Blood and bone marrow changes

Agranulocytosis is defined by a peripheral neutrophil blood count of less than 200 cell/mm^3, but when the fall in neutrophil count is non-progressive and remains above 200 cell/mm^3, neutropenia is considered to be present. The total white count is reduced to about 1000 cells/mm^3. The bone marrow may show either hypoplastic changes, usually involving the granulocytic precursors, or, in the early or recovery phases, hypoplasia of the granulocytic precursors with a shift to the left.

In-vitro tests are of limited value in identifying the causal drug. The leucocyte agglutination test, for example, gives positive results in cases of amidopyrene sensitivity, but it is less helpful with chlorpropamide, chlorpromazine, quinine, phenylbutazone and sulphonamides. It is most likely to give positive results in the early phases of the disease. Leucocyte cytotoxic antibody tests have limited application. Sometimes a bone marrow culture may help to identify the causal drug.

Pathogenesis

Pisciotta (1982) has described three types of agranulocytosis due to phenothiazines. One involves the sudden destruction of large number of leucocytes in the peripheral blood due to immunological mechanisms and depending on the presence of an immunoglobulin. This antibody disappears within a few days of stopping the drug. A second type of immune-mediated agranulocytosis is associated with antibodies produced against leucocyte nucleoprotein. In a third type the agranulocytosis is due to a toxic effect of the drug on the bone marrow precursors in sensitive cases.

Drug causes

While many drugs can cause agranulocytosis, most cases are due to relatively few medications. Reports to the AMA Registry rank the most common drugs causing agranulocytosis as phenothiazines, amidopyrene and its derivatives, sulphonamides, antithyroid drugs and phenylbutazone (Huguley et al, 1966). The WHO Research Centre and the National Drugs Advisory Board in Ireland rated phenylbutazone, oxyphenbutazone and indomethacin as responsible for as many as one-third of cases of agranulocytosis (Timoney, 1978). Report from Sweden, however, show that sulphonamides, antithyroid drugs, antihistamines and phenothiazines cause most cases (Arneborn & Palmblad, 1978; 1982; Bottiger et al, 1979b). During 1966–70 dipyrone (a derivative of amidopyrene) caused so many cases that it was withdrawn from use in 1974 (Bottiger et al, 1979b).

The drugs which are discussed below include those likely to be prescribed for elderly patients.

Antirheumatic drugs

Phenylbutazone. This is a common cause of agranulocytosis. The majority of cases occur in patients over the age of 50 years and almost entirely in females. The total dose of drug given varies from 4 to 35 g (McCarthy & Chalmers, 1964). Fowler (1967) in his review concluded that phenylbutazone was more likely to cause agranulocytosis in younger patients, but aplasia in older ones. Agranulocytosis usually develops within three months of the onset of treatment. Inman (1977) in his review found that many elderly patients, especially women, were likely to develop blood dyscrasias due to phenylbutazone. Since 1984 the use of phenylbutazone in the UK has been severely restricted.

Allopurinol. This has been associated with agranulocytosis in middle-aged or elderly patients (Hawson & Bain, 1980; McInnes et al, 1981), but some of them had underlying tumours. Younger patients who have developed agranulocytosis were on a total starvation regime (Scobie et al, 1980).

Levamisole. This can cause neutropenia which is associated with antibody formation that can, therefore, be used for screening purposes (Rosenthal et al, 1977; Drew et al, 1980). Azothiaprine has been reported to cause neutropenia in middle-aged patients.

Anti-bacterial drugs

The association of sulphonamides with agranulocytosis is well known (Huguley et al, 1966; Arneborn & Palmblad, 1978; Bottiger et al, 1979b). The combination of sulphamethoxazole and trimethoprim is now accounting for a number of cases. Salter (1973), for example, reported 108 cases of granulocytopenia, of which nine cases were classified as agranulocytic. Inman (1977) reported 13 patients aged 52–84 years who developed fatal agranulocytosis with cotrimoxazole. Trimethiprim has itself recently been reported to cause pancytopenia in a 70-year-old female (Sheehan 1981).

Agranulocytosis or leucopenia has been caused by a number of other anti-infective drugs. Penicillin has been associated with leucopenia, but this most commonly occurs in the middle-aged when large doses are given for long periods (Colvin et al, 1974; Corbett et al, 1982). Penicillin and cephalosporin homologues have been associated with leucopenia in a number of patients occurring two to three weeks after starting treatment (Homayouni et al, 1979). Cefoxitin has caused an onset of leucopenia in a 78-year-old lady (Shansky & Greenlaw, 1980). Chloramphenicol can cause agranulocytosis, but this is less frequent than aplasia. Dapsone also causes agranulocytosis, but less often than haemolytic anaemia, when doses larger than 300 mg are used (McKenna & Chalmers 1958).

Antipsychotic drugs

Phenothiazines. The association of agranulocytosis with phenothiazine has been widely investigated (Pisciotta, 1969). The onset may commence gradually without warning or symptoms. The drug has to be given for at least ten days (usually 20–30 days) and in a total dosage exceeding 5 g (usually 20–30 g). Agranulocytosis is most likely to occur in ill, Caucasian, middle-aged to elderly females, who also bear the brunt of mortality (Mandel & Gross, 1968; Marcus & Mulvihill, 1978). Regular white blood counts may help in prevention but they will fail to detect patients who develop sudden agranulocytosis. Other phenothiazines, which are less frequently implicated than chlorpromazine are promazine, methozine and thioridazine (Pisciotta, 1978).

Antidepressants

Cases of agranulocytosis or granulopenia due to mianserin have been reported in patients with a median age of 67 years (McEwen, 1982; Clink & Shaw, 1982; Current Problems, 1983). Agranulocytosis has followed the use of imipramine and amitriptyline (Goodman, 1961; Gault, 1963). Lithium carbonate has been associated with lymphopenia in patients aged 20–64 years, the majority of whom were males (Perez-Cruet et al, 1978; Lapier & Stuart, 1980).

Anticonvulsants

Huguley and colleagues (1966) reported five cases of agranulocytosis due to phenytoin but did not mention the age of the patients. Gabriel and colleagues (1966), however, found no cases of agranulocytosis in their review of patient given hydantoin or oxazolidines.

There have been reports linking carbamazepine with leucopenia. Owens and colleagues (1980) reported 18 cases of leucopenia, mostly in females over the age of 45 years, as well as a case of their own in a man of 61. They considered that the development of agranulocytosis was unpredictable, was not dose-related and therefore was an idiosyncratic response, although some patients do show a significant leucopenia in the early stage of treatment. They suggested that carbamazipine should be given with care to the elderly and that the white count should be monitored frequently. Hart and Easton (1981) found a transient leucopenia occuring in the first month of treatment in 10 per cent of patients who had been given carbamazepine and that this was most likely to occur in the elderly, and in those who had a low white count before the onset of treatment. Livingston and colleagues (1967) found leucopenia in three patients out of a total of 87.

Other drugs

Cimetidine. Although leucopenia has been reported following the use of cimetidine, many of the patients had other serious illnesses and were on complex drug regimes. However, Carloss and colleagues (1980) describe a 67-year-old male who, although on other drugs, did have two repeat challenges with cimetidine resulting in leucopenia on each occasion.

Bromocriptine. Chronic administration has been associated with leucopenia in a young person (Giampietro et al, 1981).

Captopril. Heel and colleagues (1980) in a review of captopril report a number of cases of leucopenia and agranulocytosis. However many patients had complicated histories and drug regimes. Usually the white blood count returned to normal when the drug was stopped.

Chlorpropamide. A few cases of agranulocytosis have followed the use of this drug (Harris, 1971; Tucker et al, 1977).

Antithyroid drugs. Carbimazole and propylthiouracil are relatively common causes of agranulocytosis (Bottiger et al, 1979b; Arneborn & Palmblad, 1982).

Prognosis

The prognosis has improved since the introduction of antibiotics, but is still about 20–30 per cent. Poor prognosis is associated with increasing age, delay in starting treatment, the presence of other serious disease and the development of septicaemia. Those who recover usually do so within 7–14 days of the onset of symptoms. The recovery phase is indicated by a rise in the serum lysozyme concentration or the appearance of immature granulocytes in the blood. The neutrophil count may overshoot before returning to normal. While serial white blood counts are helpful in monitoring the course of the disorder, they are not necessarily useful in predicting those patients likely to develop agranulocytosis.

Treatment

Treatment has three aims. Firstly, the suspected drug must be stopped. Secondly, the bacteriological cause of the infection must be identified and treated vigorously. Antibiotics may need to be given blind until sensitivities are available — a suitable regime would be a broad-spectrum penicillin, an aminoglycoside and metronidazole. It may be necessary to isolate the patient and consider bowel sterilisation. Thirdly, the patient must be warned to avoid the drug in future.

HAEMOLYTIC ANAEMIA

The incidence of haemolytic anaemia rises with age and is now the third most common drug-induced cytopenia after thrombocytopenia and agranulocytosis (Bottiger et al, 1979b). Methyldopa caused the vast majority of cases, and the number of patients with haemolytic anaemia due to this drug doubled between 1966–70 and 1971–5. However, the authors report a tendency to prescribe less methyldopa in more recent years, perhaps because its side-effects are more widely known and also because of the greater availability of other hypotensive agents. They found that sulphonamide and dapsone were other important causes. Reports to the Irish National Drugs Advisory Board (1968–75) also show methyldopa to have caused most cases (Timoney, 1978). Primaquine, nitrofurantoin, sulphonamides, penicillin and cephalothin were other important drug causes. Deaths due to haemolytic anaemia were found to be relatively uncommon by Bottiger and colleagues (1979a)

General clinical features

The clinical features of haemolytic anaemia are those of anaemia, jaundice and malaise. Splenomegaly may or may not be found. The diagnosis is suggested by a sudden fall in haemoglobin in the absence of bleeding. The absolute reticulocyte count is increased and Heinz bodies may be seen. The bone marrow shows erythroid hyperplasia. There is an increase in unconjugated bilirubin. The lifespan of the red cell is less than the normal 120 days.

Types of haemolytic anaemia

There are two main pathogenic causes — one involves the development of antibodies, while the other results from genetically determined biochemical abnormalities of the red cell.

Haemolysis due to antibody formation

Here also there are two main causes. The commoner, auto-immune haemolysis, occurs when antibodies develop against normal red blood cells. These antibodies can be demonstrated in the serum of patients by *in vitro* tests with normal red cells without the addition of the drug. The situation is serologically similar to idiopathic auto-immune haemolytic anaemia. The other less common condition, immune heaemolysis, occurs when antibodies are directed against the drug. They cannot therefore be demonstrated *in vitro* unless the causative drug is present: thus the indirect Coombs test is negative without the drug, but positive with it. The antibody is of the IgG or IgM type and usually binds complement.

Auto-immune haemolysis. The commonest cause is methyldopa. Usually symptoms do not develop until the patient has had the drug for a least three months and when the dose exceeds 2 g a day. Although about 15 per cent of patients develop a positive Coombs test, only about 1 per cent become anaemic. The test remains positive for several weeks or months after stopping the drug. About 15 per cent of patients develop a positive ANF test. The antibody is of the IgG type.

The clinical features are like those of idiopathic auto-immune haemolytic anaemia. The severity of the anaemia varies. The prognosis in most patients is good and the anaemia responds naturally to the withdrawal of the drug or the use of steroids.

Not surprisingly perhaps, levodopa alone or in combination with a decarboxylase inhibitor has also been associated with this form of haemolytic anaemia. The direct Coombs test is positive in 10 per cent of patients on levodopa. Cases have been reported in middle-aged and elderly people, although some were also on other anti-Parkinsonian drugs (Territo et al, 1973; Lindstrom et al, 1977; Bernstein, 1979). Mefenamic acid (Ponstan) can also cause this type of anaemia in middle-aged people (Scott et al, 1968; Farid et al, 1971).

Immune haemolysis. This is a relatively rare condition which has sometimes been described in middle-aged and elderly people following the use of drugs such as sulphonamides, rifampicin, chlorpromazine, phenylbutazone, para-aminosalicylic acid, ibuprofen and chlorpropamide.

The onset is usually rapid with severe anaemia and there may be signs of intravascular haemolysis such as haemoglobinemia and haemoglobinuria. Usually there is a history of previous administration of drugs. Withdrawal of the drug leads to rapid improvement and a normal blood picture within two to three weeks.

Penicillin can cause this type of anaemia in middle-aged people (White et al, 1968). It has certain characteristic differences from other drug causes of immune haemolysis. It generally occurs when it is given for a second time in large doses (exceeding 20 mega-units a day). Anaemia develops gradually with an increasing reticulocyte count without evidence of bleeding. Intravascular haemolysis is unusual. Although the removal of the drug brings rapid cure, the direct Coombs test remains positive for many days afterwards. A somewhat different type of haemolytic anaemia due to penicillin has been described in a 69-year-old male patient by Spitzer (1981). In his patient the direct Coombs test was negative while the screening for G6PD deficiency was negative.

Cephalothin has also caused immune-type haemolytic anaemia which, unlike the penicillin type, usually develops after normal doses of the drug and within one week of starting treatment (Gralnick, 1971).

Haemolysis due to biochemical abnormality of the red cell

This is the least common cause of haemolytic anaemia in the elderly. It occurs when a drug acts on red blood cells which have a genetically determined biochemical abnormality. The commonest defect is glucose-6-phosphate dehydrogenase (G6PD) deficiency which, although most commonly seen in blacks and those from Mediterranean countries, does occur occasionally in

Caucasians. However, the amount of G6PD decreases not only with the age of the cell, but also with the age of the patient. Its activity is significantly lower in 80–90 year-old patients relative to those aged 20–30 years (Rogers et al, 1983). However, this effect might be partly explained by the medication the patients were taking.

This type of haemolytic anaemia should be considered in the patients with a current or more recent drug history and who have a negative Coombs test. Anaemia usually presents acutely and there may be signs of intravascular haemolysis. Less commonly, the patients present with chronic anaemia. No biochemical abnormalities are seen in the peripheral blood in the quiescent stage, but when haemolysis is precipitated either by a drug or by severe acute infections, diabetic keto-acidosis or renal failure, the red blood cells show anisocytosis, polychromatophilia, basophilic stippling, spherocytosis and Heinz bodies.

Drugs which might be prescribed to an elderly person which might precipitate this type of anaemia include sulphonamides, aspirin, nitrofurantoin, para-aminosalicylic acid, probenecid, quinine, primaquine and dapsone.

Prognosis

The prognosis for haemolytic anaemia is generally good, although recovery can take several weeks following withdrawal of the drug.

Treatment

There is no specific treatment other than stopping the causal drug. Steroids may be helpful. Patients must be warned to avoid the drug in future.

THROMBOCYTOPENIA

Although this is the commonest drug-induced cytopenia, it carries the lowest mortality. Up to about 20 years ago it was considered that the peak incidence of the disorder occurred in those under the age of 20 years. However, more recent evidence shows that the majority of cases occur in those over 50 years (Bottiger & Westerholm, 1972a; Bottiger et al, 1979b). There is a predominance of females.

The most common drug causes are oral diuretics (including thiazides, chlorthalidone and frusemide) and quinine/quinidine (Bottiger & Westerholm, 1972b). Bottiger and colleagues (1979b) were able to show that between 1966 and 1975 cases due to phenylbutazone decreased while those due to sulphonamides increased. These findings contrast with those of Timoney (1978) who found that indomethacin, phenylbutazone and oxyphenbutazone were implicated in nearly half the cases of thrombocytopenia reported to the Irish National Drugs Advisory Board. This group of drugs also caused more cases than any other group reported to the WHO Centre.

Clinical features

Thrombocytopenia may occur as a selective lesion, or as part of an aplastic anaemia. In the former situation patients present with gradual or sudden onset of mild or severe bleeding, initially indicated by petechiae without inflammatory reaction. These are seen at first around the mouth, but later develop on the limbs and truck. Later ecchymoses, epistaxes, bleeding into the mucosal membrane, gastrointestinal bleedings, haematuria or intracerebral haemorrhage may occur. Those patients who develop immune thrombocytopenia also have fever, aches and pains, vomiting and abdominal pain. Examination is usually unremarkable except for signs of bleeding and a positive Hess' test. However, care is required in the interpretation of this test in the elderly (Bloomer et al, 1978).

Laboratory investigations

Blood tests show that in mild cases the platelet count is less than 100 000 and less than 20 000 in severely affected patients. There is usually no neutropenia but a leucocytosis can occur following an acute bleeding episode. The bleeding time is prolonged and clot retraction is impaired. Often, bone marrow examination shows the megakaryocytes to be normal or increased in number. It may be possible to carry out tests for evidence of antibodies or platelet damage, such as platelet factor III release test and the complement fixation test.

Pathogenesis

Thrombocytopenia results from two main mechanisms — either destruction of platelets in the peripheral blood, usually due to immunological mechanisms, such as those which occur with quinine/quinidine, but occasionally due to direct toxic effects; or by a decreased production of platelets in the bone marrow (such as follows the use of heparin and paracetamol).

Drug causes

Oral diuretics

Although these drugs are common cause of thrombocytopenia, the true incidence is probably low relative to the wide prescription of these drugs: Bottiger & Westerholm (1972b) considered the incidence to be 1 in 15 000. Mild, asymptomatic cases occur in 25 per cent of patients taking chlorothiazide, and the incidence may be higher in the elderly (Hussain, 1976). The onset of symptomatic thrombocytopenia is usually gradual. Some cases appear to be due to direct toxic effects of the drug, while others are due to an immune response. The frequency with which frusemide causes thrombocytopenia is about 2 in 1000 (Lowe et al, 1979). A case due to platelet antibodies has been reported in an elderly man (Duncan et al, 1981).

Quinine/quinidine. These drugs are common causes of thrombocytopenia. Quinine is often prescribed to the elderly for night cramps, and is found in tonics and some proprietary medicines. It causes an immunological thrombocytopenia of sudden onset, with severe constitutional disturbance and bleeding. These symptoms may appear at any time the patient is taking the drug. Quinidine causes similar problems and can lead to pulmonary haemorrhage in the elderly (Libman & Goldsmith, 1972; Alperin et al, 1980; Leblanc, 1980). Recovery usually occurs with a week of stopping the drug.

Antirheumatic drugs. Although phenylbutazone, oxyphenbutazone and indomethacin were frequently reported as causes of thrombocytopenia, they are now giving rise to fewer reports, presumably due to a reduction in prescribing. Gold therapy causes thrombocytopenia in all age groups, especially when higher doses are used (Kay, 1976). It can occur both early and late in the course of therapy, but sometimes there is a time gap of 2–10 months between the last gold injection and the onset of purpura. Recovery is slow if BAL is not given in order to increase gold elimination. Causation is uncertain, but sometimes in patients who have had a low dose it appears to be due to immunological mechanisms. Cumulative toxic action is probably the cause in those patients who develop thrombocytopenia after high doses of gold.

D penicillamine, allopurinol, benoxaprofen, acetaminophen have caused thrombocytopenia in the middle-aged and elderly (Berry et al, 1976; Shoenfeld et al, 1980; Rosenbloom & Gilbert, 1981; McInnes et al, 1981; Leen et al, 1982).

Antibacterial drugs. Sulphonamides are commonly reported causes. The combination drug trimethoprim and sulphamethoxazole, follows the pattern. Salter (1973) reported that thrombocytopenia was the second most common haematological side-effect after agranulocytosis due to this combination drug, and the majority of adverse drug reactions occurred in the over-60s. Dickson (1978), in a further review, reported more cases which showed a bi-modal age distribution of the thrombocytopenia, with the second peak occurring between 60 and 69 years. The mechanism is unclear. Thrombocytopenia also occurs occasionally in elderly people due to chloramphenicol, ampicillin, ethambutol, gentamycin and rifampicin (Blajchman et al, 1970; Chen et al, 1980; Rabinowitz et al, 1982).

Other drugs. It is well known that heparin can cause thrombocytopenia. Two mechanisms are involved. Firstly, there is a delayed onset type associated with high resistance to heparin, disseminated intravascular coagulation and recurrent or denovo thromboembolic phenomena. It occurs after intravenous or subcutaneous heparin given intermittently or continuously in full or low dosage. It occurs with either bovine or porcine preparations (Ansell & Dekin, 1980). It is probably due to an immunological mechanism, since Chong and colleagues (1982) have found heparin-dependent IgG antibodies. A second type of thrombocytopenia is mild, of early onset, and patients are often symptom-free. Many cases occur in the elderly (Bell et al, 1976; Malcolm et al, 1978; Nelson et al, 1982; Chong et al, 1982).

Cases of thrombocytopenia have been reported, sometimes in middle-aged and elderly people, following the use of digoxin (Pirovino et al, 1981), chlorpropamide, imipramine, amitriptyline, doxepin (Nixon, 1972), carba-mazepam and cimetidine (Yates & Kerr, 1980; Isaacs, 1980; Glotzbach, 1982).

Prognosis

Usually the bleeding ceases shortly after the drug is withdrawn, although the platelet count may take one to two weeks to return to normal. Mortality varies and, although some series show a 10–20 per cent mortality rate, this is probably due to case selection and the true rate is probably much lower (Bottiger et al, 1979b).

Treatment

Treatment consists of stopping the suspected drug. In severe cases steroids may hasten a remission, but it is difficult to be sure how effective this therapy is, in view of the normal rapid impovement which occurs when the suspected drug is withdrawn. It is helpful to give BAL to patients with thrombocy-topenia due to gold, since it increases the drug excretion rate, which other-wise would take a considerable time to be eliminated. Platelet transfusion is usually unnecessary. Aspirin and aspirin-like compounds should be avoided in view of their action on platelets. The patient should be warned to avoid further courses of the drug.

MEGALOBLASTIC ANAEMIA

This is one of the least common side-effects due to drugs. Most cases are due to anticonvulsants or cotrimoxazole (Timoney, 1978) which act by disturb-ance of folate or vitamin B_{12} metabolism (see Chapter 4). Antimitotic drugs also cause megaloblastic changes by inhibition of DNA syntheses. These abnormalities may be potentiated by dietary deficiency.

Anticonvulsant drugs, such as diphenylhydantoin and primidone, although causing megaloblastic changes, rarely cause frank anaemia (see Chapter). Macrocytosis without anaemia is more common, occurring in about 40 per cent of patients (Reynolds & Laund, 1978). The blood changes usually occur after the patient has been on anticonvulsant drugs for several years and when doses of 200–300 mg of diphenylhydantoin are used regularly (Chanarin, 1979). Patients who develop anaemia have abnormal serum folate or red cell folate levels — those who are severely affected show blunting of mental function. Treatment is with folic acid, but this may result in an increased frequency of fits. Alternatively the anticonvulsant can be withdrawn. Barbiturates when given alone are very infrequent causes of macrocytosis.

Folate antagonists, such as trimethoprim or amethopterin cause megaloblastic marrows or anaemia (see Chapter 4). These drugs resemble folic acid and act by binding with dihydrofolate reductase and thus inhibit the conversion of dihydrofolate to tetrahydrofolate. Consequently, the deficiency is treated with folinic acid because it bypasses the dihydrofolate reductase pathway. The situation is aggravated by pre-existing folate or vitamin B_{12} deficiency (Chanarin & England, 1972). Frank anaemia due to trimethoprim appears to be fairly uncommon. Salter (1973) reported only seven cases of megaloblastic anaemia out of 194 haematological side-effects due to cotrimoxazole.

Other drugs may cause megaloblastic marrow changes. Nitrous oxide, when given for prolonged periods, as may occur in intensive care units, can cause a megaloblastic marrow to develop. The abnormality reverses on stopping exposure (Chanarin, 1980; Nunn et al, 1982). The mechanisms appears to be due to nitrous oxide inactivating vitamin B_{12} co-factor, and due to inhibition of methionine synthetase. Chronic alcoholics may develop macrocytosis or megaloblastic bone marrow due to either the direct toxic action of alcohol on the red cells, or due to dietary deficiency (see Chapter 4). Other drugs which have been found to cause megaloblastic marrows include nitrofurantoin, colchicine, metformin, phenformin, cycloserine and sulphasalazone.

SIDEROBLASTIC MARROW

In this situation the red cell precursors contain a peri-nuclear ring of iron-staining granules in the cytoplasm, due to abnormal haem development. It can be caused by isoniazid, cycloserine, chloramphenicol, alcohol and pyrazinamide, and occurs in patients after prolonged exposure.

METHAEMOGLOBINAEMIA AND SULPHAEMOGLOBINAEMIA

Both these conditions present with cyanosis, hypoxia, dyspnoea on exertion, dizziness and mental confusion. Methaemoglobinaemia occurs when the haemoglobin molecule is oxidised from the ferrous to the ferric form, making it unavailable for oxygen transfer. It is caused by phenacetin, sulphonamides, nitrities, primaquine and sulphones. It is treated with methyl blue or ascorbic acid. Sulphaemoglobinaemia is produced by the action of hydrogen sulphide on oxyhaemoglobin, making it irreversibly unavailable for oxygen transport. It is caused by phenacetin and acetanilide. There is no specific treatment.

REFERENCES

Abrams S M, Degnan T J, Vinciguerra V 1980 Marrow aplasia following topical application of chloramphenicol eye ointment. Archives of Internal Medicine 140: 576-7

Adelstein A, Loy P 1979 Fatal adverse effects of medicines and surgery. Population Trends 17: 17-22

Alperin J B, de Groot W J, Cimo P L 1980 Quinidine-induced thrombocytopenia with pulmonary haemorrhage. Archives of Internal Medicine 140: 266-7

Ansell J, Deykin D 1980 Heparin-induced thrombocytopenia and recurrent thromboembolism. American Journal of Hematology 8: 325-32

Arneborn P, Palmblad J 1978 Drug-induced neutropenia in the Stockholm region 1973-5: frequency and causes. Acta Medica Scandinavica 204: 283-6

Arneborn P, Palmblad J 1982 Drug-induced neutropenia — a survey for Stockholm 1973-8. Acta Medica Scandinavica 212: 289-92

Ashraf M, Pearson R M, Winfield D A 1982 Aplastic anaemia associated with fenoprofen. British Medical Journal 284: 1301-2

Bell W R, Tomasulo P A, Alving B M, Duffy T P 1976 Thrombocytopenia occurring during the administration of heparin. Annals of Internal Medicine 85: 155-60

Bennett L, Schlossman R, Rosenthal J, Balzova J D, Bennett A J, Rosner F 1980 Aplastic anaemia and sulendac. Annals of Internal Medicine 92: 874

Bernstein R M 1979 Reversible haemolytic anaemia after levodopa–carbidopa. British Medical Journal 1: 1461-2

Berry H, Leyanage S P, Durance R A, Barnes C G, Berger L A, Evans S 1976 Azathiopine and penicillamine in treatment of rheumatoid arthritis: a controlled trial. British Medical Journal 1: 1052-4

Blajckman M A, Lowry R C, Pettit J E, Stradling P 1970 Rifampicin induced immune thrombocytopenia. British Medical Journal 3: 24-6

Bloomer J, Morley H, Denham M J, Hodkinson H M 1978 Capillary fragility in elderly in-patients. Age and Ageing 7: 96-9

Bottiger L E, Westerholm B 1972(a) Thrombocytopenia; incidence and aetiology. Acta Medica Scandinavica 191: 535-40

Bottiger L E, Westerholm B 1972(b) Thrombocytopenia; drug-induced thrombocytopenia. Acta Medica Scandinavica 191: 541-8

Bottiger L E, Westerholm B 1973 Drug-induced blood dyscrasias in Sweden. British Medical Journal 3: 339-43

Bottiger L E, Furhoff A K, Holmberg L 1979a Fatal reactions to drugs. Acta Medica Scandinavica 205: 451-6

Bottiger L E, Furhoff A K, Holmberg L 1979b Drug-induced blood dyscrasias. Acta Medica Scandinavica 205: 457-61

Canada A T, Burka E R 1968 Aplastic anemia after indomethacin. New England Journal of Medicine 278: 743-4

Carloss H W, Tavassoli M, McMillan R 1980 Cimetidine-induced agranulocytopenia. Annals of Internal Medicine 93: 57-8

Chanarin I, England J M 1972 Toxicity of trimethoprim sulphamethoxazole in patient with megaloblastic anaemia. British Medical Journal 1: 651-3

Chanarin I, 1979 The megaloblastic anaemias, 2nd edn. Blackwell, Oxford

Chanarin I, 1980 Cobalamins and nitrous oxide: a review. Journal of Clinical Pathology 33: 909-16

Chen J H, Wiener L, Distenfeld A 1980 Immunologic thrombocytopenia. New York State Journal of Medicine 80: 1134-5

Chong B H, Pitney W R, Castaldi P A 1982 Heparin-induced thrombocytopenia. Lancet 2: 1246-8

Clink H M, Shaw W L 1982 Mianserin-induced agranulocytosis. British Medical Journal 285: 437-8

Colvin B, Rogers M, Layton C 1974 Benzylpenicillin-induced leucopenia: complication of treatment of bacterial endocarditis. British Heart Journal 36: 216-9

Corbett G Mc, Perry D J, Shaw T R D 1982 Penicillim-induced leucopenia. New England Journal of Medicine 307: 1642-3

Current Problems 1983 Mianserin (Bolvidon, Norval) Committee of Safety of Medicine no. 10

Del Giacco S G, Petrini M T , Jannelli S, Carcassi U 1981 Fatal bone marrow hypoplasia in a shepherd using chloramphenicol spray. Lancet 1: 945

Dickson H G 1978 Trimethoprim — sulphamethoxazole and thrombocytopenia. Medical Journal of Australia 2: 5–7

Dixon A St J et al 1975 Synthetic D(−) penicillamine in rheumatoid arthritis. Double-blind controlled study of a high and low dosage regimen. Annals of the Rheumatic Diseases 34: 416–21

Drew S I, Carter B M, Nathanson D S, Terasaki P I 1980 Levamisole associated neutropenia and auto-immune granulocytotoxins. Annals of the Rheumatic Diseases 39: 59–63

Duncan A, Moore S B, Barker P 1981 Thrombocytopenia caused by frusemide-induced platelet antibody. Lancet 1: 1210

Durrant S, Read D 1982 Fatal aplastic anaemia associated with mianserin. British Medical Journal 285: 437

Farid N R, Johnson R J, Low W T 1971 Haemolytic reaction to mefenamic acid. Lancet 2: 382

Fowler P D 1967 Marrow toxicity of the pyrazoles. Annals of the Rheumatic Diseases 26: 344–5

Gabriel B, Gabriel B J, Olmer J 1966 Aplasies médullaires au cours des traitments anti-épileptiques. Marseille Medical 103: 935–46

Gault J E 1963 Agranulocytosis due to amitriptylene. Lancet 1: 44–5

Giampietro O, Ferdeghini M, Petrini M 1981 Severe leukopenia and mild thrombocytopenia after bromocriptine administration. American Journal of the Medical Sciences 281: 169–172

Gill M J, Ratcliff D A, Harding L K 1980 Hypoglycaemic coma, jaundice and pure RBC aplasia following chlorpropamide therapy. Archives of Internal Medicine 140: 714–5

Girdwood R H 1971 The effect of drugs on the blood. In: Hansen G C The adverse effects of drugs. Beecham Research Laboratories, p 70–83

Glotzbach R E 1982 Cimetidine-induced thrombocytopenia. Southern Medical Journal 75: 232–4

Goodman H L 1961 Agranulocytosis associated with tofranil. Annals of Internal Medicine 55: 321–3

Gralnick H R, McGinniss M, Elton W, McCurdy P 1971 Haemolytic anaemia associated with cephalothin. Journal of the American Medical Association 217: 1193–7

Harris E L 1971 Adverse reactions to oral anti-diabetic agents. British Medical Journal. 3: 29–30

Hart R G, Easton J D 1981 Carbamazepine and haematological monitoring. Annals of Neurology 11: 309–312

Hawson G A T, Bain B J 1980 Allopurinol and agranulocytosis. Medical Journal of Australia 1: 283–4

Heel R C, Brogden R N, Speight T M, Avery G S 1980 Captopril: a preliminary review of its pharmacological properties and therapeutic efficiency. Drugs 20: 409–52

Homayouni H, Gross P A, Setra V, Lynch T J 1979 Leucopenia due to penicillin and cephalosporin homologues. Archives of Internal Medicine 139: 827–8

Huguley C M, Lea J W, Butts J A 1966 Adverse haematologic reactions to drugs. Progress in Haematology 5: 105–35

Hurwitz N 1969 Predisposing factors in adverse reaction to drugs. British Medical Journal 1: 536–9

Hussain S 1976 Disorders of hemostasis and thrombosis in the aged. Medical Clinics of North America 60: 1273–87

Inman W H W 1977 Study of fatal bone marrow depression with special reference to phenylbutazone and oxyphenbutazone. British Medical Journal 1: 1500–5

Isaacs A J 1980 Cimetidine and thrombocytopenia. British Medical Journal 1: 294

Kay A G L 1973 Depression of bone marrow and thrombocytopenia associated with chrysotherapy. Annals of Rheumatic Diseases 32: 277–8

Kay A G L 1976 Myelotoxicity of gold. British Medical Journal 1: 1266–8

Kay A G L 1979 Myelotoxicity of D penicillamine. Annals of Rheumatic Diseases 38: 232–6

Kean W F, Dwosh I L, Anastassiades T P, Ford P M, Kelly H G 1980 The toxicity pattern of D penicillamine therapy. A guide to its use in rheumatoid arthritis. Arthritis and Rheumatism 23: 158–164

Lapier G, Stewart R B 1980 Lithium carbonate and leucocytosis. American Journal of Hospital Pharmacy 37: 1525–8

Leblanc K E 1980 A second case of quinidine-induced thrombocytopenia with pulmonary haemorrhage. Archives of Internal Medicine 140: 1250–1

Leen C, Gibb A P, Brettle R P, Welsby P D 1982 Transient neutropenia and thrombocytopenia due to benoxaprofen. Lancet 1: 1302

Libman L J, Goldsmith K L G 1972 Quinidine-induced thrombocytopenia. Proceedings of the Royal Society of Medicine 65: 590

Lindstrom F D, Lieden G, Engstrom M S 1977 Dose-related levodopa-induced haemolytic anaemia. Annals of Internal Medicine 86: 298–300

Livingston S, Villameter C, Sakata Y, Pauli L L 1967 Use of carbamazepine in epilepsy. Journal of American Medical Association 200: 116–120

Lowe J, Gray J, Henry D A, Lauson D H 1979 Adverse reactions to frusemide in hospital patients. British Medical Journal 2: 360–2

McCarthy D D, Chalmers M B 1964 Haematologic complications of phenylbutazone therapy: review of the literature and report of two cases. Canadian Medical Association Journal 90: 1061–7

McEwen J 1982 Mianserin-induced agranulocytosis. British Medical Journal 285: 438

McInnes G T, Lawson D H, Jick H 1981 Acute adverse reactions attributed to allopurinol in hospitalised patients. Annals of the Rheumatic Diseases 40: 245–9

McKenna W B, Chalmers A C 1958 Agranulocytosis following dapsone therapy. British Medical Journal 1: 324–5

Malcolm I D, Wigmore T A, Steinbrecher Y P 1978 Thrombocytopenia induced by low dose subcutaneous heparin. Lancet 1: 444

Mandel A, Gross M 1968 Agranulocytosis and phenothiazines. Diseases of the Nervous System 28: 32–6

Marcus J, Mulvihill F J 1978 Agranulocytosis with chlorpromazine. Journal of Clinical Psychiatry 39: 77–9

Mauer E F 1955 Toxic effects of phenylbutazone (Butazolidin). Review of the literature and report of the twenty-third death following its use. New England Journal of Medicine 253: 404–410

Miller J L 1980 Marrow aplasia and sulindac. Annals of Internal Medicine 92: 129

Nelson P H, Moser K M, Stoner C, Moser K S 1982 Risk of complications during intravenous heparin therapy. Western Journal of Medicine 136: 189–197

Nixon D D 1972 Thrombocytopenia following doxepin treatment. Journal of the American Medical Association 220: 418

Nunn J F, Sharer N M, Gorchein A, Jones J J, Wickramasinghe S N 1982 Megaloblastic haemopoiesis after multiple short term exposure to nitrous oxide. Lancet 1: 1379–81

OPCS (Office of Population Censuses and Surveys) Mortality Statistics 1980, England and Wales. Series DH2, No 7, Table 2, p 56–7

Owens C WI, Parker N E, Nunn P P, Davies J 1980 Agranulocytosis associated with carbamazephine and a positive reaction with anti lymphoid leukaemia antiserum during recovery. Postgraduate Medical Journal 56: 665–8

Perez Cruet J, Dancey J T, Waite J 1978 Lithium effects on leucocytosis and lymphopenia In: Johnson F N, Johnson S(eds) Lithium in medical practice. MTP Press, Lancaster, England, pp 271–7

Pirovino M, Ohnhaus, E E, von Felton, A 1981 Digoxin associated thrombocytopenia. European Journal of Clinical Pharmacology 19: 205–7

Pisciotta A V 1969 Agranulocytosis induced by certain phenothiazine derivatives. Journal of the American Medical Association 208: 1862–8

Pisciotta A V 1978 Drug-induced agranulocytosis. Drugs 15: 132–43

Pisciotta A V 1982 Drug-induced agranulocytosis. Series Haematologica 67: 292–318

Rabinowitz M, Pitlik M D, Halevy J, Rosenfeld J B 1982 Ethambutol-induced thrombocytopenia. Chest 81: 765–6

Rawlins M D 1981 Adverse reactions to drugs. British Medical Journal 282: 974–6

Reynolds E H, Laundry M 1978 Haematological effects of anticonvulsant treatment, Lancet 2: 682

Rogers G P, Lichtman H C, Sheff M F 1983 Red blood cell glucose-6-phosphate dehydrogenase activity in aged humans. Journal of the American Geriatrics Society 31: 8–11

Rosenbloom D, Gilbert R 1981 Reversible flu-like syndrome, leucopenia and thrombocytopenia induced by allopurinol. Drug Intelligence and Clinical Pharmacy 15: 286–7

Rosenthal R L, Blackman A 1965 Bone marrow hypoplasia following use of chloramphenicol eyedrops. Journal of the American Medical Association 191: 136–7

Rosenthal M, Breysse Y, Dixon A, Franchimont P 1977 Levamisole and agranulocytosis. Lancet 1: 904–5

Salter A J 1973 The toxicity profile of trimethoprim (sulphamethoxazole) after four years of widespread use. Medical Journal of Australia 1, Spec. Suppl. 2: 70–4

Sanz M A, Martinez J A, Gomis F, Garcia-Borras J J 1980 Sulindac-induced bone marrow toxicity. Lancet 2: 802–3

Scobie I N, MacCuish A C, Kesson C M, McNeil I R 1980 Neutropenia during allopurinol treatment in total therapeutic starvation. British Medical Journal 1: 1163

Scott G L, Myles A B, Bacon P A 1968 Auto-immune haemolytic anaemia and mefenamic acid therapy. British Medical Journal 3: 543–5

Seidl L G, Thornton G F, Smith J W, Cluff L E 1966 Studies on the epidemiology of adverse drug reactions. Bulletin of the Johns Hopkins Hospital 119: 299–315

Shansky M Greenlaw C W 1980 Reversible acute leucopenia and cefoxitin. Annals of Internal Medicine 90: 874–5

Sheehan J 1981 Trimethoprim associated marrow toxicity. Lancet 2: 692

Shoenfeld Y, Shaklai M, Livni E, Pinkhas J 1980 Thrombocytopenia from acetaminophen. New England Journal of Medicine 303: 47

Smith P J, Swinburn W R 1980 Adverse reactions to D penicillamine after gold toxicity. British Medical Journal 2: 617

Spitzer T R 1981 Penicillin-induced haemolytic anaemia with negative direct antiglobulin tests. Lancet 1: 1361–2

Territo M C, Peters R W, Tanaka K R 1973 Auto-immune hemolytic anemia due to levodopa therapy. Journal of the American Medical Association 226: 1347–8

Timoney R E 1978 Drug-induced haematological reactions. Journal of the Irish Medical Association 71: 573–7

Tonkonow B, Hoffman R 1980 Aplastic anaemia and cimetidine. Archives of Internal Medicine 140: 1123–4

Tucker S G, Lynch J P, Ansell B F 1977 Chlorpropamide-induced agranulocytosis. Journal of the American Medical Association 238: 422

White J M, Brown D L, Hepner G W, Worlledge S M 1968 Penicillin-induced haemolytic anaemia. British Medical Journal 3: 26–9

White C M, Price J J, Hunt K M 1980 Bone marrow aplasia associated with metronidazole. British Medical Journal 1: 617

Williamson J 1979 Adverse reactions to prescribed drugs in the elderly. In: Crooks J Stevenson I H (eds) Drugs and the elderly. Macmillan, London, p 239–46

Yates V M Kerr R E L 1980 Cimetidine and thrombocytopenia. British Medical Journal 1: 1453

Index

Acetaminophen
  and aplastic anaemia, 271
  and thrombocytopenia, 280
Acetanilide, and sulphaemogloinaemia, 282
Acetazolomide, and aplastic anaemia, 268
Achlorhydria, histamine-fast,
  and atrophic gastritis, 53
  and pernicious anaemia, 51
Acquired haemolytic anaemias, 110–126, *see
  also named types.*
  and chemical agents, 112, 113
  classification, 110, 111
  and infectious agents, 111, 112, 113–114
  and physical agents, 112, 113
Activated partial thromboplastin time, 181,
  182, 183
Acute leukaemias, *see also named types.*
  classification, 188, 189
  clinical features at diagnosis, 192
  and cytotoxic drugs, 196–198
  mortality and age, 188, 190
  and multiple myeloma, 226
  treatment, 195–202
    cytotoxic drugs, 196–198
    following remission, 201–202
    platelet transfusions, 200–201
    pyrexia, 200
    of relapse, 202
    remission rate, 199
    suppertive care, 198–201
Acute liver disease, and normocytic anaemia,
  65
Acute lymphoblastic leukaemias,
  classification, 188, 189
  mortality and age, 188, 190
  treatment, 197–198
Acute myeloid leukaemia
  biological features, 191
  classification, 188, 189
  clinical features at diagnosis, 192, 193
  mortality and age, 188, 190
  treatment, 197–202
    following remission, 201–202
    of relapse, 202

    remission rate, 199
Acute recurrent deep-vein thrombosis
  diagnosis, 162, 166–171
  treatment, 184
Acyclovir, and chronic lymphocytic
  leukaemia, 205
Addison's disease, and anaemia, 65, 76
Adriamycin
  and acute leukaemia, 198
  metabolism, 196
  in multiple myeloma, 223
  and non-Hodgkin lymphoma, 260, 262
Adult T-cell leukaemias
  classification, 190
  clinical features at diagnosis, 195
  treatment, 205
Aetiocholanolone, and aplastic anaemia, 90
Ageing, and blood, normal changes with, 1–3
Agranulocytosis, 93, 94, 95, 271–275
  blood changes, 272
  bone marrow changes, 272
  clinical features, 271
  drugs causing, 272–275
  pathogenesis, 272
  prognosis, 275
  treatment, 275
Alcohol, and sideroblastic marrow, 282
Alcoholism
  and macrocytosis, 44, 59
  and thrombocytopenia, 95
Allopurinol
  and acute leukaemia, 201
  and agranulocytosis, 273
  and chronic myeloid leukaemia, 203
  and polycythaemia rubra vera, 239
  and thrombocytopenia, 280
Amethoplerin, and megaloblastic anaemia,
  282
Amidopyrene, and agranulocytosis, 272
Amitriptyline
  and agranulocytosis, 274
  and thrombocytopenia, 281
Amphotericin B, and acute leukaemia,
  pyrexia, 200

Ampicillin, and thrombocytopenia, 280
Anaemia, *see also named types*.
  of chronic disorders, 65–73, *see also named disorders*.
    clinical features, 67
    definition, 65
    pathogenesis, 66–67
    treatment, 67
  classification, automated, 69
  definition, 64
  incidence, 64
  and multiple myeloma, 212
  and myelofibrosis, 239, 240, 241, 242
  prevalence, 100–101
  prevention, 106–107
  and screening, requirements for, 100–106, 107
    and special risk patients, 105–106
  severity, 64
  and Waldenstrom's macroglobulinaemia, 230
Analgesics
  and aplastic anaemia, 66
  and non-Hodgkin lymphoma, 263
Androgen therapy
  and aplastic anaemia, 90
  and myelofibrosis, 242
  and paroxysmal nocturnal haemoglobinuria, 126
Angular stomatitis, and iron deficiency, 30
Ankylosing spondilitis, and normocytic anaemia, 71
Anthracyclin
  and acute leukaemia, 198, 201
  and hairy cell leukaemia, 205
Antibacterial drug
  and agranulocytosis, 273
  and aplastic anaemia, 268–269
  and thrombocytopenia, 280
Antibiotics
  and acute leukaemia, pyrexia, 200
  and aplastic anaemia, 66, 90
  and chronic lymphocytic leukaemia, 204
  and megaloblastic anaemia
    following gastrectomy, 55
    and tropical sprue, 58
  and non-Hodgkin lymphoma, 263
  and platelet dysfunction, 145
Antibodies
  and ageing, changes in, 1–2
  and atrophic gastritis, 53
  and pernicious anaemia, 49–50
Anticoagulants, and gastrointestinal blood loss, 28
Anticoagulation therapy
  and acute recurrent deep-vein thrombosis, 165, 167, 168, 169, 184
  and deep-vein thrombosis
    prophylaxis, 173, 174, 175, 176
    treatment, 180–183
  and pulmonary embolism, treatment, 180–183
Anticonvulsants
  and agranulocytosis, 274
  and aplastic anaemia, 66
  and macrocytosis, 44, 58–60
  and megaloblastic anaemia, 58–60, 281
  mode of action, 59–60
  and neutropenia, 94
Antidepressants
  and agranulocytosis, 274
  and aplastic anaemia, 270
  and macrocytosis, 44, 45
Anti-emetic drugs, and acute leukaemia, 201
Anti-epileptic drugs, and aplastic anaemia, 270
Antihistamines
  and aplastic anaemia, 84
  and polycythaemia rubra vera, 239
Antilymphocyte globulin, and red cell aplasia, 93
Antipsychotic drugs, and agranulocytosis, 274
Antirheumatic drugs
  and agranulocytosis, 273
  and aplastic anaemia, 269
  and thrombocytopenia, 280
Antithymocyte globulin, and aplastic anaemia, 90–91
Antithyroid drugs
  and agranulocytosis, 272, 275
  and aplastic anaemia, 66, 84, 270
Aplasia, and bone marrow examination, 19
Aplastic anaemia, 64–65, 80
  aetiology, 82–85
  blood changes, 267–268
  bone marrow changes, 268
  clinical features, 85–87, 267
  differential diagnosis, 87–88
  drugs causing, 66, 268–271
  incidence, 81
  management, 88–91
  and paroxysmal nocturnal haemoglobinuria, 111, 124–126
  pathogenesis, 66
  pathophysiology, 81–82
  prognosis, 87, 271
  treatment, 271
Arachidonic acid, and platelet activation, 134–135
Ascorbic acid, and iron-deficiency anaemia, 36
Asparaginase, metabolism, 197
Aspirin
  and essential thrombocytopenia, 243
  and gastrointestinal blood loss, 28, 29
  and haemolytic anaemia, 278
  and iron deficiency anaemia, 102, 106
  and platelet dysfunction, 144
  and thrombocytopenia, 281

Atrophic gastritis, 52–54
  and hypothyroidism, 75
  and pernicious anaemia, 49, 52
    comparison, 53
Atrophic glossitis, and iron deficiency, 30
Auto-antibodies
  and immune-haemolytic anaemia
    cold reactive, 115, 117–119
    drug-induced, 119–122
    warm reactive, 114–116
  platelet, 142
  production, and haemolysis, 112
Auto-immune disease, *see also named diseases.*
  and aplastic anaemia, 82, 85
  and pernicious anaemia, 106
  and red cell aplasia, 92, 93
Auto-immune haemolytic anaemia
  and chronic lymphocytic leukaemia, 193,
    204
  and cold reactive antibodies, 111, 115,
    117–119
  drug-induced, 111, 115, 119–122, 276–277
  and megaloblastic anaemia, 60–61
  and Systemic Lupus Erythematosus, 71
  and warm-reactive antibodies, 111, 114–117
    diagnosis, 114–116
    treatment, 116–117
Automated blood counting, and
  haematological evaluation
  and anaemia of chronic disease, 105
  and aplastic anaemia, 86
  and iron-deficiency anaemia, 32, 105
  and megaloblastic anaemia, 46–47, 105
  normal values, 17–18
  of peripheral blood smear, 14
  and pernicious anaemia, 105
  platelets, 9–11, 18
    and disorders, classification using, 6–8
  red cells, 4–5, 18
    and disorders, classification using, 6–8
  and thalassaemia, 105
  white cells, 13–14, 18
Automated white cell differential, 13–14
5-azacytidine, metabolism, 197
Azathioprine
  and auto-immune haemolytic anaemia, 117
  and macrocytosis, 44
  and red cell aplasia, 93

Bacteria
  and acquired haemolytic anaemias, 114
  infection
    and aplastic anaemia, 84
    and normocytic anaemia, 65, 68–69
    and megaloblastic anaemia, 46, 55–56
Behaviour, and iron deficiency, 31
Benign monoclonal gammopathy, 209, 228
Benoxaprofen, and thrombocytopenia, 280
Benzene, and aplastic anaemia, 66, 83

Bleeding, *see also* Blood coagulation
  and coagulation defects, 146–147
  disorders, *see* Haemostasis, Platelets
  and haematological evaluation, 16
  and liver disease, 148–149
  and multiple myeloma, 212, 216–217
  and plasminogen activator, 154–155
  and platelet function disorder, 140–146
  test time for, 141
  aand vascular disorders, 153–154
  and vitamin K deficiency, 147–148
Blood
  changes, in healthy elderly subjects, 1–3
  clotting, *see* Blood coagulation
  coagulation
    and anticoagulants, 148
    clotting reactions, 136–139
    congenital, 147
    defects, 146–147
    disseminated intravascular, 141–142,
      149–151
    extrinsic pathway, 135–139
    factors, inhibitors, 152–153
    inhibitors, 138
    intrinsic pathway, 135–139
    and multiple myeloma, 217
    screening tests, 146
    and vitamin K deficiency, 147–148
Blood counting, automated, *see* Automated
  blood counting
Blood transfusion
  and aplastic anaemia, 89, 90
  and chronic renal failure, anaemia, 75
  and clotting factor deficiency, 151
  and megaloblastic anaemia, 62
  and non-Hodgkin lymphoma, 263
  and paroxysmal nocturnal
    haemoglobinuria, 111, 124–126
  and thrombocytopenia, 151
B-lymphocyte
  and ageing, changes in, 2
  function, 50
  maturation
    assessment, methods, 209–210
    and malignancy, targets, 210
    stages, 209–210
  and multiple myeloma, 209–211
Bone marrow
  and ageing, changes in, 1
  biopsy
    and Hodgkin's disease, 252, 253
    and lymphoma, 250
  and chronic liver disease, anaemia, 72, 73
  examination
    and anaemia of chronic disorders, 65, 66
    indications, 18
    and iron-deficiency anaemia, 34
    and megaloblastic anaemia, 46, 47
    value of, 18–19

failure
    definition, 81
    pancytopenia due to, 80–98
and hypothyroidism, anaemia, 75
and iron storage, 24
and megaloblastic anaemia
    and anticonvulsants, 58, 59
    and chronic haemolytic states, 61
    and chronic myelofibrosis, 61
and multiple myeloma, 208–211, 218–219
transplantation, and acute leukaemia,
    treatment, 201–202
Bromocriptine, and leucopenia, 275
Busulphan
    and aplastic anaemia, 270
    and chronic myeloid leukaemia, 203
    metabolism, 197
    and myelofibrosis, 242
    and polycythaemia rubra vera, 238, 239

Captopril, and leucopenia, 275
Carbamazepam, and thrombocytopenia, 281
Carbamazepine
    and aplastic anaemia, 270
    and leucopenia, 274
Carbimazole
    and agranulocytosis, 275
    and aplastic anaemia, 66, 270
Carcinoma, see also Lymphoma
    gastric, see Gastric carcinoma
    and normocytic anaemia, 65, 68
    and thrombocytopenia, 95
Cefotaxime, and acute leukaemia, pyrexia,
    200
Cephaloridine, and aplastic anaemia, 90
Cephalosporin
    and drug-induced immune haemolytic
        anaemia, 115, 120, 122
    and leucopenia, 273
Cephalothin, and immunohaemolytic
    anaemia, 276, 277
Chemotherapy
    and acute leukaemias, 195–202
    and chronic leukaemias, 203–205
    and Hodgkin's disease, 252, 253, 255–257
    and non-Hodgkin's lymphoma, 258–259,
        260, 262, 263
    and preleukaemia, 203
    and smouldering leukaemia, 203
Chlorambucil
    and chronic lymphocytic leukaemia, 204
    and hairy cell leukaemia, 205
    and macrocytosis, 44
    metabolism, 197
    and non-Hodgkin lymphoma, 260, 262
    and polycythaemia rubra vera, 238, 239
Chloramphenicol
    and agranulocytosis, 273
    and aplastic anaemia, 66, 83–84, 268
    and sideroblastic marrow, 282

and thrombocytopenia, 280
Chlorpromazine
    and agranulocytosis, 274
    and haemolytic anaemia, 277
Chlorpropamide
    and agranulocytosis, 275
    and aplastic anaemia, 66, 270–271
    and haemolytic anaemia, 277
    and thrombocytopenia, 281
Cholestyramine, and polycythaemia rubra
    vera, 239
Chlorthalidine, and thrombocytopenia, 278,
    279
Chronic haemolytic states, and megaloblastic
    anaemia, 46, 60–61
Chronic leukaemias, see also named types
    classification, 188, 190
    clinical features at diagnosis, 192–195
    mortality and age, 188, 190
    and splenectomy, 97
    treatment, 203–205
Chronic liver disease
    and anaemia, 64, 72–75
    and clotting factors, 148–149
    and plasminogen activator, 154–155
    and platelet dysfunction, 143, 144, 148–149
    and vitamin K deficiency, 147–148
Chronic lymphocytic leukaemia
    biological features, 191
    and B- lymphocyte maturation, 210
    classification, 188, 190
    clinical features at diagnosis, 193–194
    mortality and age, 188, 190
    treatment, 204–205
Chronic myelofibrosis, and megaloblastic
    anaemia, 61
Chronic myeloid leukaemia
    acute phase, 203–204
    chronic phase, 203
    classification, 188, 190
    clinical features at diagnosis, 193
    mortality and age, 188, 190
    treatment, 203–204
Chronic renal failure
    and multiple myeloma, 213–214
    and normocytic anaemia, 65, 73–75
        aetiology, 74
        clinical features, 74
        treatment, 74–75
    and platelet dysfunction, 143
Cimetidine
    and aplastic anaemia, 271
    and leucopenia, 275
    and polycythaemia rubra vera, treatment,
        239
    and thrombocytopenia, 281
Coagulation, and haematological evaluation,
    16–17
Coagulation factor deficiency, see Blood
    coagulation

Cobalamin, *see also* Cobalamin deficiency
  and ageing, changes in, 3
  and anaemia, preventative treatment,
    106–107
  and megaloblastic anaemia, treatment, 56,
    58, 62
Cobalamin deficiency
  and atrophic gastritis, 53–54
  aand co-trimoxazole, 60
  diagnosis, 47–48
  and gastric atrophy, 53–54
  and hypothyroidism, 75, 76
  and macrocytosis, megaloblastic, 44
  and megaloblastic anaemia, 46, 47–56, 58
    following gastrectomy, 54, 55
  nutritional, 56
  and pernicious anaemia, 46, 49, 51, 52
  and tropical sprue, 46, 58
Coeliac disease, and megaloblastic anaemia,
  46, 57–58
Colchicine, and megaloblastic anaemia, 282
Cold agglutin syndrome, 115, 117–119
  clinical features, 118
  treatment, 118–119
Compensated haemolytic disease, 109
'Coombs' test, and auto-immune haemolytic
  anaemia, 115–116, 276
Corticosteroids
  and Addison's disease, anaemia, 76
  and anaemia of chronic disorders, 67
    Felty's syndrome, 70
    rheumatoid arthritis, 69–70
    Systemic Lupus Erythematosus, 71
  and aplastic anaemia, 90, 91
  and auto-immune haemolytic anaemia,
    116–117
  and chronic lymphocytic leukaemia, 204
  and neutropenia, 95
  and paroxysmal nocturnal
    haemoglobinuria, 126
  and red cell aplasia, 93
  and thrombocytopenia, 281
Co-trimoxazole
  and agcanulocytosis, 273
  and megaloblastic anaemia, 60, 281
Cyancobalamin, and pernicious anaemia, 52
Cyclophosphamide
  and adult T-cell leukaemia, 205
  and aplastic anaemia, 91, 270
  and auto-immune haemolytic anaemia, 117
  and chronic lymphocytic leukaemia, 204,
    205
  and hairy cell leukaemia, 205
  metabolism, 197
  and multiple myeloma, 223
  and non- Hodgkin lymphoma, 260, 262
  and polycythaemia rubra vera, 238
  and prolymphatic leukaemia, 205
  and red cell aplasia, 93

Cycloserine
  and megaloblastic anaemia, 282
  and sideroblastic marrow, 282
Cytopenia, *see also named types*
  and bone marrow failure, 80–98
    isolated, 91
  drug-induced, 266
Cytosine arabinoside
  and acute leukaemia, 198, 201, 202
  and macrocytosis, 44
  metabolism, 196
Cytostatics, and aplastic anaemia, 268
Cytotoxic drugs
  and acute leukaemias, 196–198
  and aplastic anaemia, 270
  and auto-immune haemolytic anaemia, 116
  and chronic leukaemias, 203–205
  and macrocytosis, 44
  and preleukaemia, 203
  and red cell aplasia, 91
  and smouldering leukaemia, 203

Daunorubicin
  and acute leukaemia, 198
  metabolism, 196
Deep-vein thrombosis, 157–185
  acute recurrent, *see* Acute recurrent
    deep-vein thrombosis.
  calf, treatment, 183
  diagnosis
    clinical, 158
    objective tests, 158–165
    practical approach for, 163–165
  prevalence, 157
  prognosis, 165
  prophylaxis, 173–176
  and pulmonary embolism, *see* Pulmonary
    embolism,
  recurrent leg symptoms following, 165–173
  treatment, 180–184
Deoxyuridine supression test, and
  megaloblastic anaemia, 59
Dermatomyositis, and normocytic anaemia,
  72
Dextran, and deep-vein thrombosis,
  prophylaxis, 174, 175
Digoxin, and thrombocytopenia, 281
Diphenylhydantain
  and aplastic anaemia, 270
  and megaloblastic anaemia, 59, 60, 281
2–3 diphosphoglyceric acid, in red cell
  and chronic renal failure, anaemia, 74
  and iron deficiency, 30
Dipyrone, and agranulocytosis, 272–273
Disseminated intravascular coagulation,
  141–142
  and blood transfusion, 151
  causes, 149–151
  management, 150–151

screening tests, 150
Diuretics, and thrombocytopen, 278, 279–280
Doppler ultrasound
    and deep-vein thrombosis, 162–163, 165
    and post-phlebitic syndrome, 172
Doxepin, and thrombocytopenia, 281
Drug-induced blood dyscrasias, 265–282, *see
    also named disorders.*
Drug-induced immune haemolytic anaemia,
    111, 115, 119–122
    type, 119, 120
Drug reaction, adverse
    incidence, 266–267
    mortality, 266–267
    types, 265–266
Drugs, *see also named types.*
    and aplastic anaemia, 82, 83–84
    and haemolytic anaemia, 111, 112, 113, 115
        in glucose-6-phosphate dehydrogenase
            deficiency, 124
    and iron-deficient anaemia, 28–29, 102
    and macrocytosis, 44, 45
    and megaloblastic anaemia, 46
    and neutropenia, 94
    and platelet dysfunction, 144, 145
    and red cell aplasia, 93
Dysproteinaemia, and platelet dysfunction,
    144

EDTA, and automated blood counting, 10, 11
Epilepsy, and anaemia, 106
Epipodophyllotoxin
    and acute leukaemia, 202
    metabolism, 197
Erythropoietin
    and anaemia of chronic disorders, 67
        rheumatoid arthritis, 69
    secretion, and normocytic anaemia, 73–75
        and Addison's disease, 76
        and hypopituitarism, 76
    secretion
        and hypothyroidism, 75–76
        and renal failure, 73–75
Ethambutol, and thrombocytopenia, 280
External pneumatic compression, and
    deep-vein thrombosis, prophylaxis,
    173–174, 175, 176

Factor VIII complex, 132–133
Fanconi's anaemia, 82
Felty's syndrome
    and normocytic anaemia, 70
    and splenectomy, 70
Fenprofen, and aplastic anaemia, 269
Ferritin, in serum, measurement,
    and anaemia of chronic disorders, 67
    and iron-deficiency anaemia, evaluation,
        32–34, 35
    and iron storage, and ageing, 24, 33

Ferrous sulphate, and iron-deficiency
    anaemia, 35, 36
Fibrin, 136–139
Fibrinolytic enzyme system, 136
5- fluorouracil, and macrocytosis, 44
Folate, *see* Folic acid.
Folic acid
    and chronic haemolytic states, 61
    and chronic myelofibrosis, 61
    and coeliac disease, 58
    deficiency
        and anticovulsants, 46, 58–60
        and chronic haemolytic states, 60–61
        and chronic myelofibrosis, 46, 61
        and coeliac disease, 46, 57–58
        and co-trimoxazole, 60
        diagnosis, 48
        and macrocytosis, megaloblastic, 44
        and megaloblastic anaemia, 46, 48, 56,
            57, 58, 60, 62, 281, 282
        and myelofibrosis, 242
        nutritional, 46, 56, 57
        and rheumatoid arthritis, 69
    and megaloblastic anaemia, 62
        and anticonvulsants, 59
        following gastrectomy, 55
Free erythrocyte protoporphyrin, and iron
    deficiency anaemia, 35
Frusemide
    and megaloblastic anaemia, 62
    and thrombocytopenia, 278, 279–280

Gardia lamblia, and tropical sprue, 58
Gastrectomy, following megaloblastic
    anaemia, 54–55, 106
Gastric atrophy, 52–54
    and pernicious anaemia, 49
    comparison, 52
Gastric carcinoma
    and gastrectomy, following megaloblastic
        anaemia, 54–55
    and iron-deficiency anaemia, 102
    and pernicious anaemia, 52
Gastric surgery
    anaemia following, 106
    and iron-deficiency anaemia, 28
Gastrointestinal blood loss, and
    iron-deficiency anaemia, 102
    causes, 28–29, 106
    treatment, 37
Gentamycin
    and acute leukaemia, pyrexia, 200
    and aplastic anaemia, 90
    and thrombocytopenia, 280
Glucose-6-phosphate dehydrogenase
    deficiency, and haemolytic anaemia, 111,
    112, 124, 126–127, 277–278
Gluten, and coeliac disease, 57, 58
Gold

and aplastic anaemia, 66, 269
and thrombocytopenia, 280

Haemodialysis, and haemolytic anaemia, 113
Haemolysis, *see also* Haemolytic anaemia.
  intravascular, evidence of, 110
  signs of, 109, 110
Haemolytic anaemia, 109–127, *see also named
  types*.
  acquired, 110–126, 276–277
  and chronic liver disease, 73
  classification, 110–112
  clinical features, 276
  definition, 109
  diagnosis, 109–110
    mistaken, 110, 111
  incidence, 275–276
  inherited, 111, 126–127, 277–278
  microangiopathic, and chronic renal failure,
    73, 74
  prognosis, 278
  and scleroderma, 71
  treatment, 278
Haemolytic-uraemia syndrome, and chronic
  renal failure, 73
Haemostasis
  control, 136–139
  failure
    diagnosis, 139
    inherited, 140
    pathogenesis, 139
    screening tests, 140
  platelet involvement, 132–139
  reactions, classification, 132
Hairy cell leukaemia
  classification, 190
  clinical features at diagnosis, 194
  and splenectomy, 97
  treatment, 205
'Ham'test, 125
Haemoglobin
  and ageing, changes in, 2, 25, 26
  and anaemia, 100–101
  H disease, and megaloblastic anaemia,
    60–61
  measurement, 4, 5, 18
    and iron-deficiency anaemia, evaluation,
      32
    and posture, 103–104
  synthesis, 22
  values, 64
Heart, and iron deficiency, effects on, 29–30
Heparin
  and deep-vein thrombosis,
    prophylaxis, 173, 174, 175, 176
    treatment, 180–181, 182, 183, 184
  and pulmonary embolism, treatment,
    180–181, 182, 183

Hepatitis virus
  and anaemia, 69
  and aplastic anaemia, 84–85
Hereditary haemorrhagic telangiectasia, 153
Herpes zoster, and chronic lymphocytic
  leukaemia, 204–205
Histamine-fast achlorhydria, *see*
  Achlorhydria.
Hodgkin's disease
  chemotherapy, 255–257
  clinical manifestations, 250–251
  diagnosis, 247
  epidemiology, 245–247, 248
  incidence, 246, 248
  mortality, 246, 248
  staging, 249, 250
  survival, 245, 246
    and staging, 252–255
    and treatment, effects on, 255–257
  treatment, and survival, 255–257
Hydantoin
  and agranulocytosis, 274
  and aplastic anaemia, 270
Hydroxobalamin, and pernicious anaemia, 52
Hydroxocobalamin, and pernicious anaemia,
  52
Hydroxydaunorubicin
  and adult T-cell leukaemia, 205
  and chronic lymphocytic leukaemia, 205
  and prolymphocytic leukaemia, 205
Hypercalcaemia, and multiple myeloma, 216
Hypersplenism, 80, 95–98
  causes, 80, 96–97
  definition, 96
  and splenectomy, 96–98
  types, 95–96
Hyperphosphatemia, and haemolytic
  anaemia, 111, 113, 115
Hyperviscosity syndrome
  and multiple myeloma, 215–216
  and Waldenstrom's macroglobulinaemia,
    230, 231
Hypopituitarism, and normocytic anaemia,
  65, 76
Hypothyroidism
  and macrocytosis, 44–45
  and normocytic anaemia, 65, 75–76
  and pernicious anaemia, 52, 106

Ibuprofen, and haemolytic anaemia, 277
Idiopathic haemochromatosis, and
  iron-deficiency anaemia, 37
^{125}I-fibrinogen leg scanning
  and acute deep-vein thrombosis, 166, 167,
    168, 169, 170
  and deep-vein thrombosis, 160–162, 163,
    164, 165
    prophylaxis, 174, 175, 176

Imipramine
  and agranulocytosis, 274
  and macrocytosis, 44
  and thrombocytopenia, 281
Immune response, and chronic lymphocytic
  leukaemia, 204–205
Immune system
  and agranulocytosis, 272
  and aplastic anaemia, 85
  and iron deficiency, 31
  and pernicious anaemia, 49–50
  and red cell aplasia, 92, 93
  and Systemic Lupus Erythematosus, 71
Immunoglobulin, and ageing, changes, 2
Immunoglobulin A myeloma, and platelet
  dysfunction, 144
Immunohaemolytic anaemia
  classification, 111, 115
  and cold-reactive antibodies, 111, 115,
    117–119
  drug-induced, 111, 115, 119–122, 277
  and warm-reactive antibodies, 111, 114–117
Impedance plethysmography
  and acute recurrent deep-vein thrombosis,
    166, 167, 168, 169, 170, 171
  and deep-vein thrombosis, 160, 161, 163,
    164–165
    prophylaxis, 174, 175
  and pulmonary embolism, diagnosis, 179,
    180
Indomethacin
  and agranulocytosis, 272
  and aplastic anaemia, 269
  and gastrointestinal blood loss, 28
  and thrombocytopenia, 278, 280
Infection
  and acquired haemolytic anaemias, 111,
    112, 113–114, 115
  and aplastic anaemia, 82, 84–85
  and chronic lymphocytic leukaemia,
    204–205
  and cold agglutinin syndrome, 117
  and multiple myeloma, 217
  and normocytic anaemia, 65, 68–69
Inherited haemolytic anaemia, 111, 126–127
  and glucose-6-phosphate dehydrogenase,
    124, 126–127, 277–278
Iron
  absorption, 22–23, 28
  and anaemia, prevention, 107
  -deficient erythropoiesis, 21
  dietary, importance, 22–23, 27
  excretion, 23–24
  and megaloblastic anaemia, following
    gastrectomy, treatment, 55
  metabolism, 21–22
    and anaemia of chronic disorders, 66–67,
      69
    and rheumatoid arthritis, 69, 70

metalloproteins, 21
  and rheumatoid arthritis, anaemia,
    treatment, 69
  storage, 24
    depletion, 21
  supply, evaluation, 34–35
Iron binding capacity, and iron-deficiency
  anaemia, evaluation, 34–35
Iron deficiency, see also Iron-deficiency
  anaemia.
  and anaemia of chronic liver disease, 72, 73
  causes, 27–29
  degress of, 6, 7
  effects of, 29–31
  and hypothyroidism, 75, 76
  and pernicious anaemia, 52
  prevalence, 24–27
  stages of, 21
Iron-deficiency anaemia
  aetiology, 27–29, 106
  and bone marrow examination, 19
  causes, 102, 106
  clinical features, 31
  diagnosis, 35, 105
  effects of, 29–30
  and gastrectomy, 54
  laboratory evaluation, 32–35
  prevalence, 24–27
  prevention, 107
  screening, 101–102, 103
  treatment, 35–37, 101–102
Iron-deficient erythropoiesis, 32
Iron dextran, and iron-deficiency anaemia,
  36–37
Isoniazid, and sideroblastic marrow, 282

Koilonychia, and iron deficiency, 30

Laparotomy
  and Hodgkin's disease, 252, 253, 255
  and lymphoma, 250
  and non-Hodgkin lymphoma, 262

Leucopenia
  drug-induced, 273, 274
  and Felty's syndrome, 70
  and hypopituitarism, 76
Leukaemias, 188–205, see also named types.
  and age, 188, 190
  and ankylosing spondilitis, 71
  biological features, 190–191
  classification, 188, 189–190
  clinical features at diagnosis, 192–195
  definition, 188
  incidence, 188
  and macrocytosis, 44, 45
  mortality and age, 188, 190
  and platelet dysfunction, 143
  and thrombocytopenia, 95

treatment, 195–206
Levadopa
  and auto-immune haemolytic anaemia, 277
  and drug-induced haemolytic anaemia, 122
Levamisole, and agranulocytosis, 273
Lithium carbonate, and lymphopenia, 274
Liver
  and aplastic anaemia, 84–85
  disease
    acute, *see* Acute liver disease.
    chronic, *see* Chronic liver disease.
    'spur cell' anaemia in, 124
  and iron storage, 24
Lymphocyte
  and ageing, changes in, 2
  function, 50
Lymphography
  and Hodgkin's disease, 252
Lymphoma, 245–263, *see also named types.*
  diagnosis, 247–249
  epidemiology, 245–247, 248
  and normocytic anaemia, 65, 68
  staging, 249, 250
  and thrombocytopenia, 95
Lung scan, and pulmonary embolism,
    diagnosis, 177–178, 179, 180

Macrocytic anaemia
  causes, 72
  and chronic liver disease, 72
Macrocytosis
  megaloblastic, causes, 44, 28–282
  and megaloblastic anaemia, 46–47
  normoblastic
    and anticonvulsants, 44, 58–60
    causes, 43–45, 58–60
  physiological, 44
M-AMSAand acute leukaemia, 202
  metabolism, 197
Mean cell haemoglobin (MCH), 5, 18, 43
  and anaemia of chronic disorders, 66
  and normocytic anaemia, 64, 65
Mean cell haemoglobin concentration
    (MCHC), 5, 6, 18
Mean cell volume (MCV)
  and anaemia of chronic disease, 105
  and iron-deficiency anaemia, evaluation, 32
  and macrocytosis, normoblastic, 44, 45
  and anticonvulsants, 58–59
  mean value, 43
  and megaloblastic anaemia, 46, 105
    and coeliac disease, 58
    and co-trimoxazole, 60
    following gastrectomy, 54
  and normocytic anaemia, 64, 65
  and pernicious anaemia, 52
  and red cell disorders, 6, 7, 8, 9
Mean platelet volume (MPV), 10, 18
  sequential changes of, 12–13

Mefanamic acid
  and auto-immune haemolytic anaemia, 277
  and drug-induced immune haemolytic
    anaemia, 122
Megaloblastic anaemia, 43–62, *see also*
    Pernicious anaemia.
  blood transfusion in, 62
  and bone marrow examination, 19
  causes, 44, 46, 49–62, 106, 281–282
  diagnosis, 45–48
  drug-induced, 281–282
  and epilepsy, 106
  and gastrectomy, 106
  and intestinal bacterial flora, abnormal,
    55–56
  and rheumatoid arthritis, 69
Melphalan
  and aplastic anaemia, 270
  and essential thrombocythaemia, 243
  and macrocytosis, 44
  in multiple myeloma, 223
6-mercaptopurine
  and aplastic anaemia, 270
  metabolism, 196
Metformin, and megaloblastic anaemia, 282
Methaemoglobinaemia, 282
Methoin, and aplastic anaemia, 66
Methotrexate
  and aplastic anaemia, 270
  and macrocytosis, 44
  metabolism, 197
α-methyldopa
  and drug-induced immune haemolytic
    anaemia, 115, 120, 121–122
  and macrocytosis, 45
Methylphenylethl-hydantoin, and aplastic
    anaemia, 270
Methylprednisolone, and aplastic anaemia,
    270
Methylprednisolone, and aplastic anaemia, 91
Metronidazole, and aplastic anaemia, 269
Mianserin
  and agranulocytosis, 274
  and aplastic anaemia, 270
Microangiopathic haemolytic anaemia, 111,
    123–124
Microcytic anaemia, and chronic liver disease,
    72
Monoclonal gammopathies of uncertain
    significance, *see* Benign monoclonal
    gammopathy.
Multiple myeloma
  aetiology, 209–211
  clinical features, 211–218
  diagnostic criteria, 229
  historical aspects, 208
  incidence, 208–209
  laboratory investigations, 218–221
  pathogenesis, 209–211

and plasma cell kinetics, 211
prognosis, 221–222
staging, 221–223
treatment, 223–228
  and acute leukaemia, 226
  combination, 223–224
  complications, 226
  and hypercalcaemia, 226–227
  and infections, 227
  plasma exchange, 227
  radiotherapy, 227
  and renal failure, 226
  resisitance, 225
Muscle performance, and iron deficiency,
  30–31
Myelofibrosis, 143, 239–242
  clinical features, 240–241
  course, 241
  haematological findings, 241
  prognosis, 241
  treatment, 242
'Myeloma kidney', 213–214
Myeloproliferative disorders, 143, see also
  Platelets, Thrombocytopenia,
Myxoedema
  and macrocytosis, normoblastic, 44–45

Neoplasia
  and macrocytosis, 44, 45
  and thrombocytopenia, 95
Nervous system, and multiple myeloma,
  214–215
Neutropenia
  causes, 93–94
  definition, 93
  drug-induced, 94
  Felty's syndrome, 70
  management, 94–95
Nitrofurantoin
  and haemolytic anaemia, 276, 278
  and megaloblastic anaemia, 282
Nitrous oxide, and megaloblastic anaemia,
  282
Non-Hodgkin lymphoma
  and B-lymphocyte maturation, 210
  diagnosis, 247–249
  epidemiology, 245–247, 248
  incidence, 246, 248, 257–258
  mortality, 246, 248, 258
  and splenectomy, 97
  staging, 249, 250
    and survival, 259–260
  survival, 259–263
  treatment, 258–259, 260
    and survival, 259–263
Non-steroidal anti-inflammatory drug
  and iron-deficiency anaemia, 28–29, 102,
  106

and normocytic anaemia, 71
aand polycythaemia rubra vera, 239
Normocytic anaemia, 64–76
  and bone marrow failure, 65, 81–98, see also
    Bone marrow failure.
  of chronic disorders, 64–73, see also named
    disorders.
  definition, 64
  and impaired erythropoietin secretion, 65,
    73–76
    chronic renal failure, 65, 73–75
    endocrine disorders, 65, 75–76
  and multiple myeloma, 218

Oestrogen, and thrombocytopenia, 95
Oncovin, see Vincristine.
Oxazolidines
  and agranulocytosis, 274
  and aplastic anaemia, 270
Oxymethalone, and aplastic anaemia, 90
Oxyphenbritazone, and aplastic anaemia, 66
Oxyphenbutazone
  and agranulocytosis, 272
  and aplastic anaemia, 268, 269
  and thrombocytopenia, 278, 280

Packed cell volume (PVC), 4–5, 18
  and iron deficiency anaemia, evaluation, 32
  and polycythaemia
    relative, 242–243
    rubra vera, 32
    secondary, 239
Pancytopenia, causes, 80-98, see also named
  types and disorders
Para-aminosalicyclic acid, and haemolytic
  anaemia, 277, 278
Paraproteins
  in multiple myeloma, 209, 219–220
  in Waldenstromes macroglobulinaemia, 230
Paroxysmal cold haemoglobinuria, 115, 117
Paroxysmal nocturnal haemoglobulinuria,
  111, 124, 126
Partial thromboplastin time, and
  haematological evaluation, 16
Penicillamine
  and aplastic anaemia, 269
  and thrombocytopenia, 280
Penicillin
  and aplastic anemia, 269
  and drug-induced immunohaemolytic
    anaemia, 115, 119, 120
  and haemolytic anaemia, 276
  and immunohaemolytic anaemia, 276
  and leucopenia, 273
  and neutropenia, 94
Peptic ulcer disease, and iron deficient
  anaemia, 28, 29
Peripheral Blood Smear, and haematological

evaluation, 14–15
platelets, 15
red cells, 14–15
white cells, 15
Pernicious anaemia, 46, *see also* Megaloblastic
anaemia
and atrophic gastritis, comparison, 53
causes, 49–50
clinical features, 50–51
definition, 48
diagnosis, 51, 105
frequency, 49
screening, 102, 103
treatment, 52, 102
Phenacetin
and methaemoglobinaemia, 282
and sulphaemoglobinaemia, 282
Phenformin, and megaloblastic anaemia, 282
Phenobarbital, and megaloblastic anaemia, 59
Phenothiazine
and agranulocytosis, 271, 272, 274
and neutropenia, 94
Phenylbritazone, and aplastic anaemia, 66
Phenylbutazone
and agranulocytosis, 271–272, 273
and aplastic anaemia, 268, 269
and haemolytic anaemia, 277
and iron-deficiency anaemia, 102
and thrombocytopenia, 278, 280
Phenytoin
and agranulocytosis, 274
and aplastic anaemia, 66
Phosphorus, radioactive
and essential thrombocythaemia, treatment,
243
and polycythaemia rubra vera, treatment,
238, 239
Piperacillin, and acute leukaemia, pyrexia,
200
Plasma cells, *see named types*
Plasminogen, 136–139
activator, and bleeding, 154–155
inhibitors, 155
Platelet activating factor, 134
Platelet
activation, 132–135
adhesion, 132
aggregation, and haematological evaluation,
17, 133–135
automated blood counting, 9–11, 18
and disorders, classification using, 11–12
characteristics, 133
coating factors, 132
count, 9–10, 140–141
-crit, 11
destruction, 142
disorders, 140–146
classification, 11–12

distribution width, 11
drug-induced disorders, 144–146
granule content, 133, 134, 135
and haemostasis, 132–139
and iron-deficiency anaemia, 32
life span, 142
and peripheral blood smear, 15
volume, distribution histogram, 10–11
Polycythaemia, 234–239, 242–243
classification, 234
relative, 234, 239, 240, 242–243
rubra vera, 143, 234–239
Polymylgia rheumatica, and normocytic
anaemia, 71
Post-phlebitic syndrome, 165–166
diagnosis, 163, 166, 171–172
treatment, 184
Post-cricoid oesophageal webs, and iron
deficiency, 30
Potassium
and megaloblastic anaemia, 62
perchlorate, and aplastic anaemia, 66
Prednisolone
and acute leukaemia, treatment, 198
and adult T-cell leukaemia, treatment, 205
and auto-immune haemolytic anaemia, 116
and chronic lymphocytic leukaemia,
treatment, 204, 205
and Felty's syndrome, anaemia, 70
and Hodgkin's lymphoma, 259, 260, 262
and non-Hodgkin's lymphoma, 255
and multiple myeloma, 223
and polymylgia rheumatica, anaemia, 71
and prolymphocytic leukaemia, 205
Preleukaemia
biological features, 191
classification, 188, 189–190
and macrocytosis, 44, 45
treatment, 203
Primaquine
and haemolytic anaemia, 276, 277
and methaemoglobinaemia, 282
Primethamine, and macrocytosis, 44
Primidone, and megaloblastic anaemia, 59,
281
Probenecid, and haemolytic anaemia, 278
Procarbazine, and Hodgkin's disease, 255,
256, 257
Prolymphocytic leukaemia
classification, 190
clinical features, at diagnosis, 194
treatment, 205
Propylthiouracil, and agranulocytosis, 275
Prostacyclin, 139
Prothrombin time, 182, 183
and haematological evaluation, 16
Pulmonary angiography, and pulmonary
embolism, diagnosis, 177, 178, 179, 180,

183
Pulmonary embolism
    and deep-vein thrombosis, 173
        diagnosis, 176–180
        prophylaxis, 173, 174, 175, 176
Pyrazinamide, and sideroblastic marrow, 282
    and Hodgkin's disease, 255, 259

Quinidine, and thrombocytopenia, 278, 280
Quninine, and haemolytic anaemia, 278
Quinone, and thrombocytopenia, 278, 280
Quinsy, see Peritonsillar abscess

Radiotherapy
    and Hodgkin's disease, 252, 253
    and lymphoma, 250
    and non-Hodgkin lymphoma, 258, 259, 263
Red cell aplasia, 65, 91–93
    classification, 91–92
    management, 93
    pathogenesis, 92–93
Red cell
    automated blood counting, 4–5, 18
        and disorders, classification using, 6–8
    count, 4
    disorders, classification, 6–9
    distribution width, 5, 18
        and disorders, 6, 7, 8, 9
    fragmentation syndromes, 111, 122–124
    and peripheral blood smear, 14–15
    size, and ageing, changes in, 2–3
    volume distrubution histogram, 6
        and disorders, 9
Reiter's disease, and normocytic anaemia, 72
Renal failure, chronic, see Chronic renal
    failure
Reticulocyte count, 6
Reticulocytosis, and macrocytosis, 45
Rheumatoid arthritis
    and normocytic anaemia, 69–70
    and pernicious anaemia, 106
Rifampicin
    and haemolytic anaemia, 277
    and thrombocytopenia, 280
Schistocyte, 122–123, 124
Scleroderma, and normocytic anaemia, 71
Senile purpura, 153
Serum iron, and iron-deficiency anaemia,
    34–35
Sezary syndrome
    classification, 190
    clinical features, at diagnosis, 194–195
Sickle-cell anaemia, and megaloblastic
    anaemia, 60–61
Sideroblastic anaemia, 109
Sideroblastic marrow, drug-induced, 282
Skeletal system, and multiple myeloma,

212–213
Smouldering leukaemia, 188, 190
    biological features, 191
    treatment, 203
Sodium warfarin, and deep-vein thrombosis,
    treatment, 182–183
Spinal cord compression, and multiple
    myeloma, 214–215
Spleen, functions, 95
Splenectomy
    and auto-immune haemolytic anaemia, 117
    and Felty's syndrome, 70
    and hypersplenism, 96–98
Splenomegaly
    and Felty's syndrome, 70
    and hypersplenism, 80, 96, 97
    and myelofibrosis, 240, 241, 242
Spur cell anaemia, in liver disease, 111, 124
Steroids, and megaloblastic anaemia, 61
Stipophen, and drug-induced immune
    haemolytic anaemia, 115, 119, 120, 121
Streptomycin, and drug-induced immune
    haemolytic anaemia, 115, 120, 122
Sucrose water test, 125
Sulindac, and aplastic anaemia, 269
Sulphaemoglobinaemia, 282
Sulphamethoxazole
    and agranulocytosis, 273
    and thrombocytopenia, 280
Sulphasalazine, and macrocytosis, 45
Sulphasalazone, and megaloblastic anaemia,
    282
Sulphonamides
    and agranulocytosis, 272, 273
    and aplastic anaemia, 66, 84, 268, 269
    and haemolytic anaemia, 276, 277, 278
    and methaemoglobinaemia, 282
    and thrombocytopenia, 278, 280
Systemic Lupus Erythematosus, and
    normocytic anaemia, 71

Temporal arteritis syndrome, and normocytic
    anaema, 71
Tetracycline, and megaloblastic anaemia
    following gastrectomy, 55
    and tropical sprue, 58
Thiazides, and thrombocytopenia, 95, 278
6-thioguanine
    and acute leukaemia, 198
    and chronic myeloid leukaemia, 203
    metabolism, 196
Thiouracil, and aplastic anaemia, 66, 270
Thrombocythaemia, essential, 243
Thrombocytopenia, 278–281
    acute, 142
    and bone marrow
        examination, 19

failure, 95
blood changes, 279
causes, 141
clinical features, 279
chronic, 142
drug-induced, 142, 278, 279–281
essential, 143
and haemostatic failure, 139
and hypothermia, 142
and immune platelet destruction, 142
and infectious diseases, 142
and mean platelet volume, 12–13
and multiple myeloma, 217
and normocytic anaemia, 71
pathogenesis, 279
and platelet count, 12–13
post-transfusion, 151
prognosis, 281
therapy, 145–146, 281
and Waldenstrom's macroglobulinaemia, 230
Thromboneurosis, 172–173
treatment, 184–185
Thromboxane A_2, and platelet activation, 134
Thymoma, and red cell aplasia, 92,
Thyroxine, and hypothyroidism, 75
T-lymphocyte
and ageing, changes in, 2
function, 50
Tolbutamide, and aplastic anaemia, 66
Total iron binding capacity, and iron-deficiency anaemia, 34–35
Traumatic haemolytic anaemias, 111, 122–124
Transferrin, and anaemia of chronic disorders, 67
Trimethoprin
and agranulocytosis, 273
and megaloblastic anaemia, 282
and thrombocytopenia, 280
Tropical sprue, and megaloblastic anaemia, 46, 58
Tumor, and iron-deficient anaemia, 28, 29
Tyoxidone, and aplastic anaemia, 66

Uraemia, and platelet dysfunction, 144

Vasoconstriction, 132
Vegan, and anaemia, 106, 107
Venography
and acute recurrent deep-vein thrombosis, 166, 167, 168
and deep-vein thrombosis, 159–160, 164, 165
and pulmonary embolism, diagnosis, 179, 180
and thromboneurosis, 184
Venous thromboembolism, see Deep-vein thrombosis
Vinblastine, and aplastic anaemia, 270
Vincristine
and acute leukaemia, 198
and aplastic anaemia, 270
and leukaemia
acute, 198
adult T-cell, 205
chronic lymphocytic, 204, 205
prolymphocytic, 205
metabolism, 196
and multiple myeloma, 223
and non-Hodgkin lymphoma, 259, 260, 262
Virus
and aquired haemolytic anaemias, 114
hepatitis, and anaemia, 69
infection, and aplastic anaemia, 69
Vitamin B_{12}, see Cobalamin
Vitamin K deficiency, 147–148
von Willebrand's disease, 152

Waldenstrom's macroglobulinaemia, 210, 229–230
laboratory findings, 230
prognosis, 231
treatment, 230–231
White cell
automated blood counting, 13–14, 18
count, 13
and iron-deficiency anaemia, 32
and periferal blood smear, 15
Whole-blood clotting time, and haematological evaluation, 17

Zieve's syndrome, 73